Bile Acids – Cholestasis – Gallstones

Advances in Basic and Clinical Bile Acid Research

FALK SYMPOSIUM 84

Bile Acids – Cholestasis – Gallstones

Advances in Basic and Clinical Bile Acid Research

EDITED BY

H. Fromm

Division of Gastroenterology
The George Washington University Medical Center
2150 Pennsylvania Avenue NW
Washington
DC 20039
USA

U. Leuschner

Medizinische Klinik II
Johann-Wolfgang-Goethe-Universität
Theodor-Stern-Kai 7
D-60596 Frankfurt
Germany

Proceedings of the Falk Symposium No. 84, held in Berlin, Germany, June 9–10, 1995

KLUWER ACADEMIC PUBLISHERS
DORDRECHT / BOSTON / LONDON

Distributors

for the United States and Canada: Kluwer Academic Publishers, PO Box 358, Accord Station, Hingham, MA 02018–0358, USA
for all other countries: Kluwer Academic Publishers Group, Distribution Center, PO Box 322, 3300 AH Dordrecht, The Netherlands

A catalogue record for this book is available from the British Library

ISBN 0–7923–8893–3

Library of Congress Cataloging in Publication Data

Falk Symposium (84th : 1995 : Berlin, Germany)
Bile acids, cholestasis, gallstones: advances in basic and clinical bile acid research: proceedings of the Falk Symposium no. 84, held in Berlin, Germany, June 9–10, 1995 / edited by H. Fromm, U. Leuschner.
p. cm.
Includes bibliographical references and index.
ISBN 0–7923–8893–3 (casebound : alk. paper)
1. Cholestasis — Congresses. 2. Gallstones — Congresses. 3. Bile acids — Therapeutic use — Congresses. 4. Bile — Secretion — Congresses.
I. Fromm, Hans, M.D. II. Leuschner, U. III. Title
[DNLM: 1. Bile Acids and Salts — physiology — congresses.
2. Cholelithiasis — physiopathology — congresses. 3. Cholelithiasis — therapy — congresses. 4. Liver Diseases — therapy — congresses. 5. Ursodeoxycholic Aci — therapeutic use — congresses. WI 703
F191bcc 1995]
RC854. C45F35 1995
616.3′6—dc20
DNLM/DLC
for Library of Congress 95–25461
CIP

Copyright

Published in the United Kingdom by Kluwer Academic Publishers, PO Box 55, Lancaster, UK.

Kluwer Academic Publishers BV incorporates the publishing programmes of D. Reidel, Martinus Nijhoff, Dr W. Junk and MTP Press.

Typeset by EXPO Holdings, Malaysia.

Printed and bound in Great Britain by Hartnolls Ltd., Bodmin, Cornwall.

Contents

List of Principal Authors

W. F. Balistreri
Division of Pediatric
Gastroenterology/Nutrition
Children's Hospital Medical Center
3333 Burnet Avenue
Cincinnati
OH 45229-3039
USA

N. Busch
Medizinische Klinik III
Klinikum der RWTH Aachen
D-52057 Aachen
Germany

M. C. Carey
Harvard Medical School
Gastroenterology Division
Brigham and Women's Hospital
75 Francis Street
Boston
MA 02115
USA

A. D. Cooper
Director, Research Institute
Palo Alto Medical Foundation
860 Bryant Street
Palo Alto
CA 94301
USA

K. A. Einarsson
Division of Gastroenterology and
Hepatology K63
Huddinge University Hospital
S-14186 Huddinge
Sweden

C. Ell
Medizinische Klinik 1 mit Poliklinik
Universität Erlangen-Nürnberg
Krankenhausstr. 12
D-91054 Erlangen
Germany

B.-G. Ericzon
Transplantationskirugklin
Huddinge sjukhus
S-14186 Huddinge
Sweden

H. Fromm
Division of Gastroenterology
The George Washington University
Medical Center
2150 Pennsylvania Avenue NW
Washington
DC 20037
USA

S. Güldütüna
Medizinische Klinik II
Johann-Wolfgang-Goethe-Universität
D-60590 Frankfurt am Main
Germany

A. Hellstern
Medizinische Klinik III
Johann-Wolfgang-Goethe-Universität
D-60590 Frankfurt am Main
Germany

A. F. Hofmann
Division of Gastroenterology
Department of Medicine (0813)
University of California, San Diego
La Jolla
CA 92093-0813
USA

D. Keppler
Abteilung Tumorbiochemie
Deutsches Krebsforschungszentrum
Im Neuenheimer Feld 280
D-69120 Heidelberg
Germany

W. Kramer
Leitung Pharma Forschung
SBU Metabolism G 838
Hoechst AG
D-65926 Frankfurt am Main
Germany

U. Leuschner
Medizinische Klinik II
Johann-Wolfgang-Goethe-Universität
D-60590 Frankfurt
Germany

H.-U. Marschall
Medizinische Klinik III
Klinikum der RWTH Aachen
D-52057 Aachen
Germany

P. J. Meier
Abteilung für klinische Pharmakologie
Medizin Klinik
Universitätsspital
Rämistr. 100
CH-8091 Zürich
Switzerland

J. D. Ostrow
Gastroenterology Section 111-G
Northwestern University Medical School
Veterans Administration Lakeside Medical Center
400 East Ontario St
Chicago
IL 60611
USA

G. R. Pape
Medizinische Klinik II
Klinikum Grosshadern der Universität München
Marchioninistr. 15
D-81377 München
Germany

G. Paumgartner
Medizinische Klinik II
Klinikum Grosshadern der Universität München
Marchioninistr. 15
D-81377 München
Germany

M. Podda
Istituto Scienze Biomediche
Ospedale S Paolo
Via di Rudini 8
I-20142 Milano
Italy

J. Reichen
Institut für Klinische Pharmakologie
Inselspital
Murtenstr. 35
CH-3010 Bern
Switzerland

E. Roda
Cattedra di Gastroenterologia
Policlinico S. Orsola
Via Massarenti 9
I-40138 Bologna
Italy

G. Salen
Division of Gastroenterology
New Jersey Medical School
185 South Orange Avenue
Newark
NJ 07103-2757
USA

C. Sama
Clinica Medica I
Policlinico S. Orsola
Via Massarenti 9
I-40138 Bologna
Italy

T. Sauerbruch
Medizinische Universitätsklinik
Allgemeine Innere Medizin
Klinikum der Universität Bonn
Sigmund-Freud-Str. 25
D-53105 Bonn
Germany

R. D. Soloway
Division of Gastroenterology
The University of Texas Medical Branch
4 106 McCullough Building -G-64
Galveston
TX 77555-0764
USA

U. Spengler
Medizinische Universitätsklinik
Allgemeine Innere Medizin
Sigmund-Freud-Str. 25
D-53105 Bonn
Germany

A. Stiehl
Medizinische Klinik
Klinikum der Universität
Bergheimer Str. 58
D-69115 Heidelberg
Germany

S. M. Strasberg
Section of Hepatobiliary-Pancreatic Surgery
Washington University School of Medicine
One Barnes Hospital
Queeny Tower Street 6107
St Louis
MO 63110
USA

G. P. van Berge Henegouwen
Department of Gastroenterology
University Hospital Utrecht
De Uithof
Box 85500
NL-3508 GA Utrecht
The Netherlands

K. Wengler
IV Medizinische Klinik, Gastroenterologie
Universitäts-Klinikum Charité
Station 1
D-10098 Berlin
Germany

Preface

This book comprises the contributions of the meeting 'Bile Acids – Cholestasis – Gallstones. Advances in Basic and Clinical Bile Acid Research' held in Berlin in June 1995. The meeting followed a symposium held in August 1992 – shortly after the reunification of Germany – in Schwerin, Mecklenburg, which aimed at integrating our Eastern European colleagues into the international community of physicians and researchers in the wide field of gastroenterology, in general, and bile acid research, in particular. The recent symposium in Berlin combined contributions of both basic and clinical research. It offered new aspects to those participants who are familiar with the topics of the conference, since the foci of research are shifting to an increasing extent under the influence of new laboratory techniques, with resulting changes in the management of gallstone disease and other hepatobiliary disorders.

We would like to thank all the speakers for their active participation at the meeting and in the publication of this book, as well as Dr. Herbert Falk for his generous support. Our thanks also go to Mrs. I. Stimler for her editorial assistance and to Kluwer Academic Publishers for the successful production of the book.

Prof. Dr. U. Leuschner **Prof. Dr. H. Fromm**

Section I
Bile Acid Synthesis and Transport

1
Cholesterol inhibits bile acid synthesis in New Zealand white and Watanabe heritable hyperlipidaemic rabbits

G. SALEN, G. XU, S. SHEFER, G. C. NESS and T. S. PARKER

INTRODUCTION

It is well known that rabbits and rats respond differently to dietary cholesterol; plasma cholesterol levels increase markedly when cholesterol is fed to rabbits while plasma cholesterol concentrations change only a little when rats consume large amounts of cholesterol in the diet[1]. This difference may be related to the effect of cholesterol on the function of hepatic LDL receptors and bile acid synthesis in the two animal species. In cholesterol-fed rabbits[2] but not rats[3,4], hepatic LDL receptors are down-regulated so that the liver in cholesterol-fed rabbits clears less LDL from the plasma. In rats, cholesterol feeding increased bile acid synthesis by up-regulating cholesterol 7α-hydroxylase activity and mRNA levels[4–7], whereas the effect of cholesterol feeding on bile acid synthesis in rabbits has not yet been entirely defined.

The Watanabe heritable hyperlipidaemic (WHHL) rabbit model was first described by Watanabe, a veterinarian at Kobe University in Japan, in 1975[8]. It is a strain of rabbit with consistently high plasma cholesterol levels associated with elevated plasma concentrations of β-very low density lipoprotein attributed to the deficiency of LDL receptors that is inherited as a dominant trait[9]. The abnormal LDL receptor gene from WHHL rabbits has been transferred to ‘DxL’, English half-lop (EHL-WW) rabbits which then manifest marked hypercholesterolaemia in homozygotes[10].

At least four mechanisms are responsible for cholesterol homeostasis and affect plasma cholesterol concentrations: (a) synthesis from acetate as regulated by the formation of mevalonic acid from HMG-CoA that is catalysed by the rate-limiting enzyme HMG-CoA reductase[11]; (b) expression of LDL receptors, especially in the liver, where more than half of the receptors are located[12]; (c) dietary intake of cholesterol[13]; and (d) the transformation of cholesterol to bile acids, the major catabolic pathway for cholesterol that is regulated by the formation of 7α-hydroxycholesterol and is catalysed by the hepatic microsomal enzyme, cholesterol 7α-hydroxylase[14].

The aim of this chapter is to evaluate the role of bile acid synthesis in cholesterol homeostasis in normocholesterolaemic NZW and hypercholesterolaemic WHHL rabbits. The effect of feeding cholesterol and its C-24 ethyl analogue, sitosterol, which blocks the intestinal absorption of cholesterol, was compared by measuring plasma and liver cholesterol concentrations, function and mRNA levels of hepatic LDL receptors and the activities and mRNA levels of HMG-CoA reductase and cholesterol 7α-hydroxylase in both rabbit groups. The results confirm that hypercholesterolaemia was associated with diminished LDL receptor function in WHHL and cholesterol-fed NZW rabbits. However, the importance of diminished bile acid synthesis in increasing plasma cholesterol concentrations was emphasized by the inhibition of the rate-controlling enzyme, cholesterol 7α-hydroxylase, in the cholesterol-treated NZW rabbits and the hypercholesterolaemic WHHL rabbits.

METHODS

Materials

Cholesterol (cholest-5-en-3β-ol), 5α-cholestane, cholestanol (5α-cholestan-3β-ol) and sitosterol (24B-ethylcholest-5-en-3β-ol) were obtained from Sigma Chemical Co., St Louis, MO, and used as standards for the measurements of sterols by capillary gas–liquid chromatography. Normal rabbit chow (Purina Mills Inc., St Louis, MO) contained less than 0.001% w/w cholesterol as determined by capillary gas–liquid chromatography. Rabbit chow containing 0.2% and 2% cholesterol and 0.2% sitosterol (the sitosterol for preparing the feeding chow was a gift of Eli Lilly Co., Indianapolis, IN) were incorporated into the normal chow by Purina Mills Inc., St Louis, MO.

Experimental plan

The experiments were carried out in 23 NZW rabbits (Hazleton Labs, Denver, PA) weighing 2.5–3 kg and 17 WHHL rabbits (EHL-WW rabbits, weighing 2.5–2.9 kg) which were bred in the Lipid Lab, Rogosin Institute, Cornell University Medical School, New York, NY[15]. The ages of these rabbits ranged from 6.5 to 7.5 months. The control rabbits (eight NZW and six WHHL rabbits) were fed normal rabbit chow. The 0.2% cholesterol chow diet (approximately 300 mg/day) was fed to four NZW and eight WHHL rabbits; the 2% cholesterol chow diet (approximately 3 g/day) was fed to five NZW rabbits and 0.2% sitosterol chow (approximately 300 mg/day) was fed to six NZW and three WHHL rabbits. The 2% cholesterol fed to WHHL rabbits caused severe toxicity and data were not used. The rabbits were fed the experimental diets for 10 days. Blood samples (2–3 ml) were taken with the anticoagulant ethylenediamine tetra-acetate (EDTA) immediately before and at the completion of the feeding period from each rabbit, for determination of plasma cholesterol concentrations and liver function tests (plasma alkaline phosphatase, glutamic–pyruvic acid transaminase and bilirubin levels). Animals were killed under anaesthesia (ketamine 20–30 mg/kg body weight combined with xylazine 2–3 mg/kg body weight intramuscularly), liver was removed and a portion was immediately frozen for measurement of microsomal activities and mRNA levels of HMG-CoA reductase and cholesterol 7α-hydroxylase, and membrane LDL receptor function and mRNA levels. The animal protocol was approved by Subcommittee on Animal Studies at VA Medical Center, East Orange, NJ and the Institutional Animal Care and Use Committee at UMD-New Jersey Medical School, Newark, NJ.

Chemical analysis

Assays for sterols

Neutral sterols were extracted with hexane from 1 ml plasma or 1 g (wet) pieces of liver after saponification in 1 N ethanolic NaOH. Trimethylsilyl ether derivatives were prepared and quantitated by capillary gas–liquid chromatography, model 5890, Hewlett-Packard, Palo Alto, CA) equipped with a 25-m fused silica CP-Sil 5-CB capillary column as described previously[16,17]. The retention times of the sterol trimethylsilyl ether derivatives relative to the internal standard, 5α-cholestane (retention time 14.62 min) were: cholesterol, 1.40; cholestanol, 1.42 and sitosterol, 1.81. For determination of free/ester cholesterol in the liver, 1 g (wet) of liver was extracted into chloroform : methanol (2 : 1). Free and ester cholesterol were then separated by the TLC method as described previously[18].

Assays for LDL receptor function were determined according to the method of Nguyen *et al.*[19–21] and Kovanen *et al.*[22]. HMG-CoA reductase and cholesterol 7α-hydroxylase were measured by the methods of Nguyen *et al.*[21] and Shefer *et al.*[23–25].

Northern analysis to measure HMG-CoA reductase, cholesterol 7α-hydroxylase and LDL receptor mRNAs, was carried out according to Xu *et al.*[16]; β-actin mRNA probe served as an internal control[26–29].

Statistical study

Baseline data were compared statistically by the unpaired Student's *t*-test. Where control values were used several times the Bonferroni correction was employed. The BMDP Statistical Software system (BMDP Statistical Software Inc., Los Angeles, CA) was used for statistical evaluations.

RESULTS

Plasma concentrations of cholesterol were 9.9 times greater ($p<0.0001$) in WHHL than in NZW rabbits fed the control diet that was virtually devoid of cholesterol (Table 1). When the chow containing 0.2% cholesterol (300 mg/day) was fed for 10 days, plasma concentrations increased about 2-fold in both rabbit groups, and rose 26 times in NZW rabbits fed 2% cholesterol (3000 mg/day) in the diet for 10 days.

Table 1 The effect of cholesterol feeding on plasma and liver cholesterol levels in NZW and WHHL rabbits

	Plasma (mg/dl)		*Liver (mg/g(% ester))*	
	NZW	*WHHL*	*NZW*	*WHHL*
Controls	33±5 (*n*=8)	326±83 (*n*=6)	2.6±0.5 (7.1) (*n*=5)	3.9±0.5 (7.1) (*n*=5)
0.2% Cholesterol[a]	68±28 (*n*=4)	742±100[b] (*n*=8)	9.3±0.7[c] (57.1) (*n*=4)	4.9±1.0 (29.4) (*n*=5)
2% Cholesterol[a]	871±259[d] (*n*=5)		25.5±2.7[c] (68.3) (*n*=5)	N/A
0.2% Sitosterol[a]	19±2[d] (*n*=6)	447±8 (*n*=3)	2.3±0.5 (6.2) (*n*=5)	3.4±0.5 (6.8) (*n*=3)

Data presented as means ± SD.
[a] Rabbits were fed 0.2% or 2% cholesterol or 0.2% sitosterol respectively for 10 days.
[b] $p<0.001$ compared to the control value for WHHL rabbits.
[c] $p<0.001$ compared to the control value for NZW rabbits.
[d] $p<0.01$ compared with the control value for NZW rabbits.
N/A = Not available.

When 0.2% sitosterol was fed for 10 days, plasma cholesterol concentrations declined 42% ($p<0.01$) in NZW rabbits but did not decrease in the hypercholesterolaemic WHHL rabbits compared to their respective control groups. It is noteworthy that, despite the large intake (300 mg/day), the plasma sitosterol concentration remained low, i.e. less than 1 mg/dl in the NZW rabbits (data not shown).

Liver cholesterol concentrations in NZW and WHHL rabbits are presented as mg/g liver. Hepatic cholesterol concentrations were 50% higher ($p<0.005$) in the WHHL as compared to NZW rabbits fed the same, almost cholesterol-free, control diet. When 0.2% and 2% cholesterol were fed, liver cholesterol rose 3.6- and 9.8-fold ($p<0.001$), respectively, in NZW rabbits but increased only 26% (*p* not significant) in WHHL rabbits with 0.2% cholesterol in the diet for 10 days. The proportion of hepatic esterified cholesterol increased with hepatic cholesterol in both groups. Sitosterol feeding did not change hepatic cholesterol levels significantly in the NZW or WHHL rabbits.

Measurements of hepatic microsomal total HMG-CoA reductase and cholesterol 7α-hydroxylase activities are reported in Table 2. In both NZW and WHHL rabbits fed the cholesterol-deficient control diet, HMG-CoA reductase activities were similar, although plasma and liver cholesterol concentrations were greater in WHHL rabbits. Feeding cholesterol, as expected, inhibited HMG-CoA reductase activities in both rabbit groups. Total enzyme activity was reduced 18% (*p* not significant) with 0.2% cholesterol, but decreased 68% ($p<0.001$) with 2% cholesterol feeding in NZW and 64% ($p<0.05$) with 0.2% cholesterol in WHHL rabbits. In contrast, dietary sitosterol (0.2%), which acts in the intestine to block cholesterol absorption, increased hepatic HMG-CoA reductase activity 2.5 times ($p<0.05$) in the NZW rabbits, but produced only a small rise in enzyme activity in the WHHL rabbits.

Hepatic microsomal cholesterol 7α-hydroxylase activity was almost 3-fold ($p<0.0001$) higher in the NZW than WHHL rabbits at baseline when fed the cholesterol-deficient control diet. Unexpectedly, both 0.2% and 2% cholesterol in the diet progressively reduced cholesterol 7α-hydroxylase activity ($p<0.01$)

Table 2 Effect of cholesterol feeding on hepatic total HMG-CoA reductase and cholesterol 7α-hydroxylase activity in rabbits

	HMG-CoA reductase (pmol/mg⁻¹ min⁻¹)[a]		*Cholesterol 7α-hydroxylase (pmol/mg⁻¹ min⁻¹)*[a]	
	NZW	*WHHL*	*NZW*	*WHHL*
Controls	28±3 (*n*=6)	36±17 (*n*=5)	34±8 (*n*=8)	12±2 (*n*=6)
0.2% Cholesterol[b]	23±7 (*n*=4)	13±7[e] (*n*=8)	20±4[c] (*n*=4)	13±3 (*n*=8)
2% Cholesterol[b]	9±4[d] (*n*=5)	N/A	16±6[c] (*n*=5)	N/A
0.2% Sitosterol[b]	70±25[e] (*n*=3)	48±7 (*n*=3)	28±4 (*n*=3)	15±1 (*n*=3)

[a] Means ± SD.
[b] Rabbits were fed 0.2% or 2% cholesterol or 0.2% sitosterol respectively for 10 days.
[c] $p<0.001$ compared to the control value for NZW rabbits.
[d] $p<0.05$ compared to the relevant control values.
[e] $p<0.01$ compared to the control value for NZW rabbits.
N/A = Not available.

by 41% and 53% respectively in the NZW rabbits, but did not change the already low activity in the WHHL rabbits. When sitosterol was fed, cholesterol 7α-hydroxylase activity was not inhibited, and remained at baseline levels in NZW and WHHL rabbits.

Hepatic HMG-CoA reductase mRNA levels as measured by Northern blot analysis and densitometeric scanning were similar in both NZW and WHHL rabbits when fed the control cholesterol-deficient diet (Table 3). Moreover, enzyme mRNA levels did not decrease in both rabbit groups when cholesterol was added to the diet, despite the drop in HMG-CoA reductase activity (Table 2) and comparable elevated plasma cholesterol concentrations (Table 1).

Hepatic cholesterol 7α-hydroxylase mRNA levels were 10 times greater and corresponded to higher enzyme activity in NZW than WHHL rabbits fed the control cholesterol-deficient diet ($p<0.05$). Unexpectedly, 2% cholesterol feeding inhibited cholesterol 7α-hydroxylase mRNA levels 79% ($p<0.05$) in NZW rabbits, whereas in WHHL rabbits the initially low mRNA levels rose slightly with 0.2% cholesterol feeding.

Receptor-mediated hepatic LDL binding and mRNA levels are reported in Table 4. As expected, WHHL rabbits fed the control diet showed 36% less

Table 3 Effect of cholesterol feeding on hepatic HMG-CoA reductase and cholesterol 7 α-hydroxylase mRNA levels in rabbits

	HMG-CoA reductase mRNA[a]		*Cholesterol 7α-hydroxylase* m*RNA*[a]	
	NZW	*WHHL*	*NZW*	*WHHL*
Controls	0.55±0.37 (*n*=4)	0.48±0.06 (*n*=3)	29.1±15.6 (*n*=3)	2.8±0.4 (*n*=3)
0.2% Cholesterol[b]		0.48±0.19 (*n*=5)		7.2±2.2 (*n*=3)
2% Cholesterol[b]	0.48±0.04 (*n*=5)		6.2±3.7[c] (*n*=4)	

[a]Relative densitometric units (means±SD) corrected by recovery of the internal standard, β-actin.
[b]Rabbits were fed 0.2% or 2% cholesterol respectively for 10 days.
[c]$p<0.05$ compared to relevant control values.

Table 4 Effect of cholesterol feeding on hepatic LDL receptor-mediated binding and mRNA levels in rabbits

	Hepatic receptor-mediated LDL binding (ng/mg protein)		*Hepatic LDL receptor mRNA*[a]	
	NZW	*WHHL*	*NZW*	*WHHL*
Control	175±29 (n=7)	112±25 (n=6)	0.61±0.02 (n=3)	0.45±0.06 (n=3)
0.2% Cholesterol[b]	115±32 (n=4)	108±32 (n=6)		0.55±0.09 (n=5)
2% Cholesterol[b]	89±36[c] (n=5)		0.55±0.18 (n=5)	
0.2% Sitosterol[b]	228±40 (n=3)	110±58 (n=3)		

Data presented as means±SD.
[a]Relative densitometric units corrected by recovery of the internal standard, β-actin.
[b]Rabbits were fed 0.2% or 2% cholesterol or 0.2% sitosterol respectively for 10 days.
[c]p<0.01 compared to the control values for NZW rabbits.

(p<0.005) receptor-mediated LDL binding than NZW rabbits. When NZW rabbits were fed 0.2% and 2% cholesterol diets, receptor-mediated LDL binding declined 34% and 49% (p<0.01), respectively. In contrast, 0.2% cholesterol feeding to WHHL rabbits did not further decrease receptor-mediated LDL binding. Sitosterol feeding, in distinction, stimulated LDL receptor binding in NZW rabbits consistent with the decrease in plasma cholesterol concentrations (Table 1). In comparison, WHHL rabbits failed to express additional LDL receptors when fed sitosterol.

In both rabbit groups fed the control cholesterol-deficient diet, similar amounts of LDL receptor mRNA were present, and did not decrease with dietary cholesterol feeding (Table 4). Thus, WHHL and cholesterol-fed NZW rabbits show decreased hepatic LDL receptor binding despite unchanged mRNA levels.

Normal values for plasma alkaline phosphatase, glutamic–pyruvic acid transaminase and bilirubin were present in the NZW and WHHL rabbits on the control cholesterol-deficient diet, and remained normal with cholesterol feeding. The weights of the animals were similar before and after treatment in all groups. Liver histology showed only increased deposition of fat without hepatocyte destruction, inflammation, or disruption of the architecture when cholesterol was fed for 10 days to both rabbit groups.

DISCUSSION

The major new discovery in this study was the demonstration that hepatic cholesterol 7α-hydroxylase activity and mRNA levels were substantially higher in NZW than WHHL rabbits[30]. Since bile acid synthesis represents the major catabolic path for the elimination of cholesterol, reduced cholesterol 7α-hydroxylase activity and mRNA levels in the WHHL rabbits signify diminished bile acid synthesis, and provide an additional mechanism for the development of hypercholesterolaemia in these animals. In a recent study by Krause *et al.*[31], endogenous hypercholesterolaemia was produced in NZW rabbits by feeding low-fat, cholesterol-free diets that contained casein as the sole protein source. In these hypercholesterolaemic rabbits mRNA levels of cholesterol 7α-hydroxylase were also reduced. However, it is not clear whether the low levels of cholesterol 7α-hydroxylase in the baseline chow-fed WHHL rabbits represent a primary defect that is coupled to the inherited deficiency of LDL receptor function or is secondary to feedback suppression by the enlarged plasma and hepatic cholesterol pools. In this regard it is noteworthy that hepatic HMG-CoA reductase was equally active in the NZW and WHHL control rabbits. Thus the larger hepatic cholesterol pool did not inhibit hepatic cholesterol biosynthesis in the WHHL rabbits, although cholesterol 7α-hydroxylase was suppressed. This suggests that newly synthesized cholesterol, in this case, was not involved in the inhibition of cholesterol 7α-hydroxylase activity. However, feeding 0.2% cholesterol significantly inhibited HMG-CoA reductase activity in both NZW and WHHL rabbits. This suggests that HMG-CoA reductase activity is regulated by a hepatic cholesterol pool that is sensitive to dietary cholesterol.

Feeding 2% dietary cholesterol to NZW rabbits unexpectedly inhibited cholesterol 7α-hydroxylase activity and reduced mRNA levels substantially, as well as down-regulating LDL receptor function, and was associated with elevated plasma cholesterol concentrations that were as high as seen in WHHL rabbits. Liver cholesterol was also markedly enhanced. Thus the absorbed dietary cholesterol accumulated in the liver and suppressed LDL receptor expression and also probably inhibited cholesterol 7α-hydroxylase activity and reduced mRNA levels in the NZW rabbits. As a result, marked plasma hypercholesterolaemia developed. Some 30 years earlier, Hellström[32] reported that cholesterol feeding to adult male albino rabbits resulted in a reduction in turnover and faecal elimination of deoxycholic acid as measured by isotope dilution techniques, and this is consistent with our idea that cholesterol inhibits cholesterol 7α-hydroxylase (Table 2) and bile acid synthesis.

It seems likely that the larger hepatic cholesterol pool plays a role in the inhibition of cholesterol 7α-hydroxylase, since liver cholesterol concentrations were elevated at baseline in WHHL and cholesterol-fed NZW rabbits. That feeding 2% cholesterol to NZW rabbits suppressed cholesterol 7α-hydroxylase activity and mRNA levels to the baseline levels found in WHHL rabbits, but 0.2% cholesterol feeding did not further decrease the enzyme activity and mRNA levels in WHHL rabbits, suggests that the baseline enzyme levels in WHHL rabbits might be at the minimum for cholesterol 7α-hydroxylase. However, it is important to note that in NZW rabbits 0.2% cholesterol inhibited cholesterol 7α-hydroxylase activity 41%, which was still significantly higher than minimum levels in the WHHL rabbits, although hepatic cholesterol levels in these cholesterol-fed NZW rabbits were nearly twice as large as in WHHL rabbits. Therefore, a metabolically active pool of cholesterol that regulates cholesterol 7α-hydroxylase probably exists in the liver, but cannot be defined only by measuring total hepatic cholesterol concentrations.

The inhibitory effects of dietary cholesterol on cholesterol 7α-hydroxylase in NZW rabbits is unexpected, and opposite to the effect of cholesterol feeding in Sprague-Dawley rats[4–7]. Both cholesterol 7α-hydroxylase activity and mRNA levels were stimulated several-fold, and bile acid outputs were increased, in the cholesterol-fed rats. Plasma cholesterol levels did not rise in rats, although cholesterol accumulated mostly as esters in the liver. Apparently, cholesterol-fed rats respond differently, and are able to convert excess dietary cholesterol to bile acids without raising plasma concentrations. Similar results to cholesterol-fed rats have been reported by Poorman *et al.*[33] to occur in specially bred hypercholesterolaemia-resistant rabbits. In these animals the baseline activity and mRNA levels of cholesterol 7α-hydroxylase were much higher than in normal NZW rabbits, and were not inhibited by cholesterol feeding. One point is clear: in rabbits, dietary cholesterol does not up-regulate bile acid synthesis by causing intestinal bile acid malabsorption, as has been suggested to occur in the cholesterol-fed rat, by Björkhem *et al.*[34]. However, it is important to emphasize that about 90% of plasma cholesterol is transported by HDL in the rat as compared to only 50% in the rabbit[35]. Thus, the return of cholesterol to the liver in different lipoprotein fractions may ultimately determine its utilization as substrate for bile acid synthesis.

When 0.2% sitosterol was added to the diet, plasma cholesterol levels declined 42% (p<0.01) in the NZW but not in the WHHL rabbits. Apparently sitosterol, which is poorly absorbed, competitively blocks intestinal cholesterol absorption and decreases the return to the liver. Consequently, hepatic LDL receptor expression is up-regulated and HMG-CoA reductase activity, stimulated (Table 2), but the increase of LDL receptors may be greater than the input of newly synthesized cholesterol by the liver in the NZW rabbits fed sitosterol. As a result plasma cholesterol levels decline significantly. In contrast, receptor-deficient WHHL rabbits are unable to increase the number of LDL receptors when fed sitosterol; consequently, plasma cholesterol levels did not decrease.

With respect to the expression of LDL receptors, WHHL rabbits show low receptor-mediated binding but normal amounts of mRNA, consistent with an inherited translational abnormality of receptor protein. Not only is binding deficient, but the internalization of the receptor-bound cholesterol may also be impaired to account for the high level of plasma cholesterol. The higher cholesterol concentrations circulating in the plasma and increased hepatic cholesterol concentrations in the WHHL rabbits do not suppress hepatic HMG-CoA reductase activity or mRNA levels. However, feeding cholesterol to both rabbit groups strongly down-regulated HMG-CoA reductase activity without decreasing mRNA levels. Thus, dietary cholesterol probably inhibits HMG-CoA reductase post-transcriptionally in rabbits, as has been reported to occur in rats fed cholesterol[4,5,28]. In NZW rabbits the dietary cholesterol also inhibits hepatic LDL receptor function without changing LDL receptor mRNA levels. Both HMG-CoA reductase and LDL receptors in NZW rabbits appear to be coordinately regulated and respond similarly to dietary cholesterol at a post-transcriptional level. This point is supported by the sitosterol feeding experiment, in which decreasing the return of intestinal cholesterol to the liver stimulated hepatic HMG-CoA reductase activity and tended to increase the expression of LDL receptors in the NZW rabbits.

Recently, Rudel *et al.*[36] reported that dietary cholesterol inhibited cholesterol 7α-hydroxylase activity and mRNA levels in African green monkeys. The authors related the down-regulation of cholesterol 7α-hydroxylase to the accumulation of dietary cholesterol in the liver, and suggested that reduced bile acid synthesis might decrease cholesterol absorption to limit the further uptake of dietary cholesterol. The effect of dietary cholesterol on cholesterol

7α-hydroxylase in the African green monkeys is similar to the results of this study in NZW rabbits fed cholesterol. Both these experiments emphasize the role of increased hepatic cholesterol concentrations to diminish cholesterol 7α-hydroxylase that contributes to hypercholesterolaemia in these two species.

The inhibitory effect of dietary cholesterol on cholesterol 7α-hydroxylase (bile acid synthesis) in rabbits might help us to explain why some humans are so sensitive to dietary cholesterol and increase plasma concentrations. These subjects might respond to dietary cholesterol like NZW rabbits with diminished bile acid synthesis contributing to elevated plasma cholesterol levels and a reduction in LDL receptors. Alternatively, other people respond to dietary cholesterol like rats, where bile acid synthesis is stimulated and plasma cholesterol levels do not rise. Identifying these individuals should help clarify their atherosclerosis risk, and may make more sensible recommendations for dietary treatment. Nevertheless, these studies suggest that diminished cholesterol 7α-hydroxylase and bile acid synthesis are related to elevated hepatic cholesterol concentrations and, together with reduced LDL receptors, increase plasma cholesterol levels when cholesterol is fed to NZW rabbits or where LDL receptors are abnormal in WHHL rabbits.

Acknowledgements

This work was supported by VA Research Service, and US Public Health Service Grants, HL 17818, DK 26756, and HL 18094.

References

1. Beynen AC, Katan MB, Van Zutphen LFM. Hypo- and hyperresponders: individual differences in the response of serum cholesterol concentration to changes in diet. In: Paoletti R, Kritchevsky D, editors. Advances in lipid research, vol. 22. San Diego, CA: Academic Press; 1987:115–71.
2. Kovanen PT, Brown MS, Basu SK, Bilheimer DW, Goldstein JL. Saturation and suppression of hepatic lipoprotein receptor: a mechanism for the hypercholesterolemia of cholesterol-fed rabbits. Proc Natl Acad Sci USA. 1981;78:1396–400.
3. Koelz HR, Sherrill BC, Turley SD, Dietschy JM. Correlation of low and high density lipoprotein binding in vivo with lipoprotein degradation in the rat. J Biol Chem. 1982;257:8061–72.
4. Spady DK, Cuthbert JA. Regulation of hepatic sterol metabolism in the rat. J Biol Chem. 1992;267:5584–91.
5. Shefer S, Nguyen LB, Salen G *et al.* Differing effects of cholesterol and taurocholate on steady state hepatic HMG-CoA reductase and cholesterol 7α-hydroxylase activities and mRNA levels in the rat. J Lipid Res. 1992;33:1193–200.
6. Pandak WM, Li YC, Chiang YL *et al.* Regulation of cholesterol 7α-hydroxylase mRNA and transcriptional activity by taurocholate and cholesterol in the chronic biliary diverted rat. J Biol Chem. 1991;266:3416–21.
7. Jelinek DF, Andersson S, Slaughter CA, Russell DW. Cloning and regulation of cholesterol 7α-hydroxylase, the rate-limiting enzyme in bile acid biosynthesis. J Biol Chem. 1990;265:8190–7.
8. Kondo T, Watanabe Y. A heritable hyperlipemic rabbit. Exp Anim. 1975;24:89–94.
9. Watanabe Y. Serial inbreeding of rabbits with hereditary hyperlipidemia (WHHL-rabbit). Atherosclerosis. 1980;36:261–8.
10. Richards T, Horlock H, Gallagher P. Atherosclerosis in modified WHHL rabbits. Anim. Tech. 1986;37:1–6.
11. Goldstein JL, Brown MS. Progress in understanding the LDL receptor and HMG-CoA reductase, two membrane proteins that regulate the plasma cholesterol. J Lipid Res. 1984;25:1450–61.

12. Brown MS, Goldstein JL. Lipoprotein receptors in the liver: control signals for plasma cholesterol traffic. J Clin Invest. 1983;72:743–7.
13. Ross AC, Zilversmit DB. Chylomicron remnant cholesteryl esters as the major constituent of very low density lipoproteins in plasma of cholesterol-fed rabbits. J Lipid Res. 1977;18:169–81.
14. Shefer S, Hauser S, Berkersky I, Mosbach EH. Biochemical site of regulation of bile acid biosynthesis in rat. J Lipid Res. 1970;11:404–11.
15. Donnelly TM, Kelsey SF, Levine DM, Parker TS. Control of variance in experimental studies of hyperlipidemia using the WHHL rabbit. J Lipid Res. 1991;32:1089–98.
16. Xu G, Salen G, Shefer S *et al.* Different feedback regulation of hepatic cholesterol and bile acid synthesis by glycodeoxycholic acid in rabbits. Gastroenterology. 1993;105:1192–9.
17. Nguyen LB, Shefer S, Salen G, Horak I, Tint GS, McNamara DJ. The effect of abnormal plasma and cellular sterol content and composition on low density lipoprotein uptake and degradation by monocytes and lymphocytes in sitosterolemia with xanthomatosis. Metab Clin Exp. 1988;37:346–51.
18. Salen G, Ahrens EH, Grundy SM. Metabolism of β-sitosterol in man. J Clin Invest. 1970;49:952–67.
19. Havel RJ, Eder HA, Bragdon JH. The distribution and chemical composition of ultracentrifugally separated lipoproteins in human sera. J Clin Invest. 1955;34:1345–53.
20. Goldstein JL, Basu SK, Brown MS. Receptor-mediated endocytosis of low density lipoprotein in cultured cells. Methods Enzymol. 1983;98:241–60.
21. Nguyen LB, Shefer S, Salen G *et al.* A molecular defect in hepatic cholesterol biosynthesis in sitosterolemia with xanthomatosis. J Clin Invest. 1990;86:923–31.
22. Kovanen PT, Brown MS, Goldstein JL. Increased binding of low density lipoprotein to liver membranes from rats treated with 17-ethinyl estradiol. J Biol Chem. 1979;254:11367–73.
23. Shefer S, Salen G, Batta AK. Methods of assay. In: Fears R, Sabine JM, editors. Cholesterol 7α-hydroxylase (7α-monooxygenase). Boca Raton, FL: CRC Press;1986:43–9.
24. Lowry OH, Rosebrough NJ, Farr AL, Randall RJ. Protein measurement with the Folin phenol reagent. J Biol Chem. 1951;193:265–75.
25. George R, Davis PJ, Luong L, Poznansky NJ. Cholesterol-mediated regulation of HMG-CoA reductase in microsomes from human skin fibroblasts and rat liver. Biochem Cell Biol. 1990;68:674–9.
26. Chomozynski R, Sacchi N. Single step method of RNA isolation by acid guanidinium thiocyanate–phenol–chloroform extraction. Anal Biochem. 1987;162:156–9.
27. Aviv N, Ledder P. Purification of biologically active globin mRNA by chromatography on oligothymidylic acid-cellulose. Proc Natl Acad Sci USA. 1972;69:1408–12.
28. Ness GC, Keller RK, Pendelton LC. Feedback regulation of hepatic 3-hydroxy-3-methyl glutaryl coenzyme A reductase activity by dietary cholesterol is not due to altered mRNA levels. J Biol Chem. 1991;266:14854–7.
29. Horton JD, Cuthbert JA, Spady DK. Dietary fatty acids regulate hepatic low density lipoprotein (LDL) transport by altering LDL receptor protein and mRNA levels. J Clin Invest. 1993;92:743–9.
30. Dietschy JM, Kita T, Suckling KE, Goldstein JL, Brown MS. Cholesterol synthesis in vivo and in vitro in the WHHL rabbit, an animal with defective low density lipoprotein receptors. J Lipid Res. 1983;24:469–80.
31. Krause BR, Pape ME, Kieft K *et al.* ACAT inhibition decreased LDL cholesterol in rabbits fed a cholesterol-free diet. Arterioscler Thromb. 1994;14:598–604.
32. Hellström K. On the bile acid and neutral fecal steroid excretion in man and rabbits following cholesterol feeding. Acta Physiol Scand. 1965;63:21–35.
33. Poorman JA, Buck RA, Smith SA, Overturf ML, Loose-Mitchell DS. Bile acid excretion and cholesterol 7α-hydroxylase expression in hypercholesterolemia-resistant rabbits. J Lipid Res. 1993;34:1675–85.
34. Björkhem I, Eggertson G, Andersson U. On the mechanism of stimulation of cholesterol 7α-hydroxylase by dietary cholesterol. Biochim Biophs Acta. 1991;1085:329–35.
35. Spady DK, Dietschy JM. Sterol synthesis in vivo in 18 tissues of the squirrel monkey, guinea pig, rabbit, hamster, and rat. J Lipid Res. 1983;24:303–15.
36. Rudel L, Decheiman C, Wilson M, Scobey M, Anderson R. Dietary cholesterol and down-regulation of cholesterol 7α-hydroxylase and cholesterol absorption in African green monkeys. J Clin Invest. 1994;93:2463–72.

2
Conjugation of bile acids

H.-U. MARSCHALL, H. MATERN, J. SJÖVALL and S. MATERN

INTRODUCTION

The primary bile acids cholic acid (CA) and chenodeoxycholic acid (CDCA) are synthesized from cholesterol in the liver. The initial and rate-limiting step in bile acid biosynthesis is 7α-hydroxylation of cholesterol[1]. The conversion of 7α-hydroxycholesterol to bile acids involves saturation of the steroid nucleus, epimerization of the 3β-hydroxy group, introduction of a 12α-hydroxy group for biosynthesis of CA and oxidative cleavage of the side-chain of the C_{27} steroid yielding a C-24 carboxylic acid[1–3].

Following their formation as glycine and taurine conjugates in the liver, the primary bile acids CA and CDCA undergo several metabolic alterations[4]. These are hydrolysis of conjugates, oxidation, isomerization and elimination of ring hydroxyl groups, introduction of new hydroxyl groups and several conjugation reactions both in the liver and in extrahepatic organs such as the small and large intestine and the kidney. One might distinguish hydroxylation and side-chain oxidation of cholesterol to form bile acids as phase I biotransformations from subsequent conjugation as a phase II biotransformation.

AMIDATION

Prior to secretion into bile, approximately 99% of CA and CDCA are conjugated at C-24 through an amide bond with the amino acids glycine or taurine (Fig. 1) catalysed by the bile acid-CoA : amino acid *N*-acyltransferase[5]. The proportion of glycine to taurine conjugates in humans[6] is usually about 3 to 1, whereas taurine is preferred in other animals that may also form aminoacyl amidates with ornithine, arginine, β-alanine or ciliatine[4]. Conjugation with glycine or taurine converts a weak acid into a strong acid. The pK_a of glycine-conjugated bile acids is 3.9, and that of taurine conjugates[7] <1. This type of conjugation also lowers the CMpH (critical micellation pH) which is between pH 6 and pH 8 for unconjugated bile acids[8]. In addition, conjugation with glycine or taurine also prevents the formation of insoluble calcium salts[9]. Thus, *N*-acyl amidation with

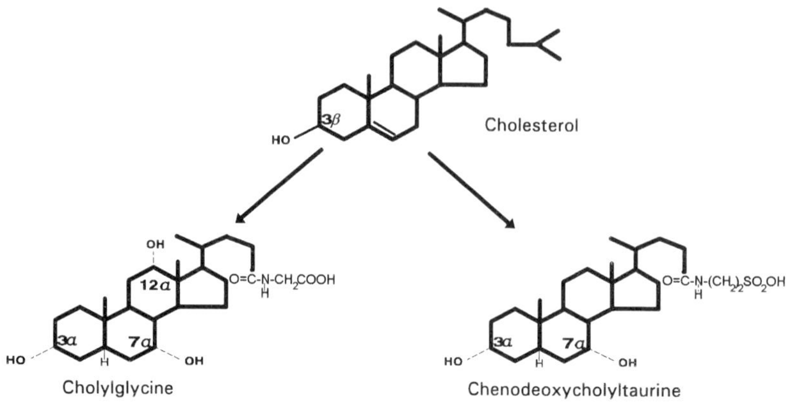

Fig. 1. Formation of cholylglycine and chenodeoxycholyltaurine from cholesterol

glycine or taurine is essential for maintaining bile acids soluble in the aqueous milieu of bile and gut[10]. It has recently been recommended to use the term cholylglycine rather than glycocholate, to indicate correctly the structure of the bile acid aminoacyl amidate[11].

After biliary secretion the bile acids are absorbed by non-ionic passive diffusion along the entire length of the intestine, unconjugated bile acids being passively absorbed in particular in the colon. Glycine or taurine conjugates of bile acids, however, are absorbed actively in the distal ileum[10,12]. The hamster ileal sodium-dependent bile acid transporter has recently been cloned and characterized[13]. Approximately 95% of biliary secreted bile acids are taken up by the intestine and returned to the liver in portal-venous blood, where the concentration of bile acids is more than 10 times higher than in systemic blood[14]. The liver extracts bile acids from the portal vein, but also from the arterial blood supply[15]. The bile acid pool of 2–3 g circulates three to 10 times a day and, at least in health, only small amounts of bile acids are excreted by the kidney after entering the systemic circulation[10].

In cholestatic liver diseases, in particular in extrahepatic cholestasis, the enterohepatic circulation is impaired and bile acids accumulate in the liver. In spite of decreased synthesis of bile acids due to negative feedback inhibition[2], levels of bile acids increase both in the liver and the systemic circulation, and alternative metabolic pathways of bile acids emerge with qualitative and quantitative changes of bile acid metabolism[16,17]. These include hepatic hydroxylation of primary and secondary bile acids at C-1 and C-6 with excretion of the products in urine[18], and alternative or additional conjugation reactions besides the amidation with glycine or taurine (Fig. 2).

SULPHATION

In cholestasis, sulphates of bile acids are formed catalysed by hepatic and extrahepatic 3′-phosphoadenosyl-5′-phosphosulphate: sulphotransferases (PAPS)[19].

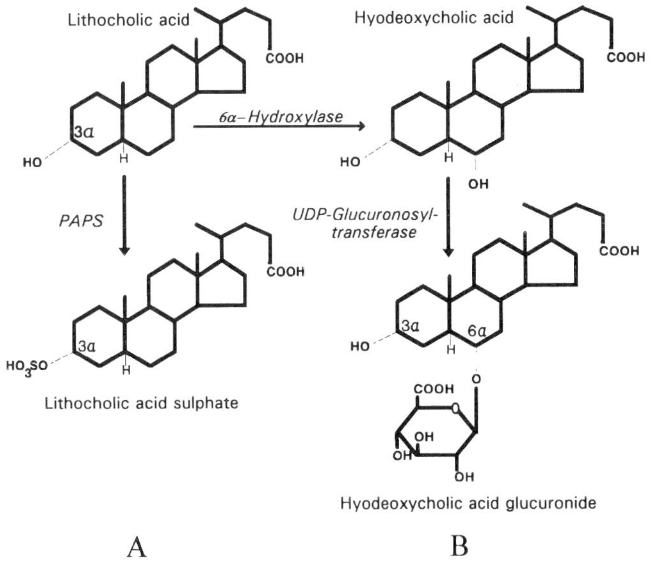

Fig. 2 Conjugation and possible detoxication of lithocholic acid. **A**: By sulphation catalysed by 3′-phosphoadenosyl-5′-phosphosulphate : sulphotransferases (PAPS); **B**: by 6α-hydroxylation followed by 6α-glucuronidation catalysed by UDP-glucuronosytransferases

A steroid sulphotransferase from human liver cytosol was characterized catalysing the sulphation of steroid hormones as well as lithocholic acid (LCA) and 6-hydroxylated bile acids[20], emphasizing the close relationship of bile acid and steroid hormone metabolism. Sulphation is the major detoxication step for the toxic bile acid LCA in humans[21], yielding a water-soluble conjugate which can be eliminated in urine (Fig. 2). Sulphation occurs at the C-3 position; however, disulphates of bile acids carrying two or more hydroxyl groups were found as very minor compounds in cholestatic urine[22].

GLUCURONIDATION

In 1974, glucuronides of bile acids were detected in urine and serum of cholestatic patients[23,24], thus establishing the first glycosidic conjugation pathway of bile acids *in vivo*. Glucuronides are found together with sulphated bile acids in cholestatic urine[23–28] and serum[29–31], sulphates almost always exceeding glucuronides in amounts. A major part of urinary bile acid glucuronides are hydroxylated at C-6[32,33]. Hyodeoxycholic acid (HDCA) is a 6α-hydroxylated bile acid (Fig. 2) and is glucuronidated at the C-6 position, whereas bile acids lacking a 6α-hydroxy group, such as CDCA, are glucuronidated at the C-3 position[33]. *In vitro*, UDP-glucuronosyltransferase activity catalysing the formation of bile acid glucuronides has been identified in microsomal preparations of human liver[34,35] and extrahepatic organs[36,37] and the highly efficient glucuronidation of HDCA *in vitro* was shown to occur at the C-6 position[38–40].

Whereas the related enzyme from rat liver catalyses the glucuronidation of both CDCA and some steroid hormones[41,42], a specific HDCA-UDP-glucuronosyltransferase was recently isolated from human liver[43]. Cloning and stable expression in cell culture of the cDNA was possible[44,45], and evidence was given that the recombinant UDP-glucuronosyltransferase 2B4 may correspond to the purified isoenzyme from human liver[46]. Recently a new radioassay for the estimation of UDP-glucuronosyltransferase activities was developed[47]. All bile acid glucuronides found in humans *in vivo* are hydroxyl-linked glucuronides. *In vitro*, however, human[48] and rat[49,50] liver microsomes also catalyse the formation of monohydroxylated side-chain carboxyl-linked glucuronides.

A possible detoxication of LCA by phase I and phase II biotransformation reactions includes 6α-hydroxylation of LCA followed by 6α-glucuronidation of the HDCA formed[32,33,39,51–53]. This mechanism (Fig. 2) is supported by the preference of glucuronidation for 6-hydroxylated bile acids and data on the glucuronidation of LCA. Using human liver microsomes a low activity of UDP-glucuronosyltransferases towards LCA was observed[39], and animal studies on the formation and metabolism of LCA glucuronide indicated that this conjugate is even more cholestatic and toxic than LCA itself[54–59]. These findings are evidence against glucuronidation as a primary detoxification mechanism for LCA. However, hydroxylation of bile acids at C-6 occurs in cholestasis[18,22,33,60–63] and HDCA can be formed by 6α-hydroxylation of LCA[4,60]. The possible coupling of 6α-hydroxylation of LCA with 6α-glucuronidation of the HDCA formed is further supported by clinical studies using phenobarbital for induction of liver enzymes in children with cholestasis[64,65]. In these studies an increased urinary excretion of bile acid glucuronides was observed combined with a fall of serum bile acid levels. In addition, stimulation of cytochrome P450-I-A2 in healthy humans by oral administration of the antibiotic rifampin[66] was followed by a significantly increased excretion of the glucuronide HDCA and a diminished excretion of the sulphate of LCA[67].

GLUCOSIDATION

In 1984, glucosidation of bile acids was first observed *in vitro*. This reaction is catalysed by a nucleotide-sugar-independent bile acid glucosyltransferase from microsome preparations of human liver[68] and extrahepatic organs[69], and human liver and kidney tumours[70]. Sugar-nucleotide-independent glucosidation of bile acids uses dolichyl phosphoglucose as the sugar donor[68], which is also an intermediate for other glucose transfer reactions in the liver[71]. The UDP-glucose dolichyl-phosphate glucosyltransferase synthesizing dolichyl phosphoglucose and the sugar-nucleotide-independent bile acid glucosyltransferase are both microsomal enzymes[69,72,73]. This is also the case for the recently described bile acid β-glucosidase[74], which is the first hepatic enzyme to hydrolyse bile acid conjugates. Thus, an intracellular cycling of bile acid glucosides can be envisaged, and bile acid glucosidation might be part of the intracellular transport of bile acids (Fig. 3).

In normal human urine the bile acid glucosides have been identified using enzymatically synthesized reference compounds[75]. Bile acid glucosides are

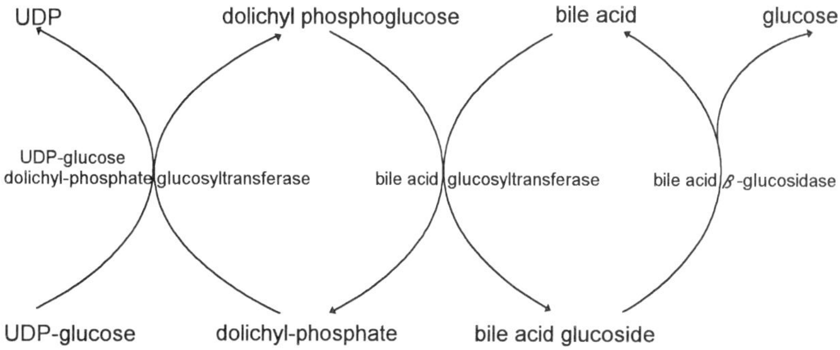

Fig. 3 Scheme of glucosidation and deglucosidation of bile acids

excreted preferably as glycine amidates in similar amounts as bile acid glucuronides[76], i.e. approximately 0.4 μmol/day. In cholestasis, excretion of bile acid glucosides increases to a much lesser extent as excretion of glucuronides[77]. Thus, glucosidation is unlikely to be a detoxication pathway of bile acids. No structural preferences for the formation of these conjugates have been observed, and the position of conjugation with glucose was found to be at C-3[78].

Recently a UDP-sugar-dependent glucosyltransferase from human liver microsomes was also characterized[79]. The role of this enzyme is even less defined. It is noteworthy that this kind of glucosidation was so far only observed *in vitro* in the case of the 6-*O*-glucosidation of HDCA. This particular conjugate has as yet not been found *in vivo*.

The chemical synthesis of 3-, 6- and 7-glycosides including the glucoside, glucuronide and *N*-acetylglucosaminide of hyodeoxycholic and ursodeoxycholic acids and related compounds has recently been described[80,81].

N-ACETYLGLUCOSAMINIDATION

In 1989, bile acid *N*-acetylglucosaminidation was described as the third glycosidic conjugation pathway in humans[76]. Daily urinary excretion rates of 0.3 0.8 μmol for these compounds were measured thus in the range of glucosides and glucuronides[76]. In contrast to the latter, conjugation with *N*-acetylglucosamine was shown to be a highly selective pathway for 7β-hydroxylated bile acids[82] such as ursodeoxycholic acid (Fig. 4). All bile acids conjugated with *N*-acetylglucosamine *in vivo* carried a hydroxyl group in 7β-position[82]. Glycosidic conjugation was studied in patients with cholestasis using stable isotope-labelled bile acids[83]. After oral administration of pharmacological doses of ^{13}C-labelled CDCA or HDCA to patients with cholestasis no *N*-acetylglucosamine conjugates were found; in the case of HDCA large amounts of HDCA 6α-glucuronide[82] as previously found using ^{14}C-labelled HDCA[84]. After administration of ^{13}C-labelled UDCA, however, 32% of this acid was excreted in urine conjugated with *N*-acetylglucosamine[82]. *N*-Acetylglucosaminides of UDCA, and of its metabolite iso-UDCA even constituted of 50% of all urinary conjugates

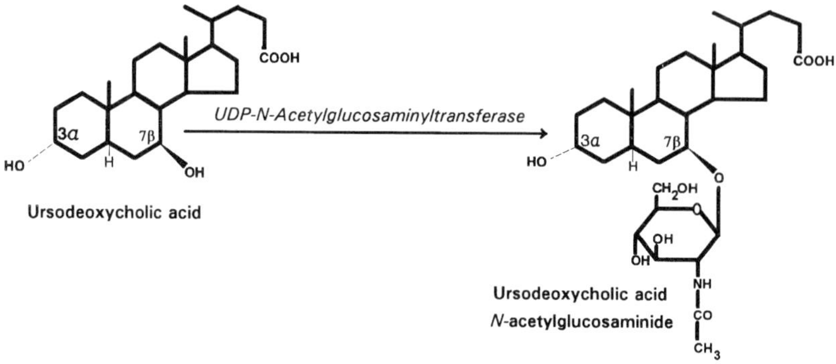

Fig. 4 7*β*-*N*-Acetylglucosaminidation of ursodeoxycholic acid

after oral administration of 3 × 250 mg UDCA/10 days to healthy volunteers. The double conjugate of UDCA with *N*-acetylglucosamine and glycine was the major compound[85]. The finding that *N*-acetylglucosaminides are the major urinary metabolites of orally administered UDCA has recently been confirmed both in health[86] and in cholestatic liver disease[87].

The selectivity of conjugation was further confirmed by the *in vitro* formation of *N*-acetylglucosaminides of 7*β*- but not of 7*α*-hydroxylated bile acids[88]. The highest activities of UDP-*N*-acetylglucosaminyltransferase both from human kidney and liver microsomes were observed towards iso-UDCA[82]. The characteristic 7*β*-position of conjugation with *N*-acetylglucosamine was confirmed both *in vitro*[78] and *in vivo*[85]. Thus, *N*-acetylglucosaminidation seems to be a metabolic pathway for UDCA and its isomers excreted in urine. It remains to be studied if this conjugation is related to the physiological and therapeutic effects of UDCA observed in patients with primary biliary cirrhosis[89]. It could be speculated that UDCA, by competing for the hepatic UDP-*N*-acetylglucosamine, could reduce the availability of this intermediate for other reactions, such as formation of glycoproteins, and thereby affect important biological functions, e.g. of cell membranes.

References

1. Björkhem I. Mechanisms of bile acid biosynthesis in mammalian liver. In: Danielsson H, Sjövall J, editors. Sterols and bile acids. Amsterdam: Elsevier; 1985:231–78.
2. Vlahcevic ZR, Heuman DM, Hylemon PB. Regulation of bile acid synthesis. Hepatology. 1991;13:590–600.
3. Russel DW, Setchell KDR. Bile acid biosynthesis. Biochemistry. 1992;31:4737–49.
4. Elliott WH. Metabolism of bile acids in liver and extrahepatic tissues. In: Danielsson H, Sjövall J, editors. Sterols and bile acids. Amsterdam: Elsevier; 1985:303–29.
5. Killenberg PG, Jordan JT. Purification and characterization of bile acid-CoA : amino acid *N*-acyltransferase from rat liver. J Biol Chem. 1978;253:1005–10.
6. Sjövall J. Bile acids in man under normal and pathological conditions. Bile acids and steroids 73. Clin Chim Acta. 1960;5:33–41.
7. Fini A, Roda A. Chemical properties of bile salts. IV. Acidity constants of glycine-conjugated bile acids. J Lipid Res. 1987;28:755–9.
8. Hofmann AF, Mysels KJ. Bile acid solubility and precipitation *in vitro* and *in vivo*: the role of conjugation, pH and Ca^{2+} ions. J Lipid Res. 1992;33:617–26.

9. Gu J-J, Hofmann AF, Ton-Nu H-T, Schteingart CD, Mysels KJ. Solubility of calcium salts of unconjugated and conjugated natural bile acids. J Lipid Res. 1992;33:635–46.
10. Carey MC, Calahane MJ. The enterohepatic circulation. In: Arias IM, Jakoby WB, Popper H, Schachter D, Shafritz DA, editors. The liver: biology and pathobiology, 2nd edn. New York: Raven Press; 1988:573–616.
11. Hofmann AF, Sjövall J, Kurtz G *et al.* A proposed nomenclature for bile acids. J Lipid Res. 1992;33:599–604.
12. Marcus SN, Schteingart CD, Marquez ML *et al.* Active absorption of conjugated bile acids *in vivo*. Kinetic parameters and molecular specificity of the ileal transport system in the rat. Gastroenterology. 1991;100:212–21.
13. Wong MH, Olkers P, Craddock AL, Dawson PA. Expression cloning and characterization of the hamster ileal sodium-dependent bile acid transporter. J Biol Chem. 1994;269:1340–7.
14. Angelin B, Björkhem I, Einarsson K, Ewerth S. Hepatic uptake of bile acids in man. Fasting and postprandial concentrations of individual bile acids in portal venous and systemic blood serum. J Clin Invest. 1982;70:724–31.
15. Hofmann AF. Bile acids. In: Arias IM, Boyer JL, Fausto N, Jakoby WB, Schachter D, Shafritz DA, editors. The liver: biology and pathobiology, 3rd edn. New York: Raven Press; 1994:677–718.
16. Matern S, Gerok W. Pathophysiology of the enterohepatic circulation of bile acids. Rev Physiol Biochem Pharmacol. 1979;85:126–204.
17. Radominska A, Treat S, Little J. Bile acid metabolism and the pathophysiology of cholestasis. Sem Liv Dis. 1993;13:219–34.
18. Bremmelgaard A, Sjövall J. Hydroxylation of cholic, chenodeoxycholic, and deoxycholic acids in patients with intrahepatic cholestasis. J Lipid Res. 1980;21:1072–81.
19. Palmer RH. The formation of bile acid sulfates: a new pathway of bile acid metabolism in humans. Proc Natl Acad Sci USA. 1967;58:1047–50.
20. Radominska A, Comer KA, Zimniak P, Falany J, Iscan M, Falany CN. Human liver steroid sulphotransferase sulphates bile acids. Biochem J. 1990;272:597–604.
21. Cowen AE, Korman MG, Hofmann AF, Cass OW. Metabolism of lithocholate in healthy man. I. Biotransformation and biliary excretion of intravenously administered lithocholate, lithocholyl-glycine, and their sulfates. Gastroenterology. 1975;69:109–18.
22. Almé B, Bremmelgaard A, Sjövall J, Thomassen P. Analysis of metabolic profiles of bile acids in urine using a lipophilic anion exchanger and computerized gas–liquid chromatography–mass spectrometry. J Lipid Res. 1977;18:339–62.
23. Back P, Spaczynski K, Gerok W. Bile salt glucuronides in urine. Hoppe-Seyler's Z Physiol Chem. 1974;355:749–52.
24. Fröhling W, Stiehl A. Bile acid glucuronides: identification and quantitative analysis in the urine of patients with cholestasis. Eur J Clin Invest. 1976;6:67–74.
25. Takikawa H, Beppu T, Seyama Y. Urinary concentrations of bile acid glucuronides and sulfates in hepatobiliary disease. Gastroenterol Jpn. 1984;19:104–9.
26. Takikawa H, Beppu T, Seyama Y. Profiles of bile acids and their glucuronide and sulphate conjugates in the serum, urine, and bile from patients undergoing biliary drainage. Gut. 1984;26:38–42.
27. Stiehl A, Raedsch R, Rudolph G, Gundert-Remy U, Senn M. Biliary and urinary excrtion of sulfated, glucuronidated and tetrahydroxylated bile acids in cirrhotic patients. Hepatology. 1985;5:492–5.
28. Hedenborg G, Norman A. The nature of urinary bile acid conjugates in patients with extrahepatic cholestasis. Scand J Clin Lab Invest. 1984;44:725–33.
29. Takikawa H, Otsuka H, Beppu T, Seyama Y, Yamakawa T. Serum concentrations of bile acid glucuronides in hepatobiliary disease. Digestion. 1983;27:189–95.
30. Takikawa H, Beppu T, Seyama Y, Obinata K, Nittono H. Serum concentrations of glucuronidated and sulfated bile acids in children with cholestasis. Biochem Med. 1985;33:381–6.
31. Hedenborg G, Norman A. Fasting and postprandial serum bile acid concentration with special reference to variations in the conjugate profile. Scand J Clin Lab Invest. 1985;45:151–6.
32. Almé B, Nordén Å, Sjövall J. Glucuronides of unconjugated 6-hydroxylated bile acids in urine of a patient with malabsorption. Clin Chim Acta. 1978;86:251–9.
33. Almé B, Sjövall J. Analysis of bile acid glucuronides in urine. Identification of $3\alpha,6\alpha,12\alpha$-trihydroxy-5β-cholanoic acid. J Steroid Biochem. 1980;13:907–16.

34. Matern H, Matern S, Schelzig Ch, Gerok W. Bile acid UDP-glucuronosyltransferase from human liver. Properties and studies on aglycone specificity. FEBS Lett. 1980;118:251–4.
35. Matern H, Matern S, Gerok W. A rapid and sensitive method for the assay of UDP-glucuronosyltransferase activity toward bile acids. Anal Biochem. 1983;133:417–24.
36. Matern S, Matern H, Farthmann EH, Gerok W. Hepatic and extrahepatic glucuronidation of bile acids in man. Characterization of bile acid uridine 5′-diphosphate-glucuronosyltransferase in hepatic, renal, and intestinal microsomes. J Clin Invest. 1984;74:402–10.
37. Parquet M, Pessah M, Saquet E, Salvat C, Raizman A, Infante R. Glucuronidation of bile acids in human liver, intestine and kidney. An *in vitro* study on hyodeoxycholic acid. FEBS Lett. 1985;189:183–7.
38. Marschall HU, Matern H, Egestad B, Matern S, Sjövall J. 6α-Glucuronidation of hyodeoxycholic acid by human liver, kidney and small bowel microsomes. Biochim Biophys Acta. 1987;921:392–7.
39. Radominska-Pyrek A, Zimniak P, Irshaid YM, Lester R, Tephly TR, Pyrek JSt. Glucuronidation of 6α-hydroxy bile acids by human liver microsomes. J Clin Invest. 1987;80:234–41.
40. Parquet M, Pessah M, Saquet E, Salvat C, Raizman A. Effective glucuronidation of 6α-hydroxylated bile acids by human hepatic and renal microsomes. Eur J Biochem. 1988;171:329–34.
41. Matern H, Matern S, Gerok W. Isolation and characterization of rat liver microsomal UDP-glucuronosyltransferase activity toward chenodeoxycholic acid and testosterone as a single form of enzyme. J Biol Chem. 1982;257:7422–9.
42. Kirkpatrick RB, Falany CN, Tephly TR. Glucuronidation of bile acids by rat liver 3-OH androgen UDP-glucuronyltransferase. J Biol Chem. 1984;259:6176–80.
43. Matern H, Lappas N, Matern S. Isolation and characterization of hyodeoxycholic acid: UDP-glucuronosyltransferase from human liver. Eur J Biochem. 1991;200:393–400.
44. Fournel-Gigleux S, Jackson MR, Wooster R, Burchell B. Expression of a human liver cDNA encoding a UDP-glucuronosyltransferase catalysing the glucuronidation of hyodeoxycholic acid in cell culture. FEBS Lett. 1989;243:119–22.
45. Fournel-Gigleux S, Sutherland L, Sabolovic N, Burchell B, Siest G. Stable expression of two human UDP-glucuronosyltransferase cDNAs in V79 cell cultures. Mol Pharmacol. 1991;39:177–83.
46. Pillot T, Ouzzine M, Fournel-Gigleux S *et al.* Glucuronidation of hyodeoxycholic acid in human liver. Evidence for a selective role of UDP-glucuronosyltransferase 2B4. J Biol Chem. 1993;268:25636–42.
47. Matern H, Heinemann H, Matern S. Radioassay of UDP-glucuronosyltransferase activities toward endogenous substrates using labelled UDP-glucuronic acid and an organic solvent extraction procedure. Anal Biochem. 1994;219:182–8.
48. Irshaid YM, Radominska A, Zimniak P, Zimniak A, Lester R, Tephly TR. Glucuronidation of monohydroxylated short chain bile acids by human liver microsomes and purified human liver UDP-glucuronosyltransferases. Drug Metabol Dispos. 1991;19:173–9.
49. Radominska-Pyrek A, Zimniak P, Chari M, Golunski E, Lester R, Pyrek JSt. Glucuronides of monohydroxylated bile acids: specificity of microsomal glucuronyltransferase for the glucuronidation site, C-3 configuration, and side chain length. J Lipid Res. 1986;27:89–101.
50. Zimniak P, Radominska A, Zimniak M, Lester R. Formation of three types of glucuronides of 6-hydroxy bile acids by rat liver microsomes. J Lipid Res. 1988;29:183–90.
51. Matern H, Marschall HU, Wietholtz H, Matern S. Glucuronidation and glucosidation of bile acids in normal tissues and carcinoma of man. In: Siest G, Magdalou J, Burchell B, editors. Cellular and molecular aspects of glucuronidation. London: Colloque INSERM/John Libbey Eurotext; 1988:173:141–9.
52. Matern H, Marschall HU, Wietholtz H, Matern S. Bile acid glycosylation in man: efficiency of glucosidation versus glucuronidation and formation of dolichyl phosphoglucose as the natural co-substrate of bile acid glucosidation. In: Paumgartner G, Stiehl A, Gerok W, editors. Trends in bile acid research. Dordrecht: Kluwer; 1989:93–7.
53. Matern S, Marschall HU, Wietholtz H, Matern H. Pathways of bile acid glycosylation in health and disease. In: Paumgartner G, Stiehl A, Gerok W, editors. Bile acids as therapeutic agents. Dordrecht: Kluwer; 1991:123–6.
54. Kuipers F, Radominska A, Zimniak P *et al.* Defective biliary secretion of bile acid 3-*O*-glucuronides in rats with hereditary conjugated hyperbilirubinemia. J Lipid Res. 1989;30:1835–45.

55. Little JM, Zimniak P, Shattuck KE, Lester R, Radominska A. Metabolism of lithocholic acid in the rat: formation of lithocholic acid 3-*O*-glucuronide *in vivo*. J Lipid Res. 1987;31:615–22.
56. Takikawa H, Narita T, Sano N, Yamanaka M. Glucuronidation of bile salts by their high-dose infusion into rats. Hepatology. 1991;13:1222–8.
57. Takikawa H, Ohki H, Sano N, Kasama T, Yamanaka M. Cholestasis induced by lithocholate and its glucuronide: their biliary excretion and metabolism. Biochim Biophys Acta. 1991;1081:39–44.
58. Oelberg DG, Chari MV, Little JM, Adcock EW, Lester R. Lithocholate glucuronide is a cholestatic agent. J Clin Invest. 1984;73:1507–14.
59. Oelberg DG, Little JM, Adcock EW, Lester R. Intestinal absorption of bile acid glucuronides in rats. Dig Dis Sci. 1988;33:1110–15.
60. Trülzsch D, Roboz J, Greim H *et al.* Hydroxylation of taurolithocholate by isolated human liver microsomes. I. Identification of metabolic product. Biochem Med. 1974;9:158–66.
61. Summerfield JA, Billing BH, Shackleton CHL. Identification of bile acids in the serum and urine in cholestasis. Evidence for 6α-hydroxylation of bile acids in man. Biochem J. 1986;154:507–16.
62. Marschall HU, Matern H, Schill A, Schumacher B, Lehnert W, Mater S. Metabolism of stable isotope labeled bile acids in extrahepatic cholestasis and liver cirrhosis of man: 6α-hydroxylation of [24-^{13}C]chenodeoxycholic and of [24-^{13}C]ursodeoxycholic acids. In: Baillie TA, Jones LR, editors. Third International Symposium on Isotopically Labelled Compounds. Amsterdam: Elsevier: 1989:699–700.
63. Nakashima T, Sano A, Seto Y *et al.* Unusual trihydroxy bile acids in the urine of patients treated with chenodeoxycholate, ursodeoxycholate or rifampicin and those with cirrhosis. Hepatology. 1990;11:255–60.
64. Back P. Phenobarbital-induced alterations of bile acid metabolism in cases of intrahepatic cholestasis. Klin Wochenschr. 1982;60:541–9.
65. Stiehl A, Becker M, Czygan P *et al.* Bile acids and their sulphated and glucuronidated derivatives in bile, plasma, and urine of children with intrahepatic cholestasis: effects of phenobarbital treatment. Eur J Clin Invest. 1980;10:307–16.
66. Wietholtz H, Zysset T, Marschall HU, Generet K, Matern S. The influence of rifampin treatment on caffeine clearance in healthy man. J Hepatol. 1995;22:78–81.
67. Wietholtz H, Marschall HU, Sjövall J, Matern S. Stimulation of bile acid 6α-glucuronidation by rifampin. (Submitted).
68. Matern H, Matern S, Gerok W. Formation of bile acid glucosides by a sugar nucleotide-independent glucosyltransferase isolated from human liver microsomes. Proc Natl Acad Sci USA. 1984;81:7036–40.
69. Matern H, Matern S. Formation of bile acid glucosides and dolichyl phosphoglucose by microsomal glucosyltransferases in liver, kidney and intestine of man. Biochim Biophys Acta. 1987;921:1–6.
70. Matern H, Fiebig HH, Matern S. Glycoside conjugation in microsomes from hepatic and renal carcinoma of man. Hepatology. 1987;7:931–6.
71. Behrens NH, Leloir LF. Dolichol monophosphate glucose: an intermediate in glucose transfer in liver. Proc Natl Acad Sci USA. 1970;66:153–9.
72. Matern H, Bolz R, Matern S. Isolation and characterization of UDP-glucose dolichyl-phosphate glucosyltransferase from human liver. Eur J Biochem. 1990;190:99–105.
73. Cartung G, Matern S, Matern H. The submicrosomal localization of uridine 5′-diphosphate-glucose dolichyl-phosphate glucosyltransferase and bile acid glucosyltransferase in the human liver. J Hepatol. 1994;20:32–40.
74. Matern H, Gartzen R, Matern S. β-Glucosidase activity towards a bile acid glucoside in human liver. FEBS Lett. 1992;314:183–6.
75. Marschall HU, Egestad B, Matern H, Matern S, Sjövall J. Evidence for bile acid glucosides as normal constituents in human urine. FEBS Lett. 1987;213:411–14.
76. Marschall HU, Egestad B, Matern H, Matern S, Sjövall J. *N*-Acetylglucosaminides: a new type of bile acid conjugate in man. J Biol Chem. 1989;264:12989–93.
77. Wietholtz H, Marschall HU, Reuschenbach R, Matern H, Matern S. Urinary excretion of bile acid glucosides and glucuronides in extrahepatic cholestasis. Hepatology. 1991;13:656–62.
78. Marschall HU, Griffiths WJ, Zhang *et al.* The positions of conjugation of bile acids with glucose and *N*-acetylglucosamine *in vitro*. J Lipid Res. 1994;35:1599–610.

79. Radominska A, Little JM, Pyrek JS *et al.* A novel UDP-Glc-specific glucosyltransferase catalyzing the biosynthesis of 6-*O*-glucosides of bile acids in human liver microsomes. J Biol Chem. 1993;268:15127–35.
80. Niwa T, Koshiyama T, Goto J, Nambara T. Synthesis of *N*-acetylglucosaminides of unconjugated and conjugated bile acids. Steroids. 1992;52:522–9.
81. Iida T, Tazawa S, Oshima Y, Niwa T, Goto J, Nambara T. Analysis of conjugated bile acids in human biological fluids. Synthesis of hyodeoxycholic acid 3- and 6-glycosides and related compounds. Chem Pharm Bull. 1994;42:1479–84.
82. Marschall HU, Matern H, Wietholtz H, Egestad B, Matern S, Sjövall J. Bile acid *N*-acetylglucosaminidation. *In vivo* and *in vitro* evidence for a selective conjugation reaction of 7β-hydroxylated bile acids in man. J Clin Invest. 1992;89:1981–7.
83. Matern S, Marschall HU, Schill A *et al.* Synthesis of ^{13}C-labeled chenodeoxy, hyodeoxy, and ursodeoxycholic acids for the study of bile acid metabolism in liver disease. Clin Chim Acta. 1991;203:77–90.
84. Sacquet E, Parquet M, Riottot M *et al.* Intestinal absorption, excretion, and biotransformation of hyodeoxycholic acid in man. J Lipid Res. 1983;24:606–13.
85. Marschall HU, Griffiths WJ, Götze U *et al.* The major metabolites of ursodeoxycholic acid in human urine are conjugated with *N*-acetylglucosamine. Hepatology. 1994;20:845–53.
86. Yamaga N, Hiromi K. Conjugation types of 7β-hydroxylated bile acids detected in healthy human urine. J Biochem. 1994;114:1123–6.
87. Kimura A, Yoneda M, Nakamura K, Akiyama K, Makino I. Urinary bile acid *N*-acetylglucosaminides during ursodeoxycholate (UDCA) treatment in patients with hepatobiliary disease. Gastroenterology. 1994;106:A917 (abstract).
88. Matern H, Bolz R, Marschall HU, Sjövall J, Matern S. Bile acid *N*-acetylglucosaminides. Formation by microsomal *N*-acetylglucosaminyltransferases in human liver and kidney. FEBS Lett. 1990;270:11–14.
89. Poupon RE, Balkau B, Eschwège E, Poupon R and the UDCA–PBC study group. A multicenter, controlled trial of ursodiol for the treatment of primary biliary cirrhosis. N Engl J Med. 1991;324:1548–54.

3
Molecular biology of hepatocellular bile acid transport

P. J. MEIER

INTRODUCTION

Bile acids or bile salts are quantitatively the major solutes in bile, and undergo efficient enterohepatic circulation. To maintain this vital physiological process liver parenchymal cells must continuously transport bile salts from portal blood plasma into bile. This vectorial transhepatocellular movement of bile salts is a concentrative transport process driven by a distinct set of primary (i.e. ATP-dependent), secondary (i.e. Na^+-gradient-dependent) and tertiary (i.e. OH^- or HCO_3^--dependent anion exchange) active transport systems at the sinusoidal (or basolateral) and canalicular (or apical) plasma membrane domains of hepatocytes (Fig. 1)[1–3].

BASOLATERAL BILE SALT UPTAKE

Sinusoidal bile salt uptake is mediated by Na^+-dependent and Na^+-independent transport systems[4]. For Na^+-dependent bile salt uptake the driving force is mediated by the prevailing out-to-in Na^+-gradient generated by the basolateral Na^+K^+-ATPase (Fig. 1). This Na^+-dependent portion of hepatocellular bile salt uptake has been well characterized in multiple experimental models, including the isolated perfused rat liver, isolated and cultured hepatocytes, and basolateral plasma membrane vesicles. Its biochemical and physiological properties have been competently reviewed and are summarized in Table 1. All these hepatocellular Na^+-dependent bile salt transport characteristics can be mediated by a single Na^+/taurocholate co-transporting polypeptide (Ntcp), that represents a glycoprotein with an apparent molecular mass of ~51 kDa in isolated basolateral rat liver plasma membranes. After *in-vitro* deglycosylation its apparent molecular weight decreased to 33 500, which corresponds to the size of the unglycosylated protein previously obtained after *in-vitro* translation of Ntcp-cRNA[5]. Ntcp is selectively localized to the basolateral plasma membrane domain of hepatocytes, and is not present in biliary epithelial cells. Ntcp is expressed only

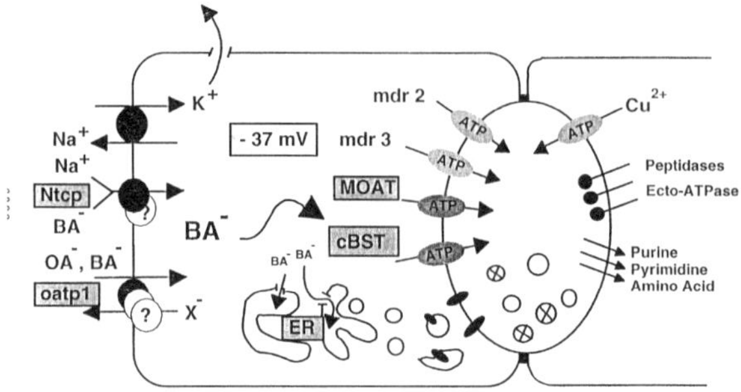

Fig. 1 The bile salt transport polarity of rat hepatocytes. Two sinusoidal bile salt uptake systems have been cloned (left): a Na^+/taurocholate co-transporting polypeptide *(*Ntcp*)* and a Na^+-independent organic anion transporter *(*Oatp1*)*. The latter transports a large variety of differently charged substrates and most probably corresponds to the previously suggested 'multispecific bile salt transporter'. While the presence of additional Na^+/bile salt co-transporters is uncertain, additional and probably more specific sinusoidal Na^+-independent organic anion transporters must be present to account for the known physiology of hepatocellular organic anion uptake *(*white circles with ?*)*. The endoplasmic reticulum (ER) localizes a potential sensitive taurocholate transport pathway, the molecular nature and exact physiological significance of which are not yet known. Among the five known ATP-dependent canalicular efflux pumps, two are involved in the secretion of bile salts into bile. The 'canalicular bile salt transporter' (cBST) mediates secretion of monovalent bile salts, and the 'multispecific organic anion transporter' (MOAT) also accepts divalent bile salt-sulphates and -glucuronidates as transport substrates. Parenthetically, the multidrug resistance gene products mdr2 and mdr3 mediate canalicular secretion of phosphatidylcholine and organic cations (and steroids), respectively. In addition to the secretory and excretory mechanisms the canalicular membrane also localizes several Na^+-dependent uptake systems to reabsorb precious cellular constituents including nucleotide precursors and amino acids. Other abbreviations: BA^-, monovalent bile salt anions; OA^-, amphipatic organic anions; X^- unidentified organic anions; ○, intracanalicular lipid vesicles, ⊗, mixed micelles

in differentiated mammalian hepatocytes, and its mRNA was first detected between 18 and 21 days of gestation in developing rat liver[6]. Ntcp expression transiently decreases after partial hepatectomy[7], and its mRNA is lost to virtually undetectable levels within 72 h in primary cultures of rat hepatocytes[8]. Functionally, Ntcp preferentially mediates Na^+-dependent transport of conjugated bile salts such as taurocholate, and to a lesser degree also of unconjugated bile salts such as cholate[9]. Ntcp-mediated Na^+-dependent taurocholate

Table 1 Biochemical and physiological properties of the Na^+-dependent bile salt uptake pathway in hepatocytes

1. Preferential transport of conjugated bile salts
2. Electrogenic Na^+/bile salt co-transport with a Na^+-taurocholate stoichiometry of greater than 1 : 1
3. K_m for taurocholate between 15 and 56 μmol/l
4. Stimulation by low concentration of bovine serum albumin
5. Possible broad substrate specificity
6. Only present in differentiated mammalian hepatocytes
7. Ontogenic expression on day 20 of gestation in fetal rat liver
8. Down-regulation during pregnancy and up-regulation in the *post-partum* period

uptake could be stimulated by low concentrations of bovine serum albumin[10] and exhibited apparent K_m values between 25 and 42 μmol/l in various eukaryotic expression systems[9]. In stably transfected CHO cells Ntcp also mediated uptake of oestrone-3-sulphate[11], which is structurally very similar to conjugated bile salts. In female rats hepatic expression of Ntcp is increased in the *post-partum* period in a prolactin-dependent manner[12]. Parenthetically, similar Na^+/taurocholate co-transporting polypeptides have also been cloned from human liver[13] and hamster ileum[14].

In addition to Ntcp the microsomal epoxide hydrolase (mEH) has also been proposed to mediate Na^+-dependent bile salt uptake into hepatocytes[15]. However, this issue remains controversial, and the suggested bile salt transport function of mEH remains to be definitely established in mammalian hepatocytes.

The hepatocellular mechanism(s) of Na^+-independent bile salt uptake is (are) less well understood than its (their) Na^+-dependent counterpart. However, in lower vertebrates such as the little skate (*Raja erinacea*), and the rainbow trout, only Na^+-independent bile salt transport mechanisms are present in hepatocytes[16,17]. In addition, in mammalian hepatocytes Na^+-independent transport accounts for most of the uptake of unconjugated bile salts such as cholate[18]. Although part of this Na^+-independent bile salt uptake portion may represent non-ionic diffusion[18], the demonstration of saturability with increasing substrate concentrations strongly indicates the involvement of carrier-mediated transmembrane transport[18]. Several potential mechanisms have been proposed, including multispecific sulphate anion exchange[19], OH^-/cholate anion exchange[20] and dicarboxylate/cholate anion exchange[18]. However, none of these putative Na^+-independent bile salt carriers has been characterized on the molecular level, and their definite role in overall hepatocellular bile salt uptake remains to be determined.

Recently, an *organic anion transporting polypeptide (Oatp 1)* consisting of 670 amino acids has been cloned from rat liver (Fig. 1)[21,22]. It most probably represents a glycoprotein with 10–12 transmembrane spanning domains and with an apparent molecular weight[22] of 74 000. Oatp1 is also selectively confined to the basolateral plasma membrane domain[23]. It can mediate chloride-dependent extraction of BSP from albumin[21] as well as chloride-independent high-affinity (K_m ~1.5 μmol/l) BSP uptake in the absence of albumin[22]. In addition, Oatp1 mediates Na^+-independent uptake of taurocholate (K_m ~50μmol/l) and cholate, and can be *cis*-inhibited by all natural conjugated and unconjugated bile salts as well as by a variety of non-bile salt amphipathic organic anions[24]. The driving force for Oatp1-mediated substrate transport is not yet known, but preliminary studies indicate that it could mediate bidirectional organic substrate transport across the sinusoidal membrane[25] (see Fig. 1). Hence, Oatp1 might also function as a sinusoidal 'overflow' system, that could prevent fatal intracellular accumulation of toxic bile salts and other cholephilic compounds in case of defective canalicular secretion (e.g. during cholestasis). Since specific antisense oligonucleotides, when mixed with total rat liver mRNA and injected into *Xenopus laevis* oocytes, inhibited the expression of Oatp1-mediated Na^+-independent taurocholate uptake to the extent of 80%[26], no additional Na^+-independent carrier would be required for hepatocellular uptake of this major conjugated natural bile salt. In contrast, the same antisense oligonucleotides inhibited expression of BSP uptake only to the extent of 50%[26], thus supporting the presence of additional BSP-uptake systems at the basolateral plasma membrane of rat hepatocytes[27]. Additional organic anion-transporting polypeptides are also required for the hepatocellular uptake of more water-soluble organic anions such as p-aminohippurate and various mono- and dicarboxylates[24]. To what extent these additional anion transporters are also involved in Na^+-independent hepatic uptake of unconjugated bile salts such as cholate[18] remains to be determined on the molecular level (Fig. 1).

INTRACELLULAR BILE SALT TRANSPORT

After uptake the incoming bile salts must first be prevented from leaking or being transported (e.g. via anion exchange) back into the blood plasma. For unconjugated dihydroxy-bile salts this goal is accomplished by rapid intracellular formation of CoA thioesters[28]. Taurine- and glycine-conjugated bile salts bind to cytoplasmic binding proteins and/or associate with intracellular membrane-bound compartments.

Cytosolic bile salt-binding proteins include glutathione-*S*-transferases, so called Y′-binding proteins, and to a lesser extent also the fatty acid-binding protein[29]. In rat liver, 3α-hydroxysteroid dehydrogenase (a Y′-class protein) represents the major cytosolic bile salt-binding protein[30]. In human liver the corresponding cytosolic bile salt binder is also a dihydrodiol dehydrogenase, but it lacks 3α-hyroxysteroid dehydrogenase activity[31]. In both rat and human liver the binding affinities of these Y′-proteins are highest for mono-, intermediate for dihydroxy-, and lowest for trihydroxy bile salts. Physiologically the cytosolic bile salt-binding proteins may predominantly serve to retain the bile salts within the cytosol, to prevent toxic damage to organelles.

Under basal bile flow conditions conjugated trihydroxy-bile salts are thought to reach the canalicular pole of hepatocytes predominantly via cytoplasmic diffusion, while at high bile salt loads canalicular bile flow and bile salt secretion become increasingly dependent on vesicle-mediated transport routes[32]. The exact nature of these bile salt-transporting vesicle pathways is not yet clear, but several observations suggest that they may be heterogeneous and involve several organelles, as well as as-yet-unidentified mechanisms. First, evidence for the involvement of the smooth endoplasmic reticulum (ER) and the Golgi has been provided, although a Na^+-independent bile salt transport system could so far only be identified in isolated ER (Fig. 1)[33,34]. Second, close regulatory similarities between the canalicular secretion of the fluid phase marker ‘horseradish peroxidase’ and of taurocholate have been demonstrated, suggesting a close relationship (or even identity) between transcytosis and bile salt transport[3]. Third, in addition to direct transcytosis, a second as-yet-unidentified vesicle-mediated pathway involving the Golgi apparatus has been recently proposed for transcellular transport of lithocholate and of other organic anions[35,36]. Fourth, various bile salts have been suggested to induce a tubular transformation of pericanalicular vesicles, raising the new possibility of a rapid ‘intratubular flow’ of certain organic anions across hepatocytes[37,38]. Interestingly, Golgi-derived vesicles could again be the primary target of this bile salt-induced tubular transformation[39]. However, a direct vesicle (or vesicotubular) pathway between the Golgi complex and the canalicular plasma membrane domain remains to be demonstrated in hepatocytes.

CANALICULAR BILE SALT SECRETION

Canalicular bile salt secretion represents the rate-limiting step in overall bile salt transport from blood into bile. Conjugated bile salts are concentrated more than 100-fold within bile canaliculi, thereby generating high osmotic gradients that provide the major driving force for the generation of intracanalicular bile flow ('bile salt-dependent bile flow'). Although canalicular bile salt secretion had originally been thought to be predominantly driven by the intracellular negative potential[40], several more recent studies have demonstrated primary ATP-dependent taurocholate transport in isolated canalicular membrane vesicles.

Five ATP-dependent organic substrate transporters have so far been identified at the bile canalicular front of rat hepatocytes (Fig. 1):

1. A copper transporting P-type ATPase that is probably defective in Wilson disease[41].
2. Mdr2, which mediates ATP-dependent canalicular secretion of biliary phosphatidylcholine[42].
3. Mdr3, which induces canalicular excretion of hydrophobic organic cations such as daunomycin, vinblastine and verapamil[43].
4. The 'multiorganic anion transporter (MOAT)', that transports mostly divalent organic anions such as GSSG, leukotrienes, bilirubindiglucuronide, dinitrophenylglutathione, BSP-glutathione, and p-nitrophenylglucuronide[44]. Furthermore, it also accepts sulphated and glucuronidated bile salts[45]. MOAT has recently been suggested to be represented by the 190 kDa multidrug resistance-associated protein (MRP)[46]. Alternatively, a 90-kDa protein has been isolated and shown to mediate ATP-dependent dinitrophenylglutathione transport when reconstituted into proteoliposomes[47,48]. It may be that this 90 kDa protein represents a subunit of the symmetrical *ABC*-transport protein MRP.
5. A separate bile salt transporter (cBST) is present at the canalicular membrane, that mediates ATP-dependent secretion of monovalent bile salts[49–52].

Using a combination of immunochemical and photoaffinity-labelling techniques it has been suggested that cBST may represent a 110-kDa polypeptide[49]. This glycoprotein had remarkably similar biochemical properties to the 100-kDa protein previously suggested to mediate trans-stimulatable and electrogenic taurocholate transport in isolated canalicular membrane vesicles[52]. However, in none of these studies was it possible to distinguish clearly the canalicular bile salt carrier(s) from the canalicular ecto-ATPase[53]. Transfection of COS cells with cDNA encoding the ecto-ATPase has been suggested to confer both ecto-ATPase and bile salt efflux activities[54]. Although these and other studies are suggestive that the ecto-ATPase may be somehow involved in the canalicular secretion of bile salts, its true bile salt transport function remains to be proven.

Two observations suggest that ATP-dependent and electrogenic canalicular bile salt secretions are mediated by two different mechanisms rather than by the same transporting polypeptide. First, a clear dissociation has been observed between normal electrogenic and decreased ATP-dependent bile salt transport in canalicular vesicles isolated from liver of ethinyloestradiol-treated rats[55]. Second, extensive subcellular fractionation studies involving further purification of routinely isolated canalicular membrane vesicles by free-flow electrophoresis indicated that electrogenic taurocholate transport is predominantly (if not exclusively) localized at the ER, whereas the ATP-dependent bile salt transport system remained associated with the further purified canalicular membrane subfraction as well as with an as-yet-unidentified 'precanalicular' vesicle compartment[34]. This distinct subcellular distribution of electrogenic and ATP-dependent taurocholate transport indicates the involvement of two separate bile salt carrier proteins, although the possibility that the ER-associated electrogenic transport system represents a precursor form of the ATP-dependent cBST cannot yet be excluded. Furthermore, the identification of a 'precanalicular' vesicle fraction exhibiting primary active ATP-dependent bile salt transport[34] supports the possibility that overall canalicular bile salt secretion may be regulated by canalicular fusion and retrieval of 'precanalicular' vesicles carrying a large number of ATP-dependent bile salt carriers[56].

Once secreted into bile canaliculi, the bile salts associate with phospholipids and cholesterol to form vesicles and mixed micelles. Furthermore, the bile salt composition of hepatic bile is further modified by bile ductular transport processes. Hence, while conjugated bile salts pass easily down the biliary tree, unconjugated mono- and dihydroxy bile acids are sufficiently lipophilic that they are absorbed by the biliary epithelial cells, return back to the sinusoid in protonated form via the periductular capillary plexus and are resecreted into bile by the hepatocytes. Such 'cholehepatic' cycling causes a bicarbonate choleresis because intraluminal carbonic acid donates the proton permitting passive bile acid absorption[57].

References

1. Boyer JL, Graf J, Meier PJ. Hepatic transport systems regulating pH_i, cell volume, and bile secretion. Annu Rev Physiol. 1992;54:415–38.
2. Gatmaitan ZC, Leveille-Webster CR, Arias IM. The biology of the bile canaliculus. In: Arias IM, Boyer JL, Fausto N, Jakoby WB, Schachter D, Shafritz DA, editors. The liver, biology and pathobiology. New York: Raven Press; 1994:665–76.
3. Nathanson MH, Boyer JL. Mechanisms and regulation of bile formation. Hepatology. 1991;14:551–66.
4. Frimmer M, Ziegler K. The transport of bile acids in liver cells. Biochim Biophys Acta. 1988;947:75–99.
5. Hagenbuch B, Stieger B, Foguet M, Lübbert H, Meier PJ. Functional expression cloning and characterization of the hepatocyte Na^+/bile acid cotransport system. Proc Natl Acad Sci USA. 1991;88:10629–33.
6. Boyer JL, Hagenbuch B, Ananthanarayanan M, Suchy F, Stieger B, Meier PJ. Phylogenic and ontogenic expression of hepatocellular bile acid transport. Proc Natl Acad Sci USA. 1993;90:435–8.
7. Green RM, Lipin AI, Pelletier EM *et al.* Hepatic regeneration is associated with a marked reduction in mRNA expression of the basolateral Na^+-taurocholate transporter. Gastroenterology. 1994;106:A901 (abstract).

8. Liang D, Hagenbuch B, Stieger B, Meier PJ. Parallel decrease of Na^+-taurocholate cotransport and its encoding mRNA in primary cultures of rat hepatocytes. Hepatology. 1993;18:1162–6.
9. Boyer JL, Ng OC, Ananthanarayanan M *et al.* Expression and characterization of a functional rat liver Na^+ bile acid cotransport system in COS-7 cells. Am J Physiol. 266 (Gastrointest Liver Physiol. 29) 1994;G382–7.
10. Hagenbuch B, Lübbert H, Stieger B, Meier PJ. Expression of the hepatocyte Na^+/bile acid cotransporter in *Xenopus laevis* oocytes. J Biol Chem. 1990;265:5357–60.
11. Schroeder A, Hagenbuch B, Stieger B *et al.* The rat hepatocyte Na^+/taurocholate cotransporting polypeptide (Ntcp) mediates multispecific substrate transport in stably transfected Chinese hamster ovary (CHO) cells. Gastroenterology. 1994;106:A979 (abstract).
12. Ganguly TC, Liu Y, Hyde JF, Hagenbuch B, Meier PJ, Vore M. Prolactin increases hepatic Na^+/taurocholate cotransport activity and messenger RNA *post partum*. Biochem J. 1994;303:33–6.
13. Hagenbuch B, Meier PJ. Molecular cloning, chromosomal localization and functional characterization of a human liver Na^+/bile acid cotransporter. J Clin Invest. 1994;93:1326–31.
14. Wong MH, Oelkers P, Craddock AL, Dawson PA. Expression cloning and characterization of the hamster ileal sodium-dependent bile acid transporter. J Biol Chem. 1994;269:1340–7.
15. Von Dippe P, Amoui M, Alves C, Levy D. Na^+-dependent bile acid transport by hepatocytes is mediated by a protein similar to microsomal epoxide hydrolase. Am J Physiol. 264 (Gastrointest Liver Physiol. 27) 1993;G528–34.
16. Fricker G, Hugentobler G, Meier PJ, Kurz G, Boyer JL. Identification of a single sinusoidal bile salt uptake system in skate liver. Am J Physiol. 253 (Gastrointest Liver Physiol. 16) 1987;G816–22.
17. Rabergh CMI, Ziegler K, Isomaa B, Lipsky MM, Eriksson JE. Uptake of taurocholic acid and cholic acid in isolated hepatocytes from rainbow trout. Am J Physiol. 267 (Gastrointest Liver Physiol. 30) 1994;G380–6.
18. Boelsterli UA, Zimmerli B, Meier PJ. Identification and characterization of a basolateral dicarboxylate-cholate antiport system in rat hepatocytes. Am J Physiol. (Gastrointest Liver Physiol.) 1995 (In press)
19. Hugentobler G, Meier PJ. Multispecific anion exchange in basolateral (sinusoidal) rat liver plasma membrane vesicles. Am J Physiol. 251 (Gastrointest Liver Physiol. 14) 1986;G656–64.
20. Blitzer BL, Terzakis C, Scott KA. Hydroxyl-bile acid exchange: a new mechanism for the uphill transport of cholate by basolateral liver plasma membrane vesicles. J Biol Chem. 1986;261:12042–6.
21. Jacquemin E, Hagenbuch B, Stieger B, Wolkoff AW, Meier PJ. Expression of the hepatocellular chloride-dependent sulfobromophthalein uptake system in *Xenopus laevis* oocytes. J Clin Invest. 1991;88:2146–9.
22. Jacquemin E, Hagenbuch B, Stieger B, Wolkoff AW, Meier PJ. Expression cloning of a rat liver Na^+-independent organic anion transporter. Proc Natl Acad Sci USA. 1994;91:133–7.
23. Shi XY, Ford AC, Jacquemin E *et al.* Immunologic distribution of an organic anion transport protein (oatp) in rat liver and kidney. Hepatology. 1994;20:205A.
24. Kullak-Ublick GA, Hagenbuch B, Stieger B, Wolkoff A, Meier PJ. Functional characterization of the basolateral rat liver organic anion transporting polypeptide. Hepatology. 1994;20:411–16.
25. Shi XY, Bai S, Ford AC *et al.* Stable inducible expression of a functional rat liver organic anion transport protein (oatp) in HeLa cells. Hepatology. 1994;20:174A (abstract).
26. Hagenbuch B, Scharschmidt BF, Meier PJ. Use of antisense oligonucleotides to assess the role of the cloned transporters Ntcp and oatp in Na^+-dependent and Na^+-independent hepatic uptake of taurocholate and non-bile acid organic anions. Hepatology. 1994;20:201A (abstract).
27. Torres AM, Lunazzi GC, Stremmel W, Tiribelli C. Bilitranslocase and sulfobromophthalein/bilirubin-binding protein are both involved in the hepatic uptake of organic anions. Proc Natl Acad Sci USA. 1993;90:8136–9.
28. Clayton LM, Gurantz D, Hofmann AF, Hagey LR, Schteingart CD. The role of bile acid conjugation in hepatic transport of dihydroxy bile acids. J Pharmacol Exp Ther. 1989;248:1130–7.
29. Erlinger S. Intracellular events in bile acid transport by the liver. In: Tavoloni N, Berk PD, editors. Hepatic transport and bile secretion. Physiology and pathophysiology. New York: Raven Press; 1993;467–75.

30. Stolz A, Takikawa H, Ookhtens M, Kaplowitz N. The role of cytoplasmic proteins in hepatic bile acid transport. Annu Rev Physiol. 1989;51:161–76.
31. Stolz A, Hammond L, Lou H, Takikawa H, Ronk M, Shively JE. cDNA cloning and expression of the human hepatic bile acid-binding protein. A member of the monomeric reductase gene family. J Biol Chem. 1993;268:10448–57.
32. Coleman R. Biochemistry of bile secretion. Biochem J. 1987;244:249–61.
33. Alves C, Von Dippe P, Amoui M, Levy D. Bile acid transport into hepatocyte smooth endoplasmic reticulum vesicles is mediated by microsomal epoxide hydrolase, a membrane protein exhibiting two distinct topological orientations. J Biol Chem. 1993;268:20148–55.
34. Kast C, Stieger B, Winterhalter KW, Meier PJ. Hepatocellular transport of bile acids. Evidence for distinct subcellular localization of electrogenic and ATP-dependent taurocholate transport in rat hepatocytes. J Biol Chem. 1994;269:5179–86.
35. Aoyama N, Ohya T, Chandler K, Gresky S, Holzbach RT. Transcellular transport of organic anions in the isolated perfused rat liver: the differential effects of monensin and colchicine. Hepatology. 1991;14:1–9.
36. Wilton JC, Matthews GM, Burgoyne RD, Mills CO, Chipman JK, Coleman R. Fluorescent choleretic and cholestatic bile salts take different paths across the hepatocyte: Transcytosis of glycolithocholate leads to an extensive redistribution of annexin II. J Cell Biol. 1994;127:401–10.
37. Hayakawa T, Ng OC, Ma A, Boyer JL. Taurocholate stimulates transcytotic vesicular pathways labeled by horseradish peroxidase in the isolated perfused rat liver. Gastroenterology. 1990;99:216–28.
38. Sakisaka S, Harada M, Gondo K, Yoshitake M, Tanikawa K. Tubulovesicular transport of horseradish peroxidase in isolated rat hepatocyte couplets: effects of low temperature, cytochalasin B, and bile acids. Hepatology. 1994;20:1015–23.
39. Cluett EB, Wood SA, Banta M, Brown WJ. Tubulation of Golgi membranes *in vivo* and *in vitro* in the absence of brefeldin A. J Cell Biol. 1993;120:15–24.
40. Meier PJ. Transport polarity of hepatocytes. Sem Liv Dis. 1988;8:293–307.
41. Dijkstra M, In't Veld G, van den Berg GJ, Müller M, Kuipers F, Vonk R. Adenosine triphosphate-dependent copper transport in isolated rat liver plasma membranes. J Clin Invest. 1995;95:412–16.
42. Smit JJM, Schinkel AH, Oude Elferink RPJ *et al.* Homozygous disruption of the murine *mdr2* P-glycoprotein gene leads to a complete absence of phospholipid from bile and to liver disease. Cell. 1993;75:1–20.
43. Kamimoto Y, Gatmaitan Z, Hsu J, Arias IM. The function of Gp-170, the multidrug resistance gene product in rat liver canalicular membrane vesicles. J Biol Chem. 1989;264:11693–8.
44. Zimniak P, Awasthi YC. ATP-dependent transport systems for organic anions. Hepatology. 1993;17:330–9.
45. Oude Elferink RP, Ottenhoff R, Radominska A, Hofmann AF, Kuipers F, Jansen PLM. Inhibition of glutathione-conjugate secretion from isolated hepatocytes by dipolar bile acids and other organic anions. Biochem J. 1991;274:281–6.
46. Müller M, Mejer C, Zaman GJR *et al.* Overexpression of the gene encoding the multidrug resistance-associated protein results in increased ATP-dependent glutathione *S*-conjugate transport. Proc Natl Acad Sci USA. 1994;91:13033–7.
47. Pikula S, Hayden JB, Awasthi S, Awasthi YC, Zimniak P. Organic anion-transporting ATPase of rat liver. I. Purification, photoaffinity labeling, and regulation by phosphorylation. J Biol Chem. 1994;269:27566–73.
48. Pikula S, Hayden JB, Awasthi S, Awasthi YC, Zimniak P. Organic anion-transporting ATPase of rat liver. II. Functional reconstitution of active transport and regulation by phosphorylation. J Biol Chem. 1994;269:27574–9.
49. Müller M, Ishikawa T, Berger U *et al.* ATP-dependent transport of taurocholate across the hepatocyte canalicular membrane mediated by a 110-kDa glycoprotein binding ATP and bile salt. J Biol Chem. 1991;266:18920–6.
50. Nishida T, Gatmaitan Z, Che M, Arias IM. Rat liver canalicular membrane vesicles contain an ATP-dependent bile acid transport system. Proc Natl Acad Sci USA. 1991;88:6590–4.
51. Stieger B, O'Neill B, Meier PJ. ATP-dependent bile-salt transport in canalicular rat liver plasma-membrane vesicles. Biochem J. 1992;284:67–74.

52. Ruetz S, Fricker G, Hugentobler G, Winterhalter K, Kurz G, Meier PJ. Isolation and characterization of the putative canalicular bile salt transport system of rat liver. J Biol Chem. 1987;262:11324–30.
53. Lin SH, Guidotti G. Cloning and expression of a cDNA coding for a rat liver plasma membrane ecto-ATPase. J Biol Chem. 1989;264:14408–14.
54. Sippel CJ, Suchy FJ, Ananthanarayanan M, Perlmutter DH. The rat liver ecto-ATPase is also a canalicular bile acid transport protein. J Biol Chem. 1993;268:2083–91.
55. Bossard R, Stieger B, O'Neill B, Fricker G, Meier PJ. Ethinyl-estradiol treatment induces multiple canalicular membrane transport alterations in rat liver. J Clin Invest. 1993;91:2714–20.
56. Häussinger D, Lang F, Gerok W. Regulation of cell function by the cellular hydration state. Am J Physiol. 267 (Endocrinol Metab. 30) 1994:E343–55.
57. Hofmann AF. Bile acids. In: Arias IM, Boyer JL, Fausto N, Jakoby WB, Schachter D, Shafritz DA, editors. The liver: biology and pathobiology. New York: Raven Press; 1994:677–718.

4
Effect of bile acid structure on bile flow and biliary lipid secretion

A. F. HOFMANN

OVERVIEW

Bile acid anions are actively transported across the canalicular membrane by one or more canalicular ATPases denoted by the abbreviation cBAT. In the canalicular lumen, the osmotic activity of the bile acid anions induces water and solute flow from the space of Disse across the paracellular junctions. The mixture of water and solutes induced by bile acid secretion is defined as bile acid dependent (BAD) bile flow. Other solutes, presumably mostly anions, are secreted actively by canalicular transport systems. These solutes also induce a flow of water and filtrable solutes into the canalicular lumen. That bile flow which is induced by the secretion of solutes other than bile acids is defined as bile acid independent (BAI) bile flow. The sum of BAD bile flow and BAI bile flow is defined as canalicular bile flow[1]. Solutes that are actively secreted into the canalicular lumen and induce bile flow are termed *primary solutes*. Those that enter the canalicular lumen via the paracellular junctions in response to the osmotic gradient are termed *secondary solutes*[2]. Chloride ions, which enter bile as secondary solutes, might well exchange with bicarbonate ions as a chloride/bicarbonate exchanger has been identified in the canalicular membrane[3].

The canalicular lumina form a network of fine canals lined by the external face of the apical membranes of hepatocytes. The canaliculi have a blind end at the pericentral region of the hepatic lobule. The canalicular lumen is surrounded by a cylinder of actin filaments organized in a pericanalicular spiral. The tone of these filaments prevents dilatation of the canaliculi when bile is secreted into it. Contraction of the filaments induces bile to flow in a periportal direction, countercurrent to sinusoidal blood flow[4]. The periportal end of the canaliculi coalesce into small tubes that link the canaliculi with the biliary ductules. These tubes, known as the canals of Hering, are lined with a transitional epithelium. The biliary ductule is defined as that canal possessing a true epithelial lining. The biliary ductule is surrounded by a peribiliary capillary plexus that originates from branches of the hepatic artery, and drains into the sinusoid[5].

In addition to inducing bile flow by their osmotic effects, bile acids also induce biliary lipid secretion. The lipids are predominantly phospholipid and cholesterol. The phospholipid consists mostly of phosphatidylcholine (PC) molecules, this class of zwitterionic lipids being termed lecithin in the older biliary literature. Biliary PC, in turn, consists of a fairly narrow spectrum of molecular species[6,7]. The ratio of cholesterol (C) to PC is species dependent and ranges over an order of magnitude. In the dog, the C/PC ratio is 0.02; in cholesterol gallstone patients, it is 0.33[8,9]. Biliary lipid secretion is predominantly bile acid dependent. However, in some species, there continues to be lipid secretion in the absence of appreciable bile acid secretion, suggesting that a fraction of biliary lipid secretion is bile acid independent. In addition, brefeldin, an agent that disrupts the Golgi apparatus, has been shown to decrease biliary lipid secretion in the fasting state, but not that induced by bile acid administration[10,11]. Thus, there appears to be a continuing default secretion of vesicles into bile unrelated to bile acid secretion. It is useful, therefore, to postulate that canalicular biliary lipid secretion is the sum of BAD biliary lipid secretion and BAI biliary lipid secretion.

Bile flow may be modified during passage through the biliary tract. One view is that canalicular bile is hypertonic, since a hypertonic primary secretion is diluted by an isotonic filtrate from plasma[3]. If so, water is likely to enter bile in the initial segments of the biliary ductules, since duct bile is invariably isotonic. The paracellular junctions of the ductules are much tighter than those of the canalicular membrane[12]; presumably, water enters through these or through water channels in the apical membrane. In either event, ductular water flow that is responsible for dilution of bile and rendering it isotonic is unaccompanied by an appreciable flux of 'secondary solutes'.

Additional modifications of ductular bile include secretion and absorption of solutes that is accompanied by water movement. Secretion involves bicarbonate ions (via the cystic fibrosis transmembrane conductance regulator (CFTR)), which, in turn, must cause sodium ions to enter ductular bile. Absorption involves primary and secondary solutes. Glutathione is hydrolysed by ductular γ-glutamyltranspeptidase (GGT), and the hydrolysis products absorbed[13]. Glucose is efficiently absorbed[14,15]. The absorption of glucose, and probably that of other anions, is likely to be sodium coupled. Therefore, such ductular absorption of solutes will induce the absorption of a small volume of water by the osmotic effect of the absorbed solutes. Absorption might occur in one segment of the biliary ductules, and secretion in another. Thus, hepatic (duct) bile flow can be considered to consist of four terms:

$$^{H20}J_{hepduct} = {}^{H20}J_{can.bad} + {}^{H20}J_{can.bai} + {}^{H20}J_{sec.duc} - {}^{H20}J_{abs.duc}$$

where the meanings of the above terms are self-evident from the preceding discussion. In the gallbladder, absorption occurs during interprandial fasting, and secretion is likely to occur during meals[16].

At present, it is assumed that neither secretion nor absorption of PC or cholesterol occurs during ductular passage. The validity of this assumption is not known. In the gallbladder, there is modest absorption of both PC and cholesterol during gallbladder storage[17].

In this brief essay, I will review selected aspects of BAD bile flow and BAD biliary lipid secretion, with emphasis on the influence of bile acid structure.

ZONATION AND THE ENTEROHEPATIC CIRCULATION

The concept of zonal localization (zonation) of many hepatocyte functions is well established[18] and is also pertinent to events in bile acid metabolism. Efficient intestinal absorption of secreted bile acids leads to the accumulation of a bile acid pool whose circulation increases in frequency with meals and decreases in frequency during the fasting state[19]. Bile acids absorbed from the intestine are extracted predominantly by periportal cells. The periportal hepatocytes transport the absorbed bile acids from the basolateral (sinusoidal) membrane to the apical (canalicular) membrane.

In most species, the majority of bile acids that are absorbed from the intestine and delivered to the periportal hepatocytes are likely to be conjugated bile acids that were secreted and absorbed in this chemical form. A minority of bile acids has undergone chemical modification by bacterial enzymes present in the distal intestine. It is useful to term such chemical modification as 'damage' because the products resulting from such biotransformation have physicochemical properties that are inferior to those of the primary bile acid conjugates[20]. During hepatocyte transport, such modifications are often reversed, and the reversal of damage may be termed 'repair'. Periportal hepatocytes transport and repair the majority of recycling bile acids. Periportal hepatocytes are also responsible for the majority of hepatic cholesterol biosynthesis. Periportal hepatocytes are thus responsible for most BAD bile flow and BAD biliary lipid secretion.

Pericentral cells extract and repair those bile acids not removed by the periportal cells. Overall hepatic extraction of bile acids ranges from 50–90% depending on bile acid structure, and is presumably first order[21]. Accordingly, uptake of bile acids by the periportal cells should be at least two thirds of the bile acid flux, whereas uptake by the pericentral cells should be no more than one third, if periportal and pericentral hepatocytes have the same transport kinetics. Pericentral cells are responsible for most bile acid biosynthesis in the organism with an intact enterohepatic circulation[22]. Secretion of newly synthesized bile acids by pericentral cells constitutes <5% of secreted bile acids, at least in man. With interruption of the enterohepatic circulation, bile acid synthesis increases. The site of bile acid biosynthesis changes, moving toward the portal triad[22]. In this circumstance, both pericentral and periportal cells participate in upregulated bile acid biosynthesis. The proportion of bile acid secretion that is derived from bile acid synthesis increases. With complete interruption of the enterohepatic circulation, all bile acid secretion originates from de-novo bile acid biosynthesis.

DAMAGE, REPAIR, AND DETOXIFICATION DURING THE ENTEROHEPATIC CIRCULATION OF BILE ACIDS

In most mammals, bile acids are secreted into bile in a chemical form that is optimal for aqueous solubility and detergency. With respect to the side-chain, bile acids are fully conjugated with taurine (or glycine). With respect to the nucleus, two or three hydroxy groups are present in the α configuration and the A/B ring juncture is *cis* (the hydrogen at C-5 is in the β position). (There are some uncommon exceptions to this statement: some reptiles have 5α-bile acids, and some species have 7β-hydroxy- or 7-oxo groups rather than a 7α-hydroxy group)[23].

Bile acids are absorbed by passive and active mechanisms from the small intestine[24]. Aerobic bacteria are present in the small intestine, their density increasing in the ileum. In herbivores and some carnivores, a caecum is present which contains a flora rich in anaerobic bacteria.

With respect to the side-chain, the major bacterial biotransformation is deconjugation, a process mediated by both aerobic and anaerobic bacteria. For the nucleus, damage consists of modification of the hydroxy groups. Such modifications are of two major types: dehydrogenation and 7-dehydroxylation. Dehydrogenation denotes oxidoreduction of the hydroxy groups (oxidation of an α or β hydroxy group to an oxo group, which, in turn, may be followed by reduction to an α or β hydroxy group). Oxidoreduction can occur with either conjugated or unconjugated bile acids. Dehydroxylation denotes removal of the 7-hydroxy group, a complex process that begins with CoA formation of the unconjugated bile acid and is followed ultimately by the formation of a 3-oxo-$\Delta^{4,6}$ resonating intermediate that involves both the A and B rings[25,26]. Dehydroxylation cannot occur at any other position than C-7. Dehydroxylation requires prior deconjugation because CoA formation does not occur with taurine or glycine conjugated bile acids, as CoA formation occurs more readily with weak acids than strong acids.

Deconjugation and oxido-reduction are likely to begin in the distal small intestine and continue in the large intestine. In contrast, dehydroxylation occurs only in the colon, as it is mediated by only a few species of bacteria, and such species are strict anaerobes.

As a result of this bacterial damage, a group of unconjugated bile acids (primary, hydroxy-oxo and 7-deoxy bile acids) are absorbed from the distal intestine. Conjugated hydroxy-oxo bile acids formed by bacterial damage are absorbed mostly by active mechanisms, as are the conjugated bile acids that have remained unaltered by bacterial enzymes. These fluxes of undamaged and damaged bile acids mix in the portal venous blood flow and return to the liver. The magnitude and composition of the stream of damaged bile acids that returns to the liver has been characterized in very few species. It is likely that the efficiency of bile acid absorption is greater from the small intestine than the large intestine because of the greater surface area of the small intestinal epithelium and its lower bacterial colonization compared with the large intestine[27]. Of course, newly formed 7-deoxy bile acids are absorbed solely from the colon, the site of their formation[28].

The damaged bile acids are 'repaired' or detoxified during passage through the periportal hepatocytes. Unconjugated bile acids are efficiently reconjugated. The oxo group of hydroxy-oxo bile acids is reduced stereospecifically, but the completedness and the stereospecificity of the reduction is both position and species dependent. The most important repair is at the 3 position, and involves the reduction of 3-oxo bile acids to 3α-hydroxy bile acids, as well as the epimerization of 3β-hydroxy bile acids to 3α-hydroxy bile acids. Studies with isolated vesicles have suggested that 3-oxo bile acids cannot be secreted into bile[29], although, in fact, they are found in biliary bile acids in moderate proportions in some species[30,31].

7-Oxo bile acids undergo variable reduction. In some species, reduction is mostly to the 7β-hydroxy configuration; in others, to the 7α-hydroxy configuration (c.f. Reference 32).

The fate of the two common 7-deoxy bile acids – lithocholic acid (3α-OH) and deoxycholic acid (3αOH, 12αOH) – is also species dependent. Lithocholic acid is probably 7-rehydroxylated to chenodeoxycholic acid (3αOH, 7αOH) in most species in which it is a major faecal bile acid (c.f. Reference 31). In man and chimpanzee, LCA is first *N*-acylamidated with taurine or glycine (on the side-chain) and is then partly sulphated at the 3 position[33,34]. The resulting sulpholithocholymidates are rapidly eliminated from the circulating bile acids, as they undergo little carrier-mediated absorption from the small intestine[35]. Deoxycholic acid has different fates in different species. In some species, it is partly or completely rehydroxylated (to cholic acid), and then conjugated with cholic acid. In other species, including man and rabbit, deoxycholic acid is not rehydroxylated, but merely reconjugated. Its conjugates join with those of the primary bile acids in the circulating bile acids. In a few uncommon species, deoxycholic acid is hydroxylated at a new position such as C-6 or C-16 to form a new trihydroxy bile acid which then joins with the primary bile acid conjugates in the circulating bile acids.

BILE FLOW

The undamaged and repaired bile acids, all in conjugated form, are actively secreted into the canaliculus, inducing BAD bile flow and BAD biliary lipid secretion. For some years, it has been customary to graph hepatic bile flow (vertical axis) against bile acid output in hepatic (duct) bile (horizontal axis). The slope of this line, Δ bile flow/Δ bile acid is termed the 'apparent choleretic activity' (ACA) and is expressed as μl/μmol (or ml/mmol). (Reasons for the qualifying adjective 'apparent' have been given elsewhere[36].) These units are the equivalent of reciprocal osmolarity. In isosmotic saline, there are 6.6 μl/μmol chloride anions, and, in principle, the ACA of conjugated bile acids would be expected to have a value somewhere around this. In practice, values of 8–15 μl/μmol are commonly observed.

There are at least two factors that are responsible for the ACA being greater than its theoretical value. The first is that bile acids self-associate to form simple micelles; in the presence of PC-cholesterol, they form mixed micelles. Since osmolality is a colligative property, that is, determined solely by the number of particles, micelle formation means that there will be less water per μmol bile acid. On the other hand, the formation of bile involves the paracellular entry of filtrable solutes together with water, and these are also osmotically active. This effect increases the amount of water per μmol bile acid. Experimentally, the effect of micelle formation can be eliminated by using non-micelle-forming bile acids. The ACA of dehydrocholyltaurine, a tri-oxo bile acid is about 20% higher than that of cholyltaurine (taurocholate). Under steady-state conditions, a value of 13 μl/μmol was observed for dehydrocholyltaurine compared with 11 μl/μmol for cholyltaurine[37].

In order to develop principles of BAD bile flow, the general practice is to infuse an exogenous bile acid into an anaesthetized biliary fistula rat. Such experiments are confounded by the contribution of the endogenous bile acids of the animal as well as the toxicity of the infused bile acids. In addition, there may be effects of the anaesthetic agent if it has intrinsic choleretic activity, as well as the influence of general anaesthesia per se. To mitigate these problems, investigators may flush out the intestine of the rat before commencing the bile acid infusion, or may study the animal after much of the endogenous pool has drained from the animal. Studies may also be performed in the unanaesthetized animal by using an exteriorized enterohepatic circulation with the animal tethered to a swivel arrangement[38,39] or by using an appropriate restraining cage, such as the Bollman cage[40]. Despite all these problems, such experiments give reasonably consistent results, and three types of BAD bile flow patterns may be observed: eucholeresis, hypercholeresis and cholestasis.

Eucholeresis

In eucholeresis, the infused bile acid is efficiently extracted and secreted into bile. Bile flow increases in direct proportion to the output of the infused bile acid (and/or its biotransformation products), and the ACA is 6–15 μl/μmol. If a non-micelle-forming bile acid is used, the ACA is slightly higher. Non-micelle-forming bile acids do not induce BAD biliary lipid secretion. Thus, bile flow induced by non-micelle-forming bile acids contains bile acid molecules largely in monomeric form.

Hypercholeresis

In hypercholeresis, the ACA is increased, ranging from 20–400 μl/μmol, as evidenced by the plot of bile flow against bile acid recovery having a very steep slope. Because ductular bile is always isotonic, an additional osmotically active anion must be present, and this has been shown in numerous studies to be bicarbonate. The bicarbonate concentration in rodent bile is usually 25–35 mmol/L; with hypercholeresis, [HCO_3^-] increases to 40–60 mmol/L[36]. Hypercholeresis occurs when dihydroxy bile acids (and one trihydroxy bile acid, β-muricholic acid[41]) are secreted into bile in unconjugated form. Secretion in unconjugated form occurs when the rate of hepatocyte uptake exceeds the rate of conjugation or when the structure of the side-chain is modified so that the bile acid becomes a poor substrate for bile acid conjugation. The conjugation capacity of the hepatocyte may be exceeded either by a supraphysiological rate of bile acid infusion or by inducing a taurine deficiency in the hepatocyte in those species that conjugate preferentially with taurine. Bile acids that have induced hypercholeresis include UDCA, its 23-methyl derivative, nor-UDCA, nor-CDCA, nor-DCA, and the 12β-epimer of deoxycholic acid (for primary references, see Reference 36).

When a dihydroxy bile acid is secreted into bile in unconjugated form, a substantial fraction is absorbed passively by the biliary ductular epithelium.

Absorption involves uptake of the protonated bile acid, which generates a bicarbonate anion in the lumen. The apical membranes of the biliary ductular epithelium appear to lack a Na^+/H^+ exchanger, so that the hydrogen atom that enters with the protonated bile acid is not returned to the lumen and a sodium ion is not absorbed. The absorbed bile acids pass through the ductular epithelial cell (cholangiocyte), exit via the basolateral membranes of the cholangiocyte, and are returned to the sinusoid by the plasma flow in the periductular capillary plexus. A fraction of the unconjugated bile acid is likely to undergo amidation by taurine (or glycine) during transport through the cholangiocyte[42].

Dihydroxy bile acids may not be good substrates for conjugation with glycine or taurine, but nonetheless may be conjugated (with glucuronate) during hepatocyte transport. If the hepatocyte is acidified by amiloride, glucuronidation of unconjugated bile acids increases markedly, abolishing hypercholeresis[43]. Trihydroxy bile acids, such as cholic acid, and more hydrophilic derivatives, such as its $7\beta,12\beta$-epimer, are too polar to be appreciably absorbed during passage down the biliary ductules; accordingly, they induce little or no hypercholeresis.

In principle, any rather hydrophobic organic anion that is the conjugate base of a weak acid will induce hypercholeresis if it is secreted into bile in unconjugated form. Our laboratory has recently shown that sulindac, a widely used non-steroidal anti-inflammatory agent, induces hypercholeresis in the rat[44].

Cholestasis

As first reported by Javitt[45], lithocholic acid and its conjugates, as well as other monohydroxy bile acids induce cholestasis when infused intravenously into rats[46]. Since bile flow decreases below the value of BAI bile flow, and, since the infused bile acid is poorly recovered in bile, it is likely that acute cholestasis induced by the intravenous infusion of monohydroxy bile acids results from these bile acids inhibiting the transport activity of both cBAT (the canalicular bile acid transporter) and MRP, the transporter responsible for the secretion of many other organic anions into bile (MRP is referred to as MOAT in much of the recent literature). The latter transporter has recently been cloned[47] and it should be possible to examine whether lithocholic acid (and its conjugates) interact with it in such a way as to inhibit its transport of other anions.

UDCA AND CHOLERESIS

The limited data that are available[48] suggest that UDCA is not hypercholeretic, at least in patients without liver disease. The possibility remains that some patients with liver disease will not conjugate endogenous or exogenous bile acids efficiently, and that dihydroxy bile acids (endogenous or exogenous) will induce hypercholeresis. One report has claimed that, in some patients with cholestatic liver disease, conjugation is not complete[49]; but a second report could not confirm this observation[50].

Nor-UDCA is hypercholeretic in the healthy human, based on a single observation[51]. In this unpublished study, nor-UDCA induced a bicarbonate-rich bile flow with an ACA of $50/\mu l$ being observed. Nor-UDCA was mostly conjugated with glucuronate at C-23 in ester linkage, a biotransformation pattern not observed in other mammals. This observation raises the possibility that, if UDCA were to escape efficient amidation in patients with liver disease, it would undergo glucuronidation. Were this to occur, hypercholeresis would not be induced.

UDCA administration will induce eucholeresis to the extent that it causes increased canalicular secretion of bile acids. The limited data that are available suggest that UDCA causes no, or only a modest, increase in bile acid secretion in patients with cholestatic liver disease[52,53]. The failure of exogenous UDCA to increase bile acid secretion can be explained by intestinal transport being rate limiting and homeostatically regulated by negative feedback, based on animal studies[54]. To increase canalicular secretion, it is necessary to increase cBAT transport activity by providing more substrate, if substrate is rate limiting. In principle, this can be done by infusing UDCA (as the sodium salt) into the small intestine[55] but the feasibility of this approach in the clinical situation has not been examined. If there is obstruction to bile flow in some biliary ductules, increasing canalicular function of non-obstructed biliary ductules will improve hepatic excretory function, but may or may not decrease the bile acid concentration of obstructed hepatocytes.

BILIARY LIPID SECRETION

PC secretion

Great progress has been made in understanding the broader aspects of biliary lipid secretion during the past five years. A series of studies by Verkade and his colleagues (reviewed in Reference 9) provided strong evidence that bile acids act on the luminal side of the canalicular membrane to induce BAD biliary lipid secretion. In other Dutch studies[56], the *mdr*2 canalicular ATPase was shown to be required for biliary phospholipid secretion. Crawford and his colleagues obtained electron microscopic evidence for budding of lipid vesicles from the luminal face of the canalicular lumen during BAD biliary lipid secretion[57]. It is hoped that these images are not artifacts induced by the fixation process.

Thus, according to current concepts, bile acid anions deterge PC molecules from the luminal hemileaflet of the canalicular membrane, possibly by creating zones of instability resulting from bile acids absorbing to and expanding the area of the luminal hemileaflet. A second possibility is that bile acids simultaneously deterge and solubilize PC molecules in the same manner that bile acids interact with lipolysis products generated at the surface of the oil droplets during intestinal fat digestion. Contraction of the pericanalicular filaments may serve to enhance vesicle budding in the presence of bile acids[4]. If this concept is correct, the canalicular membranes with its surrounding spiral of microfilaments is a vesicle generator.

This view of BAD biliary lipid secretion predicts that lipid coupling will be decreased by experimental manoeuvers that decrease the surface activity of bile acids. Such manoeuvers include:

1. Secretion of anions that complex with bile acid;
2. Secretion of anions that induce BAI flow, e.g. ceftriaxone[58];
3. Secretion of non-micelle-forming bile acids[37].

Agents that decrease the ratio of phospholipids to bile acids in bile have been termed 'uncoupling agents'. The observations that such uncoupling agents were devoid of activity in the MRP-deficient rat (in whom the intrahepatocyte concentration should be markedly elevated because of defective canalicular secretion by MOAT) was a strong piece of evidence in favour of the thesis that biliary lipid secretion results from interaction of bile acids with phospholipids at the luminal face of the canalicular membrane. Uncoupling agents are now considered to act within the canalicular lumen, diminishing the surface activity of bile acid monomers.

Cholesterol secretion

In contrast to the advances made in understanding BAD PC secretion, much less is known about the determinants of biliary cholesterol secretion. An elevated cholesterol/PC ratio is the fundamentally pathochemical defect in cholesterol gallstone disease; and the ability of orally administered CDCA and UDCA to decrease the cholesterol/PC ratio forms the rationale for the medical dissolution of gallstones. What can be said is that total body cholesterol metabolism does influence biliary cholesterol secretion. Biliary cholesterol secretion increases with increased cholesterol biosynthesis (as in obesity) and is decreased by pharmaceutical agents that decrease cholesterol input into the exchangeable pool. Such agents include CDCA (a weak HMG-CoA reductase inhibitor), lovostatin and its congeners (potent HMG-CoA reductase inhibitors) and UDCA, which decreases cholesterol absorption and also inhibits the usual compensatory increase in HMG-CoA reductase levels.

MICELLAR SOLUBILIZATION OF BILIARY LIPIDS

Cholesterol is dispersed in mixed micelles in hepatic bile in all species; in species that have relatively high biliary cholesterol proportions, vesicles are also present. It may well be that both vesicles and mixed micelles are present in canalicular bile in all species. The major constituent of both vesicles and micelles are PC and cholesterol. When mixed micelles form, PC molecules transfer to micellar form to a greater extent, increasing the cholesterol/PC ratio of vesicles[59]. Bile acids are present in a much higher proportion in micelles than in vesicles. Bile acid anions bind counterions weakly; polyvalent cations will be bound to a greater extent than monovalent cations.

For some three decades, the structure of the mixed micelle has been considered to be a bilayer disk surrounded by bile acid anions[60]; in this model, the hydrophobic side of the molecule rests against the hydrocarbon chain of the PC molecules. The bile acid molecule is parallel to the acyl chains of the PC molecules.

Recent work by Hjelm and his colleagues using neutron scattering[61] has led to the proposed modification of this model. In the Hjelm model, PC molecules are arranged in a radial array, so that the mixed micelles have a cylindrical shape. Bile acid molecules rest between the charged heads, their hydrophobic face pushing the zwitterionic heads apart. In this model, the bile acid molecule is perpendicular to the PC molecules. If this new view is correct, the fundamental physicochemical effect of bile acids is to transform the bilayer arrangement (lamellar phase) into cylindrical, mixed micelles. There continues to be controversy about whether a lamellar phase consisting of PC-cholesterol lamellae is also present in bile[62–64].

EPILOGUE

The relationship between BAD bile flow, BAD biliary PC secretion, biliary lipid solubilization, and bile acid structure is now fairly well understood. One clinical situation in which BAD bile flow has an inexplicably elevated ACA value is in the patient who has an external biliary fistula immediately after liver transplantation[65]. It remains unclear whether increased choleresis per se is a rational therapeutic goal in cholestatic liver disease. UDCA induces bile flow as any bile acid, but has the great advantage of being devoid of side-effects.

Biliary PC secretion serves to protect the biliary tree from the corrosive effects of bile acids and also to solubilize biliary cholesterol. A major unsolved problem is the mechanism and regulation of biliary cholesterol secretion.

References

1. Nathanson MH, Boyer JL. Mechanisms and regulation of bile secretion. Hepatology. 1991;14:551–66.
2. Hofmann AF. Overview of bile secretion. In: Schultz SG, ed. Handbook of physiology. Bethesda: American Physiological Society; 1989:549–66.
3. Meier PJ. Transport polarity of hepatocytes. Semin Liver Dis. 1988;8:293–307.
4. Tsukada N, Ackerley CA, Phillips MJ. The structure and organization of the bile canalicular cytoskeleton with special reference to actin and actin-binding proteins. Hepatology. 1995;21:1106–13.
5. McCuskey RS, Reilly FD. Hepatic microvasculature: dynamic structure and its regulation. Semin Liver Dis. 1993;13:1–12.
6. Alvaro D, Cantafora A, Attili AF *et al.* Relationship between bile salts hydrophilicity and phospholipid composition in bile of various animal species. Comp Biochem Physiol. 1986;83:551–4.
7. Van Erpecum KP, Van Berge Henegouwen GP, Stolk MF. Bile acid and phospholipid fatty acid composition in bile of patients with cholesterol and pigment gallstones. Clin Chim Acta. 1991;199:295–303.
8. Hofmann AF, Grundy SM, Lachin JM *et al.* and the National Cooperative Gallstone Study Group. Pretreatment biliary lipid composition in white patients with radiolucent gallstones in the National Cooperative Gallstone Study. Gastroenterology. 1982;83:738–52.
9. Verkade HJ, Vonk RJ, Kuipers F. New insights into the mechanism of bile acid-induced biliary lipid secretion. Hepatology. 1995;21:1174–89.
10. Berr F, Jaeger H, Walli A, Bitterle T, Wilcox H. Biliary secretion of phospholioids and aplolipoprotein A-I: Evidence for intracellular supply of phospholipids by a non-vesicular transport route. Hepatology. 1993;18:179A.
11. Alvaro D, Benedetti A, Gigliozzi A *et al.* Effect of Brefeldin A on transcytotic vesicular pathway and bile secretion: a study on the isolated perfused rat liver and isolated rat hepatocyte couples. Hepatology. 1995;21:450–9.
12. Wheeler HO, Ross ED, Bradley SE. Canalicular bile production in dogs. Am J Physiol. 1968;214:866–74.
13. Ballitori N, Jacob R, Barrett C, Boyer JL. Biliary catabolism of glutathione and differential reabsorption of its amino acid constituents. Am J Physiol. 1988;254:G1–G7.
14. Guzelian P, Boyer JL. Glucose reabsorption from bile: evidence for a biliohepatic circulation. J Clin Invest. 1974;53:526–35.

15. Lira M, Schteingart CD, Steinbach JH, Lambert K, McRoberts J. Hofmann AF. Sugar absorption by the biliary ductular epithelium of the rat: evidence for two transport systems. Gastroenterology. 1992;102:563–71.
16. Rege RV, Moore EW. Convective movement of Ca^{2+} across guinea pig gallbladder epithelium. Am J Physiol. 1992;262:G990–5.
17. Shiffman ML, Shamburek RD, Schwartz CC, Sugerman HJ, Kellum JM, Moore EW. Gallbladder mucin, arachidonic acid, and bile lipids in patients who develop gallstones during weight reduction. Gastroenterology. 1993;105:1200–8.
18. Vagenaar GT, Moorman AF, Chamuleau RA *et al.* Vascular branching pattern and zonation of gene expression in the mammalian liver. A comparative study in rat, mouse cynomolgus monkey and pig. Anat Red. 1994;239:441–52.
19. Hofmann, AF. Enterohepatic circulation of bile acids. In: Schultz SG, ed. Handbook of physiology. Bethesda: American Physiological Society; 1989;567–96.
20. Hofmann AF, Mysels KJ. Bile salts as biological detergents. Colloids Surfaces. 1988;30:145–73.
21. Hofmann AF. Bile acids. In: Arias IM, Boyer JL, Fausto N, Jakoby WB, Schachter DA, Shafritz DA, eds. The liver: Biology and pathobiology. 3rd ed. New York: Raven Press Ltd; 1994:677–718.
22. Twisk J, Hoekman MF, Mager WH *et al.* Heterogeneous expression of cholesterol 7-α hydroxylase and sterol 27 hydroxylase genes in the rat liver lobule. J Clin Invest. 1995;95:1235–43.
23. Hofmann AF, Schteingart CD, Hagey LR. Species differences in bile acid metabolism In: Paumgartner G, Beuers U, eds. Bile acids in liver diseases. Boston: Kluwer Academic Publishers. [In press].
24. Hofmann AF. Intestinal absorption of bile acids and biliary constituents: the intestinal component of the enterohepatic circulation and the integrated system. In: Johnson LR, Alpers DH, Christensen J, Jacobson ED, Walsh JH, eds. Physiology of the gastrointestinal tract. 3rd edn, vol 2. New York: Raven Press; 1994:1555–76.
25. Hylemon PB. Metabolism of bile acids in intestinal microflora. In: Danielsson H, Sjövall J, eds. Sterols and bile acids. Amsterdam: Elsevier Science Publishers; 1985:331–43.
26. Coleman JP, White WB, Egestad B, Sjövall J, Hylemon PB. Biosynthesis of a novel bile acid nucleotide and mechanism of 7-α-dehydroxylation by an intestinal Eubacterium species. J Biol Chem. 1987;262:4701–7.
27. Molino G, Hofmann AF, Cravetto C, Belforte G, Bona B. Simulation of the metabolism and enterohepatic circulation of endogenous chenodeoxycholic acid in man using a physiological pharmacokinetic model. Eur J Clin Invest. 1986;16:397–414.
28. Hofmann AF, Cravetto C, Molino G, Belforte G, Bona B. Simulation of the metabolism and enterohepatic circulation of endogenous deoxycholic acid in man using a physiological pharmacokinetic model for bile acid metabolism. Gastroenterology. 1987;93:693–709.
29. Stieger B, Zhang J, O'Neill B, Sjovall J, Meier P. Transport of 7α-hydroxy-3-oxo-4-cholenoic acid and 3β,7α-dihydroxy-5-cholenoic acid in rat liver plasma membrane vesicles. In: van Berge Henegouwen GP, van Hoek B, de Groote J, Matern S, Stockbrugger RW, eds. Cholestatic liver diseases. Boston: Kluwer Academic Publishers.
30. Cantafora A, Alvaro D, Attili AF *et al.* Hepatic 3-α dehydrogenation and 7-α dehydroxylation of deoxycholic acid in the guinea pig. Comp Biochem Physiol. 1986;85:805–10.
31. Crombie DL, Hagey LR, Lillienau J, Miyai K, Hofmann AF. Toxicity of orally administered cholyltaurine in the guinea pig: discovery of a rodent that cannot detoxify deoxycholic acid. Gastroenterology. 1992;102:A922.
32. Fromm H, Carlson GL. Hofmann AF, Farivar S, Amin P. Metabolism in man of 7-ketolithocholic acid: presursor of cheno- and ursodeoxycholic acids. Am J Physiol. 1980;239:G161–6.
33. Cowen AE, Korman MG, Hofmann AF, Cass OW. Metabolism of lithocholate in healthy man. I. Biotransformation and biliary excretion of intravenously administered lithocholate, lithcholylglycine and their sulfates. Gastroenterology. 1975;69:59–66.
34. Schwenk M, Hofmann AF, Carlson GL, Carter JA, Coulston F, Greim H. Bile acid conjugation in the chimpanzee: effective sulfation of lithocholic acid. Arch Toxicol. 1978;40:109–18.
35. Cowen AE, Korman MG, Hofmann AF, Cass OW, Coffin SB. Metabolism of lithocholate in healthy man. II. Enterohepatic circulation. Gastroenterology.1975;69:77–82.
36. Hofmann AF. The cholehepatic circulation of unconjugated bile acids: an update. In: Paumgartner G, Stiehl A, Gerok W, eds. Boston: Kluwer Academic Publishers; 1993:143–60.

37. O'Maille ERL, Hofmann AF. Relatively high biliary secretory maximum for non-micelle forming bile acids: possible significance for mechanism of secretion. Q J Exp Physiol. 1986;71:475–82.
38. Kuipers F, Havinga R, Bosschieter H, Toorop GP, Hindriks FR, Vonk RJ. Enterohepatic circulation in the rat. Gastroenterology. 1985;88:403–11.
39. Kanz MF, Whitehead RF, Ferguson AE, Kaphalia L, Moslen MT. Biliary function studies during multiple time periods in freely moving rats: A useful system and set of marker solutes. J Pharm Toxicol Meth. 1992;27:7–15.
40. Bollman, JL. A cage which limits the activity of rats. J Lab Clin Med. 1948;33:1348–51.
41. Kanai S, Kitani K, Sato Y. Bile secretory characteristics of β-muricholate and its taurine conjugates are similar to those of ursodeoxycholate in the rat. Life Sci. 1991;48:949–57.
42. Hylemon PB, Bohdan PM, Sirica AE, Heuman DM, Vlahcevic ZR. Cholesterol and bile acid metabolism in cultures of primary rate bile ductular epithelial cells. Hepatology. 1990;11:982–6.
43. Lake JR, Renner EL, Scharschmidt BF *et al.* Inhibition of Na^+/K^+ exchange in the rat is associated with decreased ursodeoxycholate hypercholeresis, decreased secretion of unconjugated ursodeoxycholate, and increased ursodeoxycholate glucuronidation. Gastroenterology. 1988;95:454–63.
44. Trang NV, Schteingart CD, Cerre C, Hofmann AF. Hepatic handling of NSAIDs: evidence for cholehepatic shunting and induction of hypercholeresis by sulindac. Hepatology. 1994;20:A660.
45. Javitt NB. Cholestasis in rats induced by taurolithocholate. Nature. 1966;210:1262–3.
46. Tuchweber B, Weber A, Roy CC, Yousef IM. Mechanisms of experimentally induced intrahepatic cholestasis. Prog Liver Dis. 1986;8:61–78.
47. Jedlitschky G, Leier I, Buchholz U, Center M, Keppler D. ATP-dependent transport of glutathione S-conjugates by the multidrug resistance-associated protein. Cancer Res. 1994;54:4833–6.
48. Knyrim K, Vakil N, Pfab R, Classen M. The effects of intraduodenal bile acid administration on biliary secretion of ionized calcium and carbonate in man. Hepatology. 1989;10:134–42.
49. Batta AK, Salen G, Mirchandani R *et al.* Effect of long-term treatment with ursodiol on clinical and biochemical features and biliary bile acid metabolism in patients with primary biliary cirrhosis. Am J Gastroenterol. 1993;88:691–700.
50. Crosignani A, Podda M, Battezzati PM *et al.* Changes in bile acid composition in patients with primary biliary cirrhosis induced by ursodeoxycholic acid administration. Hepatology. 1991;14:1000–7.
51. Zakkos S, Lira M, Clerici C *et al.* Novel metabolism and hypercholeretic effect of norursodeoxycholic acid in man. Gastroenterology. 1987;92:A1793.
52. Roda E, Mazzella G, Bazzoli F *et al.* Effect of ursodeoxycholic acid administration on biliary lipid secretion in primary biliary cirrhosis. Dig Dis Sci 1989;34:52S–58S.
53. Jazrawi RP, de Castecker JS, Goggin PM *et al.* Kinetics of hepatic handling in cholestatic liver disease. Gastroenterology. 1994;106:134–42.
54. Lillienau J, Munoz J, Longmire-Cook SJ, Hagey LR, Crombie DL, Hofmann AF. Negative feedback regulation of the ileal bile acid transport system in rodents. Gastroenterology. 1993;104:38.
55. Hofmann AF. Defective biliary secretion during total parenteral nutrition and its modulation with ursodeoxycholic acid. J Pediatr Ent Nutr. 1995;20:376–90.
56. Oude Elferink RP, Ottenhoff R, van Wijland M, Smit JJ, Schinkel AH, Groen AK. Regulation of miliary lipid secretion by mdr-2 P-glycoprotein in the mouse. J Clin Invest. 1995;95:31.
57. Crawford JM, Crawford AR, Hatch VC, Stearns RC, Barnes S Godleski JJ. Hepatocellular secretion of biliary lipid: bile salt-induced vesiculation of the canalicular membrane outer leaflet. In: Hofmann AF, Paumgartner G, Stiehl A, eds. Bile acids in gastroenterology: Basic and clinical aspects. Boston: Kluwer.
58. Xia Y, Lambert KJ, Schteingart CD, Gu J-J, Hofmann AF. Concentration and biliary secretion of ceftriaxone: inhibition of lipid secretion and precipitation of calcium ceftriaxone in bile. Gastroenterology. 1990;99:454–65.
59. Booker ML, LaMorte WW, Ahrendt SA, Lillemoe KD, Pitt HA. Distribution of phosphatidylcholine molecular species between mixed micelles and phospholipid-cholesterol vesicles in human gallbladder bile: dependence on acyl chain length and unsaturation. J Lipid Res. 1992;33:1485–92.

60. Mazer NA, Benedek GB, Carey MC. Quasielastic light scattering studies of aqueous biliary lipid systems: mixed micelle formation in bile salt–lecithin solution. Biochemistry. 1980;19:601–15.
61. Hjelm R, Thiyagarajan P, Alkan H. The organization of phosphatidylcholine and bile salt in rod-like mixed micelles. J Phys Chem. 1992;96:8653–61.
62. Somjen GJ, Marikovsky Y, Sachtel E *et al.* Phospholipid lamellae are cholesterol carriers in human bile. Biochem Biophys Acta. 1990;1042:28–35.
63. Corradini SG, Arancia G, Calcabrini A *et al.* Lamellar bodies coexist with vesicles and micelles in human gallbladder bile: Ursodeoxycholic acid prevents cholesterol crystal nucleation by increasing biliary lamellae. J Hepatol. 1995;22:642–57.
64. Cohen DE, Kaler EV, Carey MC. Cholesterol carriers in bile: are 'lamellae' involved? Hepatology. 1993;18:1522–31.
65. McCashland TM, Donovan JP, Amelsberg A *et al.* Bile acid metabolism and biliary secretion in patients receiving orthotopic liver transplants: differing effects of cyclosporin A and FK 506. Hepatology. 1994;19:1381–9.

Section II
Pathophysiological and Pharmacological Aspects of Bile Acid Secretion

5
Disturbances of hepatocellular bile salt transport as possible mechanisms of cholestasis

D. KEPPLER, R. MAYER, M. BÜCHLER, I. LEIER and G. JEDLITSCHKY

INTRODUCTION

Bile flow is determined to a large extent by the hepatobiliary elimination of bile salts. Within this process, transport of bile salts across the hepatocyte canalicular membrane is rate-determining in the hepatobiliary elimination of bile salts[1]. Moreover, two ATP-dependent bile salt export pumps, rather than potential-dependent transport, provide the decisive driving force in the canalicular membrane for bile flow[2,3]. Monoanionic bile salts, such as taurocholate, are substrates for the ATP-dependent bile salt export pump in the canalicular membrane[2–7], which is highly sensitive to inhibition by cyclosporins[2,4]. Selective inhibition of this bile salt export pump by cyclosporins may cause experimental intrahepatic cholestasis[2]. On the other hand, dianionic bile salt conjugates, such as bile salt ether glucuronides, are substrates for another ATP-dependent export pump which transports, in addition, glutathione *S*-conjugates out of cells[8–10]. This transporter is less sensitive to cyclosporin inhibition[2] and is deficient in the liver of GY/TR$^-$ mutant rats[8,9]. The contribution of this ATP-dependent conjugate export pump to bile flow seems to be quantitatively less important when compared with the ATP-dependent bile salt (taurocholate) export pump[2]. The ATP-dependent conjugate export pump has been characterized functionally[8–13] and termed a multispecific organic anion transporter (MOAT)[8], non-bile acid organic anion transporter[10], glutathione *S*-conjugate export pump[11] or leukotriene export pump[12]. The latter term refers to the endogenous glutathione *S*-conjugate leukotriene C_4 (LTC_4) which is the substrate with the highest affinity known so far for this transporter[12–14].

We demonstrated recently in human leukaemia cells overexpressing the multidrug resistance protein (MRP)[15] and in HeLa cells transfected with an *MRP* expression vector[14] that the *MRP* gene encodes the ATP-dependent export pump for LTC_4 and structurally related conjugates of lipophilic compounds with glutathione and several other anionic residues[14,15]. A similar conclusion was reached more recently by another group[16]. This high-affinity LTC_4 export pump has molecular and functional properties similar to the ATP-dependent conjugate export pump in the hepatocyte canalicular membrane[17]. In transport-deficient GY/TR$^-$ Wistar rats, which are also deficient in the canalicular secretion of dianionic bile salt ether glucuronides and sulphates[8,9], we observed that secretion of the labelled glutathione S-conjugate LTC_4 into bile was selectively reduced to less than 2% of normal and labelled leukotrienes accumulated in liver[18]. Accordingly, ATP-dependent LTC_4 transport was below detectable levels in hepatocyte canalicular membrane vesicles from transport-deficient GY/TR$^-$ rats[13]. The defect of this ATP-dependent canalicular conjugate export pump in mutant GY/TR$^-$ rats is comparable to the hereditary defect in the human Dubin–Johnson syndrome[17].

The *MRP* gene encodes a protein of 1531 amino acids belonging to the ATP-binding cassette (ABC) superfamily of membrane transport proteins[19,20], which functions as conjugate export pump[14–17]. Overexpression of this membrane glycophosphoprotein with a molecular mass ranging from 170 to 195 kDa results in the resistance of human tumour cells to a number of cytotoxic drugs[19–22] which possibly undergo conjugation. Our recent studies demonstrate for the first time the expression of the *MRP* gene-encoded conjugate export pump in human liver and of its homologue in the liver of rats[17].

RESULTS

Decisive role of ATP-dependent canalicular bile salt secretion

The selective and potent inhibition of the canalicular ATP-dependent taurocholate export pump by cyclosporin A and its non-immunosuppressive structural analogue, PSC 833, allowed for a discrimination between potential-dependent and ATP-dependent bile salt transport[2]. The comparison of the different bile salt transport systems in hepatocyte membrane vesicles and the use of the cyclosporins as tools has indicated that the ATP-dependent transporter is the only decisive one for monoanionic bile salt (taurocholate) transport across the canalicular membrane[2]. This conclusion is supported by the electrophoretic separation of the transport proteins and the demonstration that the potential-dependent transporter resides entirely in the endoplasmic reticulum[3]. Selective inhibition of ATP-dependent bile salt (taurocholate) transport by the cyclosporins strongly reduced bile flow and thus demonstrates that intrahepatic cholestasis may result from inhibition of the ATP-dependent transporter[2]. This concept questions the role of the membrane potential in bile salt transport across the canalicular membrane which was previously considered the decisive driving force[23–25].

MRP gene expression in liver

Expression of the *MRP* gene in human liver and of the *mrp* gene in rat liver was analysed by polymerase chain reaction (PCR) amplification of cDNA reverse transcribed from mRNA. PCR amplification was performed by use of primers directed to two highly conserved regions of *MRP*[17]. This resulted in two expected PCR fragments. Both fragments were amplified and visible in the mRNA preparations from human liver and liver from normal Wistar rats. However, a 347-bp fragment was not detectable in the mRNA preparations from GY/TR$^-$ mutant rat liver[17]. Subcloning and sequencing of a 182-bp fragment from normal rat liver indicated an amino acid sequence identity of 83.3% when compared with the deduced human MRP sequence[17].

Immunoblot analysis of MRP in liver membranes

Immunoblots were performed with human liver canalicular (CM) and basolateral (BLM) membrane preparations and probed with 3 polyclonal antibodies raised against 3 different sequences of MRP[22] and with a monoclonal antibody (QCRL-1) directed against MRP[26]. Each of these antibodies detected a protein of about 190 kDa in human CM and BLM[17].

Immunoblot analysis of CM and BLM from normal Wistar rat liver, using the 6KQ antibody[22], detected a protein of about 170 kDa in both membrane fractions. The apparent amount of the 190-kDa protein in human and of the 170-kDa protein in rat liver BLM was at least as high as in CM[17].

A comparison of liver plasma membrane fractions from normal Wistar and GY/TR$^-$ rats by immunoblot analysis with the 6KQ antibody revealed that there was only a very small amount, if any, of the 170-kDa protein in CM from GY/TR$^-$ liver when compared with CM from normal rat liver. In contrast, there was no significant quantitative difference between the proteins in normal and GY/TR$^-$ mutant BLM[17].

ATP-dependent transport by membrane vesicles from normal and transport-deficient liver and from MRP-overexpressing cells

Primary-active ATP-dependent transport of [^{3}H]LTC$_4$ into inside-out oriented vesicles of normal Wistar and GY/TR$^-$ CM and BLM was studied[13,17]. Significant uptake of [^{3}H]LTC$_4$ was observed only with CM vesicles from normal Wistar liver. In the other membrane vesicle preparations, transport rates were below 20% of the rate in CM from normal liver[17].

As a representative bile salt glucuronide, we analysed the ATP-dependent transport of hyodeoxycholate 6α-glucuronide in membrane vesicles from MRP-overexpressing and control cells. These studies provided clear evidence that the *MRP* gene-encoded conjugate export pump also transports bile salt ether glucuronides (Jedlitschky G., Leier I., Buchholz U., Keppler D., unpublished measurements).

DISCUSSION

Conjugation of endogenous compounds, such as bile salts and bilirubin, and of lipophilic xenobiotics with glucuronate and glutathione has long been known as a possible prerequisite for their excretion across the canalicular membrane into bile. This process has been recognized as an ATP-dependent primary-active transport[8,10,13,27,28] which is deficient in the liver of GY/TR$^-$ mutant rats[8,10,13,17].

Analyses in bile[8,9,18] and transport assays in canalicular plasma membrane vesicles from mutant and normal rat liver[8,13,17,27] have been used to define the substrate specificity of this ATP-dependent transport system for conjugates of lipophilic compounds with glutathione, glucuronate, and sulphate (for review, see Reference 8). The substrate specificities of this conjugate export pump in rat hepatocytes and the human *MRP*-gene-encoded pump are very similar (compare data in References 12,13,27 with those in Reference 14). However, subtle differences in the substrate specificities must be defined after cloning and expression of the rat *mrp* cDNA. The function of the MRP pump in the hepatobiliary excretion of conjugates is in accord with its localization to the canalicular membrane domain.

Our recent work provides the first example of a mislocalization of a hepatocyte membrane transport protein resulting in impaired hepatobiliary excretion[17]. The functional defect in the GY/TR$^-$ rat mutant is considered to be very similar to the canalicular transport defect in patients with Dubin–Johnson syndrome[8,10,17]. Studies are in progress, therefore, to examine the presence and localization of MRP in the liver of patients with Dubin–Johnson syndrome. The defect in GY/TR$^-$ rats and in Dubin–Johnson syndrome of humans affects, however, only the transport of dianionic bile salts, such as hyodeoxycholate 6α-glucuronide, and not of monoanionic bile salts, such as taurocholate. Accordingly, these mutations are not associated with marked cholestasis, although a reduction of bile flow has been observed in GY/TR$^-$ rat mutants[8,18]. As the major and critical determinant for bile flow, the ATP-dependent bile salt export pump (Figure 1) is in the focus of current research on the mechanisms of cholestasis. The regulation and the possible disturbance of ATP-dependent bile salt transport across the hepatocyte canalicular membrane can be analysed in more detail when the molecular identity of this transporter has been elucidated. At present, this has been achieved only for the ATP-dependent conjugate export pump[17] which has a broad substrate specificity and also transports bile salt glucuronides in addition to several other amphiphilic anionic conjugates.

Acknowledgements

We thank the Deutsche Forschungsgemeinschaft (grant B3/SFB 352) and the Fonds der Chemischen Industrie for support of parts of this work, and Dr. Melvin Center (Manhattan, KS, USA), as well as Drs. Roger Deeley and Susan Cole (Kingston, Ontario, Canada) for providing cell lines overexpressing MRP and antibodies directed against MRP.

References

1. Boyer JL, Graf J, Meier PJ. Hepatic transport systems regulating pH, cell volume, and the bile secretion. Annu Rev Physiol. 1992;54:415–38.
2. Böhme M, Müller M, Leier I, Jedlitschky G, Keppler D. Cholestasis caused by inhibition of the adenosine triphosphate-dependent bile salt transport in rat liver. Gastroenterology. 1994;107:255–65.
3. Kast C, Stieger B, Winterhalter KH, Meier PJ. Evidence for distinct subcellular localizations of electrogenic and ATP-dependent taurocholate transport in rat hepatocytes. J Biol Chem. 1994;269:5179–86.
4. Kadmon M, Klünemann C, Böhme M *et al.* Inhibition by cyclosporin A of adenosine triphosphate-dependent transport from the hepatocyte into bile. Gastroenterology. 1993;104:1507–14.

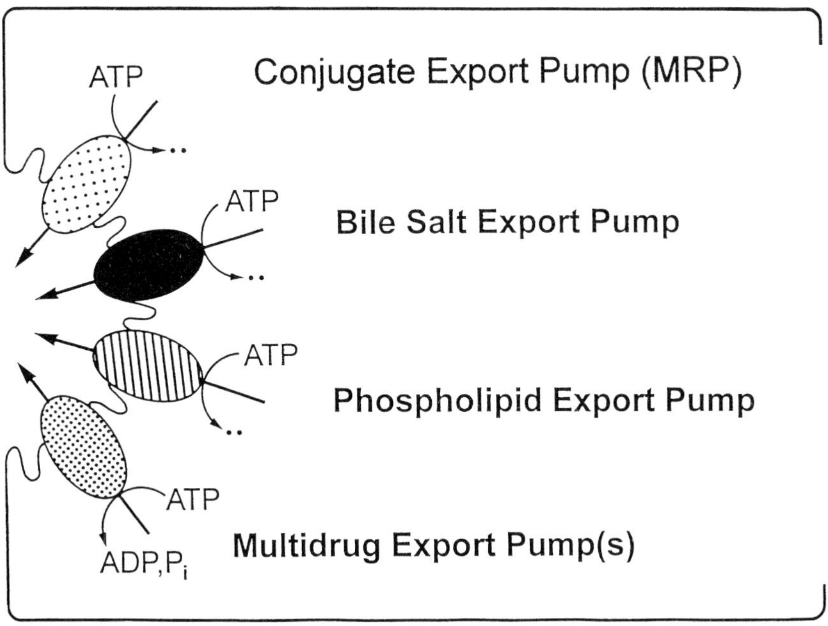

Fig. 1 Bile salt transport determined by ATP-dependent export pumps in the hepatocyte canalicular membrane. The conjugate export pump secretes several amphiphilic organic anions, including bile salt ether glucuronides, into bile. Recent work has established that this export pump is encoded by the multidrug resistance gene *(MRP)*[17]. The ATP-dependent bile salt export pump is considered rate-determining for bile flow and has been functionally well characterized[2–7], but the molecular composition and identity of this transport system is still under investigation[29]. The phospholipid export system is now known as the *mdr2* gene product[30]. There is one multidrug export pump in humans[31] and two, Mdr1a and Mdr1b, pumps in rats and mice[31–33]

5. Müller M, Ishikawa T, Berger U *et al.* ATP-dependent transport of taurocholate across the hepatocyte canalicular membrane mediated by a 110-kDa glycoprotein binding ATP and bile salt. J Biol Chem. 1991;266:18920–6.
6. Adachi Y, Kobayashi H, Kurumi Y, Shouji M, Kitano M, Yamamoto T. ATP-dependent taurocholate transport by rat liver canalicular membrane vesicles. Hepatology. 1991;14:655–9.
7. Nishida T, Gatmaitan Z, Che M, Arias IM. Rat liver canalicular membrane vesicles contain an ATP-dependent bile acid transport system. Proc Natl Acad Sci USA. 1991;88:6590–4.
8. Oude Elferink PJ, Jansen PLM. The role of the canalicular multispecific organic anion transporter in the disposal of endo- and xenobiotics. Pharmac Ther. 1994;64:77–97.
9. Kuipers F, Enserink M, Havinga R *et al.* Separate transport systems for biliary secretion of sulfated and unsulfated bile acids in the rat. J Clin Invest. 1988;81:1593–9.
10. Arias IM, Che M, Gatmaitan Z, Leveille C, Nishida T, St. Pierre M. The biology of the bile canaliculus. Hepatology. 1993;17:318–29.
11. Ishikawa T. The ATP-dependent glutathione S-conjugate export pump. TIBS. 1992;17:463–8.
12. Keppler D. Leukotrienes: biosynthesis, transport, inactivation, and analysis. Rev Physiol Biochem Pharmacol. 1992;121:1–30.
13. Ishikawa T, Müller M, Klünemann C, Schaub T, Keppler D. ATP-dependent primary active transport of cysteinyl leukotrienes across liver canalicular membrane. Role of the ATP-dependent transport system for glutathione S-conjugates. J Biol Chem. 1990;265:19279–86.
14. Leier I, Jedlitschky G, Buchholz U, Cole SPC, Deeley RG, Keppler D. The *MRP* gene encodes an ATP-dependent export pump for leukotriene C_4 and structurally related conjugates. J Biol Chem. 1994;269:27807–10.

15. Jedlitschky G, Leier I, Buchholz U, Center M, Keppler D. ATP-dependent transport of glutathione S-conjugates by the multidrug resistance-associated protein. Cancer Res. 1994;54:4833–6.
16. Müller M, Meijer C, Zaman GJR *et al.* Overexpression of the gene encoding the multidrug resistance-associated protein results in increased ATP-dependent glutathione S-conjugate transport. Proc Natl Acad Sci USA. 1994;91:13033–7.
17. Mayer R, Kartenbeck J, Büchler M, Jedlitschky G, Leier I, Keppler D. Expression of the *MRP* gene-encoded conjugate export pump in liver and its selective absence from the canalicular membrane in transport-deficient mutant hepatocytes. J Cell Biol. 1995;137–50.
18. Huber M, Guhlmann A, Jansen PLM, Keppler D. Hereditary defect of hepatobiliary cysteinyl leukotriene elimination in mutant rats with defective hepatic anion excretion. Hepatology. 1987;7:224–8.
19. Cole SPC, Bhardwaj G, Gerlach JH *et al.* Overexpression of a transporter gene in a multidrug-resistant human lung cancer cell line. Science. 1992;258:1650–4.
20. Cole SPC, Sparks KE, Fraser K *et al.* Pharmacological characterization of multidrug resistant MRP-transfected human tumor cells. Cancer Res. 1994;54:5902–10.
21. Krishnamachary N, Center MS. The MRP gene associated with a non-P-glycoprotein multidrug resistance encodes a 190-kDa membrane bound glycoprotein. Cancer Res. 1993;53:3658–61.
22. Krishnamachary N, Ma L, Zheng L, Safa AR, Center MS. Analysis of MRP gene expression and function in HL60 cells isolated for resistance to adriamycin. Oncol Res. 1994;6:119–27.
23. Inoue M, Kinne R, Tran T, Arias IM. Taurocholate transport by rat liver canalicular membrane vesicles. J. Clin Invest. 1984;73:659–63.
24. Meier PJ, Meier-Abt AS, Barrett C, Boyer JL. Mechanisms of taurocholate transport in canalicular and basolateral rat liver plasma membrane vesicles. J Biol Chem. 1984;259:10614–22.
25. Ruetz S, Hugentobler G, Meier PJ. Functional reconstitution of the canalicular bile salt transport system of rat liver. Proc Natl Acad Sci USA. 1988;85:6147–51.
26. Hipfner DR, Gauldie SD, Deeley RG, Cole SPC. Detection of the M_r 190,000 multidrug resistance protein, MRP, with monoclonal antibodies. Cancer Res. 1994;54:5788–92.
27. Akerboom TPM, Narayanaswami V, Kunst M, Sies H. ATP-dependent S-(2,4-dinitrophenyl) glutathione transport in canalicular plasma membrane vesicles from rat liver. J Biol Chem. 1991;266:13147–52.
28. Kobayashi K, Sogame Y, Hayashi K, Nicotera P, Orrenius S. ATP stimulates the uptake of *S*-dinitrophenylglutathione by rat liver plasma membrane vesicles. FEBS Lett. 1988;240:55–8.
29. Büchler M, Böhme M, Ortlepp H, Keppler D. Functional reconstitution of ATP-dependent transporters from the solubilized hepatocyte canalicular membrane. Eur J Biochem. 1994;224:345–52.
30. Smit JJM, Schinkel AH, Oude Elferink RPJ *et al.* Homozygous disruption of the murine *mdr*2 P-glycoprotein gene leads to complete absence of phospholipids from bile and to liver disease. Cell. 1993;75:451–62.
31. Gottesman MM, Pastan I. Biochemistry of multidrug resistance mediated by the multidrug transporter. Annu Rev Biochem. 1993;62:385–427.
32. Schinkel AH, Smit JJM, Van Tellingen O *et al.* Disruption of the mouse *mdr1a* P-glycoprotein gene leads to a deficiency in the blood–brain barrier and to increased sensitivity to drugs. Cell. 1994;77:491–502.
33. Silverman JA, Raunio H, Grant TW, Thorgeirsson SS. Cloning and characterization of a member of the rat multidrug resistance (mdr) gene family. Gene. 1991;106:229–36.

6
Changes in bile secretion after liver transplantation

B.-G. ERICZON, B. ANGELIN and K. EINARSSON

INTRODUCTION

Monitoring of liver function after liver transplantation is essential since it may be disturbed by various events, such as ischaemic injury to the graft, rejection episodes, and vascular thrombosis. Also, drugs, among them cyclosporine (CsA) and Tacrolimus (FK506), may interfere with the recovery of the graft. Bile secretion is a potentially useful marker of liver function, being the first reliable sign of organ functioning after hepatic transplantation.

We have performed a detailed characterization of the biliary lipid composition of bile produced after liver transplantation to study the 'normal' pattern of biliary lipid secretion from the transplanted liver and furthermore to compare the effects of CsA and FK506 on bile composition[1,2].

MATERIAL AND METHODS

Patients and surgical procedure

All together 38 patients were studied. Liver transplantations were performed orthotopically by conventional techniques including veno-venous bypass. In seven instances, a choledocho-jejunostomy was chosen for the biliary anastomosis and bile drainage was through a choledochus catheter. In the remaining cases, a choledocho-choledochostomy was performed and the bile was drained through a T-tube. The bile was continuously drained throughout the study period of a minimum of 10 days. Antibacterial prophylactics with cefotaxime and ampicillin iv was maintained for 5 days postoperatively.

Three different immunosuppressive treatment protocols were used.

Cyclosporine-based immunosuppressive protocol

The first dose of cyclosporine was administered preoperatively at a dose of 10 mg/kg orally. Thereafter, 4 mg kg^{-1} day was given as a continuous infusion.

Oral CsA was started on day 5 and was initially combined with the iv treatment. The dosage aimed at cyclosporine levels of 250–300 ng/ml in whole blood as determined by a monoclonal RIA-method. Azathioprine was given at a dose of 3 mg kg^{-1} day^{-1}, or less if leukopenia occurred.

FK506-based immunosuppressive protocol

FK506 was initially administered at a dose of 0.04 mg/kg as a continuous iv infusion for 12 h starting intraoperatively after the arterial anastomosis was completed. The same iv dose was repeated every 12 h until day 3 postoperatively, when 0.10 mg kg^{-1} $(12\ hours)^{-1}$ was given orally. It was intended that FK plasma levels after the first postoperative week would be 0.3–0.5 ng/ml. No azathioprine was administered to these patients.

OKT-3 protocol

This protocol was used in order to allow freedom from both CsA and FK506 for 10 days immediately after transplantation. OKT-3 (a monoclonal antibody against T-cells) was administered as an iv injection of 5 mg daily for 14 days. Azathioprine was given as described above.

All three groups were given corticosteroids in a similar way throughout the study period.

Analyses of bile

The volume of bile produced was monitored continuously. Bile samples (≈2 ml) were obtained for analysis of biliary lipids in the morning after an overnight fast. For determinations of cholesterol and phospholipids, a portion of the bile sample was immediately extracted with 20 volumes of chloroform/methanol (2 : 1 vol/vol). Cholesterol was determined by an enzymatic method[3] and phospholipids were determined by the method of Rouser *et al.*[4]. The total bile acid concentration was determined in another aliquot of the bile samples, using a 3α-hydroxysteroid dehydrogenase assay[5].

The individual bile acids were determined in portions of bile hydrolysed in 1 mol/L KOH at 110°C for 12 h. After acidification, the deconjugated bile acids were extracted with diethylether, and the methyltrimethylsilyl ethers were prepared and analysed by gas–liquid chromatography, using a 1% Hi-Eff BP 8 column[6].

Calculations

Data are expressed as means ± SE. The significance of differences was tested by Student's *t*-test and, for time-dependent variables, with a two-factor repeated-measures Anova (analysis of variance). Correlations were evaluated by linear regression and calculation of the correlation coefficient.

RESULTS

A patient with a typical postoperative course is illustrated in Figure 1. Bile acids, phospholipids and cholesterol were present in low concentrations during

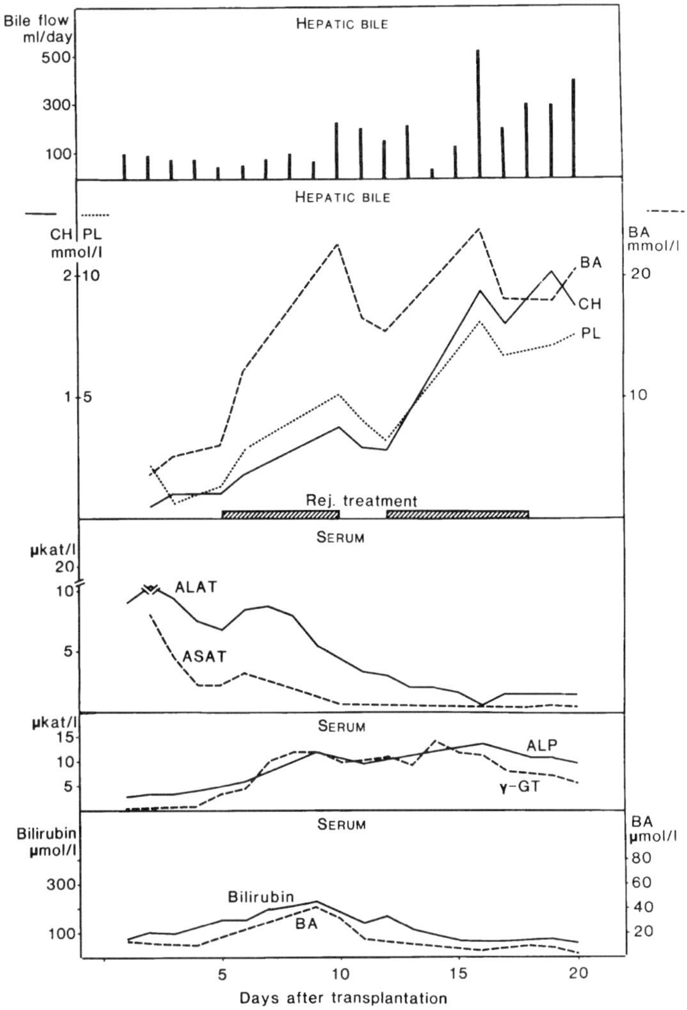

Fig. 1 Postoperative laboratory data in a patient with a typical postoperative course. CH = cholesterol; PL = phospholipids; BA = total bile acids (reference value in serum <7 μmol/L); ALAT = alanine aminotransferase (GPT; reference value <0.70 μkat/L); ASAT = aspartate aminotransferase (GOT; reference value <0.70 μkat/L); ALP = alkaline phosphate (reference value <4.2 μkat/L); γ-GT = γ-glutamyltransferase (reference value <0.50 μkat/L); bilirubin = total bilirubin (reference value <26 μmol/L)

the early postoperative days. The concentrations of all bile lipids increased steadily throughout the study period until the T-tube was clamped. The total lipid concentration in bile on days 2 and 20 was 0.35 and 1.67 g/dl respectively. Improved bile quality was reflected by increased concentration of bile acids, phospholipids and cholesterol and was seen after antirejection treatment.

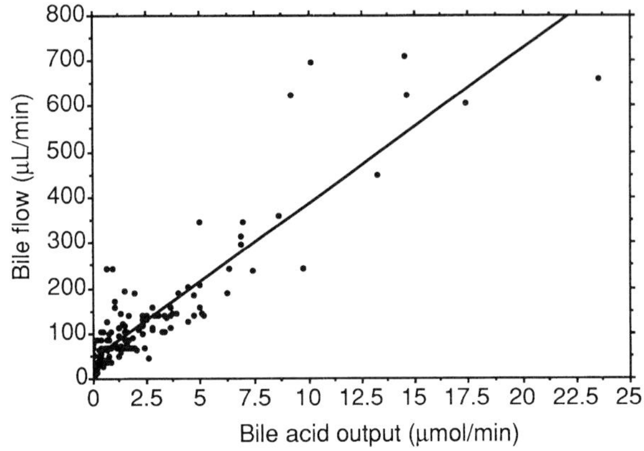

Fig. 2 Relationship between bile acid secretion rate and bile flow in liver grafts early after transplantation. Correlation coefficient = 0.89. Equation of the regression line: $y = 34.2x + 43.8$ ($p<0.0001$ for slope = 0 and intercept = 0)

The bile flow was very well correlated with the flow of bile acids (r = 0.89) but it was also possible to demonstrate a significant bile acid-independent bile flow in this model, amounting to about 44 μl/min or 63 ml/day (Figure 2). The secretion rate of cholesterol and phospholipids depended on the secretion of bile acids and no bile acid-independent secretion of cholesterol was observed.

Sixteen of the patients had been randomized to receive either FK506-based protocol or a cyclosporine-based protocol. On the first postoperative day, the mean bile flow and bile acid output were not different between the two groups. Bile flow and bile acid output then increased in both groups, but the in-

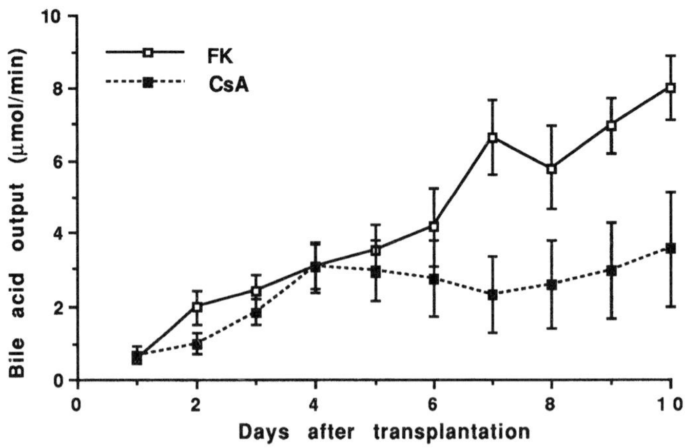

Fig. 3 Bile acid output in the subpopulation of 16 liver transplant patients who were randomized to FK506 or CsA

crease was more pronounced in patients treated with the FK506-based protocol (Figure 3).

Individual bile acids were analysed during the early postoperative course. The only bile acids regularly found in the bile of the transplanted liver with continuous biliary drainage were cholic acid and chenodeoxycholic acid. A general phenomenon was that the bile produced within the first few days after transplantation contained a greater proportion of chenodeoxycholic acid than that produced later (Figure 4). This was regardless of the immunosuppressive protocol used. Patients on FK506-based immunosuppressive protocols reached the lower plateau significantly earlier than patients on CsA-based protocols. A secondary bile acid was observed occasionally in a few patients. Small amounts of deoxycholic acid were observed but in no case could lithocholic acid or ursodeoxycholic acid be identified.

DISCUSSION

While most transplanted livers show immediate production of bile, its quality varies considerably. In our series of patients, the concentrations of the biliary lipids were low during the early postoperative days and increased during the following two weeks after transplantation to values in good agreement with those reported previously for T-tube bile in cholecystectomized subjects[7]. This most probably reflects the recovery from ischaemic damage. With a total drainage of bile, only the primary bile acids (i.e. cholic acid (CA) and chenodeoxycholic acid (CDCA)) should be present in the bile because intestinal bacteria and enteropathic recirculation are needed to convert primary bile acids to secondary bile acids. An interesting finding was that the relative proportion of CDCA decreased during the first postoperative week. We speculated that this might be

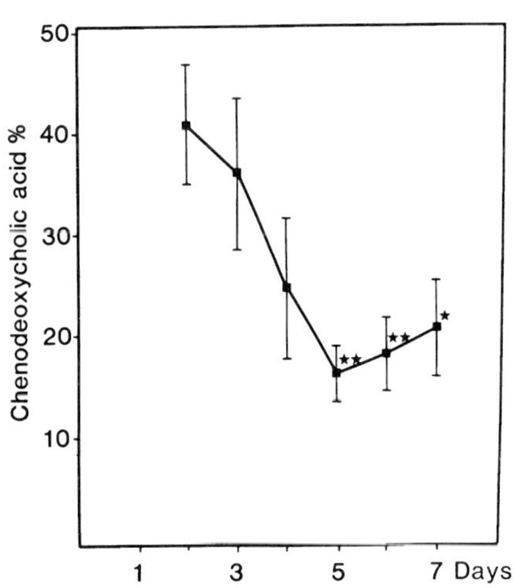

Fig. 4 Chenodeoxycholic acid as a percentage of the total bile acids in patients early after liver transplantation. Bars indicate SEM.* $p<0.05$ and ** $p<0.001$ vs day 2

caused by the postoperative bile fistula, by the recovery from hepatic ischaemia, or by an inhibiting effect of the immunosuppressants on CDCA synthesis. In our series of patients, we found that the relative reduction of CDCA during the early postoperative days was similar whether immunosuppression was maintained by OKT-3 (a monoclonal antibody), by cyclosporine A or by FK506. This finding indicates that the shift in the CDCA/CA ratio is not caused by an inhibitory effect of CsA nor FK506 on CDCA secretion. The most likely explanation of the shift in the CDCA/CA ratio observed a few days after liver transplantation is that the bile fistula, maintained by a T-tube or a choledochus catheter, renders the composition of the bile dependent entirely on de-novo synthesis. The fact that the low plateau of the CDCA level was reached earlier in those patients on FK506 treatment may explain the more rapid onset of de-novo synthesis of bile secretion in this group and may indicate a faster recovery of hepatic function. This faster recovery of hepatic function in patients with an FK506-based immunosuppressive protocol was also supported by finding that bile acid output and bile flow were significantly higher in this group of patients when compared with cyclosporine treated patients.

Bile acid independent flow is conventionally calculated by assuming that bile acid output and bile flow have a linear correlation even when bile acid output approaches zero. This linear relationship has been questioned in animals[8,9] and in man[10]; instead, a curvilinear relationship with all bile flow dependent on bile acid output has been suggested. In our patients, we were able to study this relationship when bile acid output and bile flow were extremely low. We found that bile flow increased linearly with bile acid output. In contrast to the results of Shiffman *et al.*[10], a positive intercept was found, indicating a bile acid-independent flow in these patients of approximately 44 μl/min. This is lower than results obtained in health by previous authors[11,12]. The estimation of bile acid-independent flow by extrapolating from normal bile acid output at high bile flow rate would probably give an overestimate of the bile acid-independent flow. The relationship between bile acid output and bile flow might, therefore, not be linear for a wide range of bile acid output. However, our data strongly indicate the existence of a bile acid-independent flow of bile because the relationship was studied with values very close to the *y*-axis.

Acknowledgement

This study was supported by grants from the Swedish Medical Research Council (03X-4793) and the Karolinska Institute.

References

1. Ericzon B-G, Eusufzai S, Kubota K, Einarsson K, Angelin B. Characterics of biliary lipid metabolism after liver transplantation. Hepatology. 1990;12:5:1222–8.
2. Söderdahl G, Groth C-G, Angelin B, Duraj F, Einarsson K, Ericzon B-G. FK506 improves recovery of bile secretion following orthotopic liver transplantation in man. Transplant Proc. 1995;27:1:1125.
3. Roda A, Festi D, Sama C *et al.* Enzymatic determination of cholesterol in bile. Clin Chim Acta. 1975;64:337–41.
4. Rouser G, Sidney F, Akira Y. Two dimensional thin-layer chromatographic separation of polar lipids and determination of phospholipids by phosphorus analysis of spots. Lipids. 1970;5:494–6.

5. Fausa O, Skålhegg BA. Quantitative determinations of bile acids and their conjugates using thin-layer chromatography and purified 3-alpha-hydroxy-steroid dehydrogenase. Scand J Gastroenterol. 1974;9:249–54.
6. Angelin B, Einarsson K, Leijd B. Biliary lipid composition during treatment with different hypolipidaemic drugs. Eur J Clin Invest. 1979;9:185–90.
7. Magnusson I, Einarsson K, Angelin B, Nyberg B, Bergström K, Thulin L. Effects of somatostatin on hepatic bile formation. Gastroenterology. 1989;96:206–12.
8. Balabaud C, Kron KA, Gumucio JJ. The assessment of the bile salt nondependent fraction of canalicular bile water in the rat. J Lab Clin Med. 1977;89:393–9.
9. Baker AL, Wood RAB, Moosa AR, Boyer JL. Sodium taurocholate modifies the 'bile acid independent' fraction of canalicular bile flow in the rhesus monkey. J Clin Invest. 1979;64:312–20.
10. Shiffman ML, Carithers RL, Moore EW. Bile secretion following orthotopic liver transplantation: all bile flow is dependent upon bile acid secretion (Abstract). Hepatology. 1988;8:5:1454.
11. Prandi D, Erlinger S, Glasinovic JC, Dumont M. Canalicular bile production in man. Eur J Clin Invest. 1975;5:1–6.
12. Lindblad L, Scherstén T. Influence of cholic and chenodeoxycholic acid on canalicular bile flow in man. Gastroenterology, 1976;70:1121–4.

7
Peptide delivery by coupling to bile acids

W. KRAMER, G. WESS, M. BICKEL, E. FALK, G. NECKERMANN, G. SCHUBERT and M. URMANN

INTRODUCTION

For the treatment of chronic diseases the oral route is by far the most favourable method of drug application. The potency and selectivity of many natural peptides makes them an irresistible target for drug design. The biomedical importance of peptides as drugs of the future will increase for several reasons[1].

1. Cloning of the human genome within the next decade will unveil unknown correlations of biologically active peptides to human diseases.
2. New methodologies for the synthesis of peptide libraries of high chemical diversity, and intelligent screening strategies, will allow the discovery of highly active peptides for many targets.

However, major obstacles to the successful development of biologically active peptides to a drug are the typical characteristics of peptides: (a) a low permeability to biological membranes and their negligible intestinal absorption; (b) a high susceptibility to enzymatic hydrolysis and low stability in biological fluids[2].

Proteins ingested with a meal are degraded by gastric and pancreatic proteases to amino acids and peptides, which are substrates to a whole battery of peptidases located in the brush-border membrane of the enterocyte. Only di- and tripeptides are taken up by an oligopeptide transporter in the brush-border membrane of the intestinal absorptive cells[3]. In the cytosol of the enterocyte these oligopeptides may be further degraded by cytosolic proteases to amino acids. Thus, only hydrolysis-resistant oligopeptides can leave the enterocyte in intact form across the basolateral membrane and obtain access to systemic circulation.

Starting from a biologically active peptide lead compound, a variety of possibilities have been considered to improve membrane permeability of peptides.

1. The *chemical approach* with substitution of the hydrolysis-susceptible peptide bonds such as *N*-alkylation, use of D-amino acids, cyclization or isosteres of the peptide bond[4].
2. Use of *specific formulations* such as coating of the peptides with a polymer or use of unspecific penetration enhancers or peptidase inhibitors[5–8].
3. A *physiological approach* seems possible if the respective peptide drug can be coupled to a natural ligand for which a specific endogenous transport pathway exists in the target cell and/or the intestine.

Among the multiple transport pathways in the enterocyte the largest molecules taken up by a specific mechanism are: (a) vitamin B_{12} of M_r 1335 with a receptor-mediated transcytosis; (b) bile acids with M_r of 537 for taurocholate in a Na^+/-dependent uptake mechanism; oligopeptides or β-lactam antibiotics (M_r 347 for cephalexin) taken up by a H^+/co-transport system; folate of M_r 441.

With the simple assumption that the higher the mass of the ligand, the better the endogenous transporter will tolerate the structural changes in the ligand made by the attachment of the peptide, the following three intestinal transport systems seem suited as putative shuttle systems. Vitamin B_{12} was successfully used for the absorption of proteins or peptides such as LHRH[9]. Owing to its very low transport capacity this system is preferably useful for highly active peptide and protein hormones. In contrast, the intestinal transport systems for bile acids and oligopeptides have transport capacities of more than 10 g a day. We therefore investigated these two systems in detail as putative peptide delivery systems.

INTESTINAL BILE ACID AND OLIGOPEPTIDE TRANSPORT

Intestinal bile acid absorption occurs by a secondary active transporter, the ileal bile acid transporter (IBAT) whereas the intestinal absorption of oligopeptides and orally active β-lactam antibiotics is a ternary active transport process involving the oligopeptide transporter and a Na^+/H^+ exchanger in the apical membrane, together with a Na^+/K^+-ATPase in the basolateral membrane (Fig. 1). Orally active α-amino-β-lactam antibiotics are tripeptide analogues[10], share the intestinal uptake systems for di- and tripeptides[11–16] and are taken up by the human small intestine nearly quantitatively[17].

For the characterization of these transport systems brush-border membrane vesicles from rabbit small intestine were prepared for transport measurements and photoaffinity labelling studies. The uptake of bile acids, both conjugated and unconjugated, into brush-border membrane vesicles from rabbit ileum was stimulated by an inwardly directed Na^+ gradient (Fig. 2, left panel). In contrast the uptake of the orally active α-aminocephalosporin cephalexin – a metabolically stable analogue of a tripeptide – was independent of a Na^+ gradient, but was stimulated by an inwardly directed proton gradient (Fig. 2, right panel).

Transport measurements with membrane vesicles prepared from different segments of the small intestine revealed that the H^+/oligopeptide transporter is present as the D-glucose transporter in the entire small intestine, in contrast to the bile acid transporter which is expressed only in the distal 10–12% of the small intestine[18]. From these findings of anatomical localization of intestinal

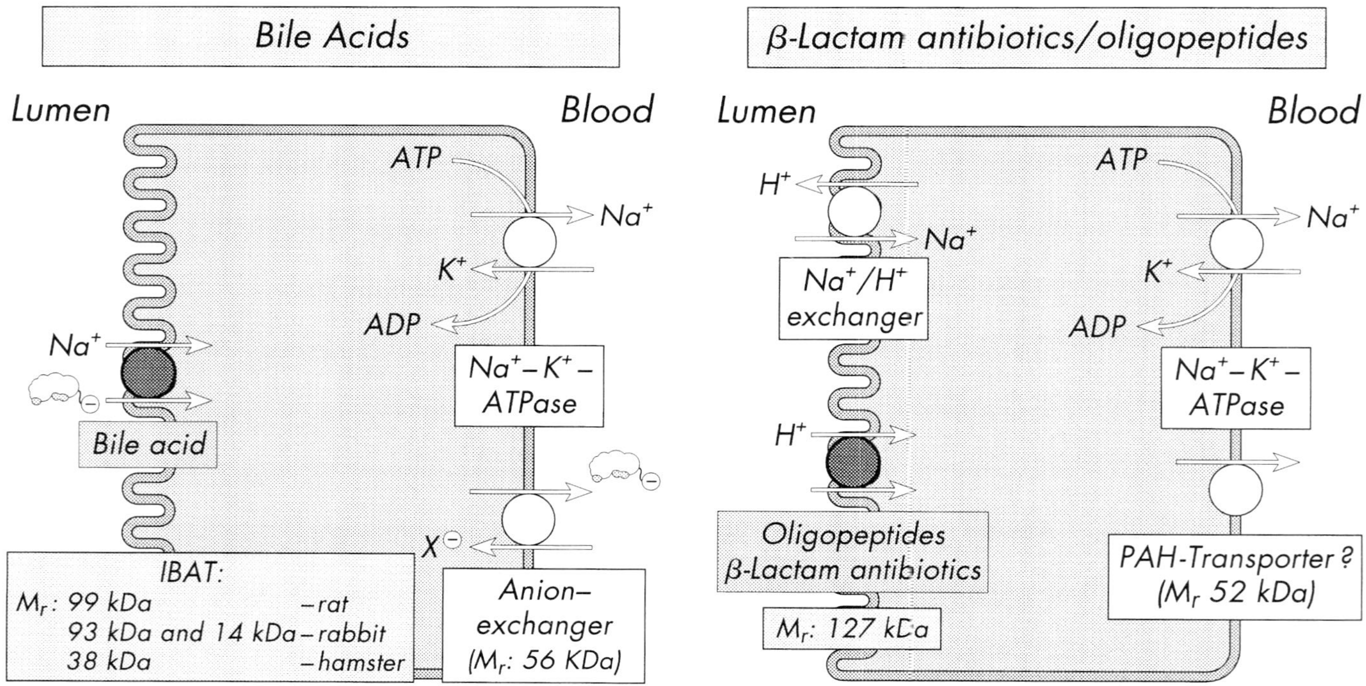

Fig. 1 Scheme for the intestinal absorption of bile acids (left panel) and oligopeptides/β-lactam antibiotics (right panel)

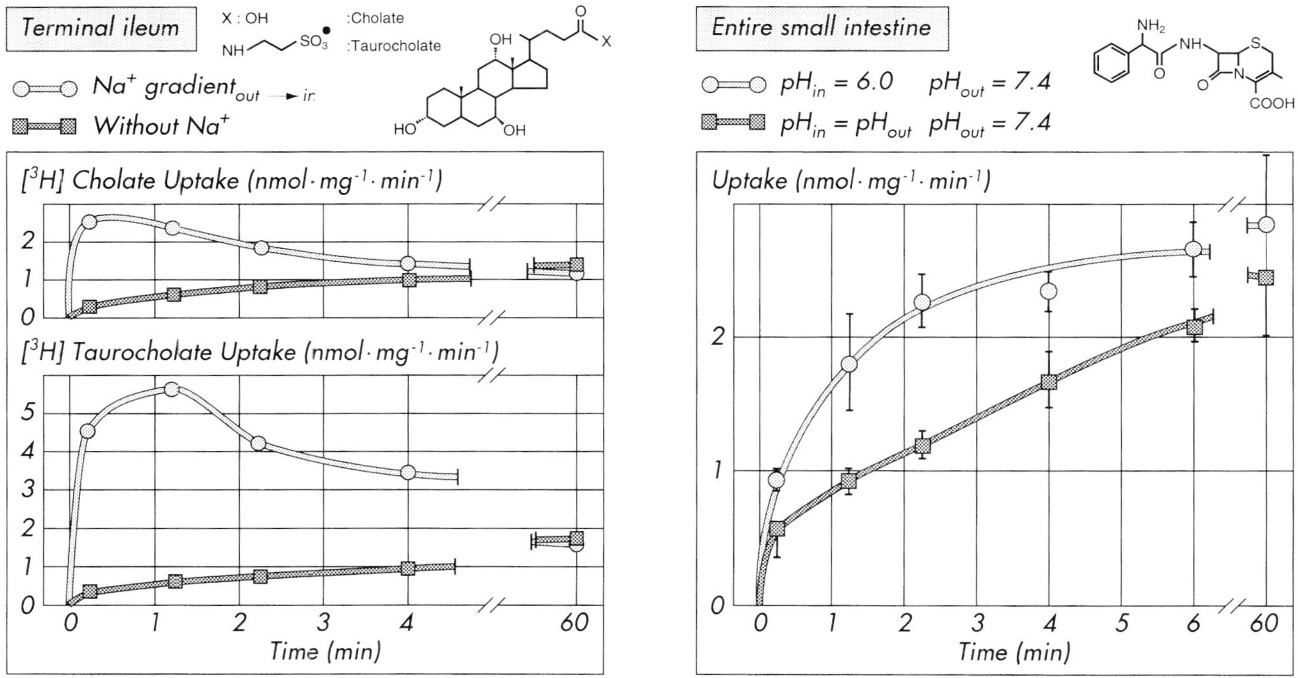

Fig. 2 Active transport of bile acids and α-amino-β-lactam antibiotics into small intestinal brush border membrane vesicles. Left panel: Uptake of 50 μmol/l (0.75 μCi) either of [^{3}H]cholate or [^{3}H]taurocholate into rabbit ileal brush-border membrane vesicles (50 μg of proteins) was measured at 30°C in the absence or presence of an inwardly directed Na^+-gradient ($[Na^+]_{out}$ = 100 mmol/l, $[Na^+]_{in}$ = 0 mmol/l at pH 7.4. Right panel: Uptake of 2 mmol/l D-cephalexin into rabbit jejunal brush-border membrane vesicles (100 μg of protein) was measured at 30°C in the absence or presence of an inwardly directed H^+-gradient (pH_{out} = 6.0, pH_{in} = 7.4)

high-capacity transporters, the oligopeptide transporter has putative advantages as a peptide delivery system because the respective peptide–ligand conjugates would be absorbed proximally in the gastrointestinal tract, and would not have to pass down to the ileum in the hostile hydrolytic luminal milieu.

To identify the putative transport proteins for bile acids and oligopeptides a variety of photolabile derivatives of bile acids, dipeptides and β-lactam antibiotics were used (Fig. 3[13–16,19–21]). Photoaffinity labelling of rabbit small intestinal brush-border membrane vesicles with these analogues and subsequent separation of membrane proteins by SDS-PAGE revealed that whereas an integral 93 kDa and a peripheral 14 kDa protein are constituents of the Na^+/bile acid cotransporter[10] (Fig. 5, left panel), an integral 127 kDa membrane protein was identified as a component of the high-capacity H^+/oligopeptide transporter from rabbit small intestine (Fig. 4, right panel)[13–16].

PEPTIDE CONJUGATES OF BILE ACIDS AND CEPHALEXIN FOR PEPTIDE DELIVERY

To investigate the potential of the bile acid and the oligopeptide transport systems as peptide delivery devices, we have attached peptides to position 3 of the steroid nucleus of modified bile acids or into position 3′ of the orally active α-aminocephalosporin cephalexin (Fig. 5[17,22–26]). The resulting cephalexin–peptide conjugates with an ester linkage between the peptide and cephalexin were extremely hydrolysis-sensitive, and were cleaved by brush-border proteases within seconds. The corresponding amides were more stable to allow transport measurements. The H^+-dependent uptake of cephalexin into rabbit small intestinal brush-border membrane vesicles was concentration-dependently and competitively inhibited by the cephalexin–peptide conjugate (Fig. 6). The bisalanyl conjugate was also taken up by the H^+/oligopeptide transport system into the vesicles.

The hydrolysis-susceptibility of a peptide conjugated to cephalexin was in any case considerably higher compared to conjugation with bile acids, presumably because the oligopeptide transporter is localized in the near vicinity of the peptide hydrolases in the brush-border membrane. Conjugation of the peptide with a bile acid, however, may prevent access of the peptide–bile acid conjugates to the brush-border peptidases and allow cellular uptake by the ileocyte. Consequently, we have synthesized peptide–bile acid conjugates with increasing chain-length of the peptide radical[17]. Additionally, model peptide conjugates with a fluorescent NBD-reporter group were synthesized, including a suicide oxaprolylpeptide inhibitor of prolyl-4-hydroxylase – a putative target for the treatment of liver fibrosis (Fig. 7). Molecular modelling demonstrates the dramatic changes of a bile acid molecule after attachment of such bulky peptide radicals shown for the NBD–nonapeptide bile acid conjugate in Fig. 8, raising the question of whether such peptide–bile acid conjugates are preferably recognized by the bile acid or by the oligopeptide transport system. To discriminate between these possibilities the influence of the peptide–bile acid conjugates on the uptake either of taurocholate or of cephalexin into ileal brush-border membrane vesicles was measured. Figure 9 shows that the inhibitory effect on

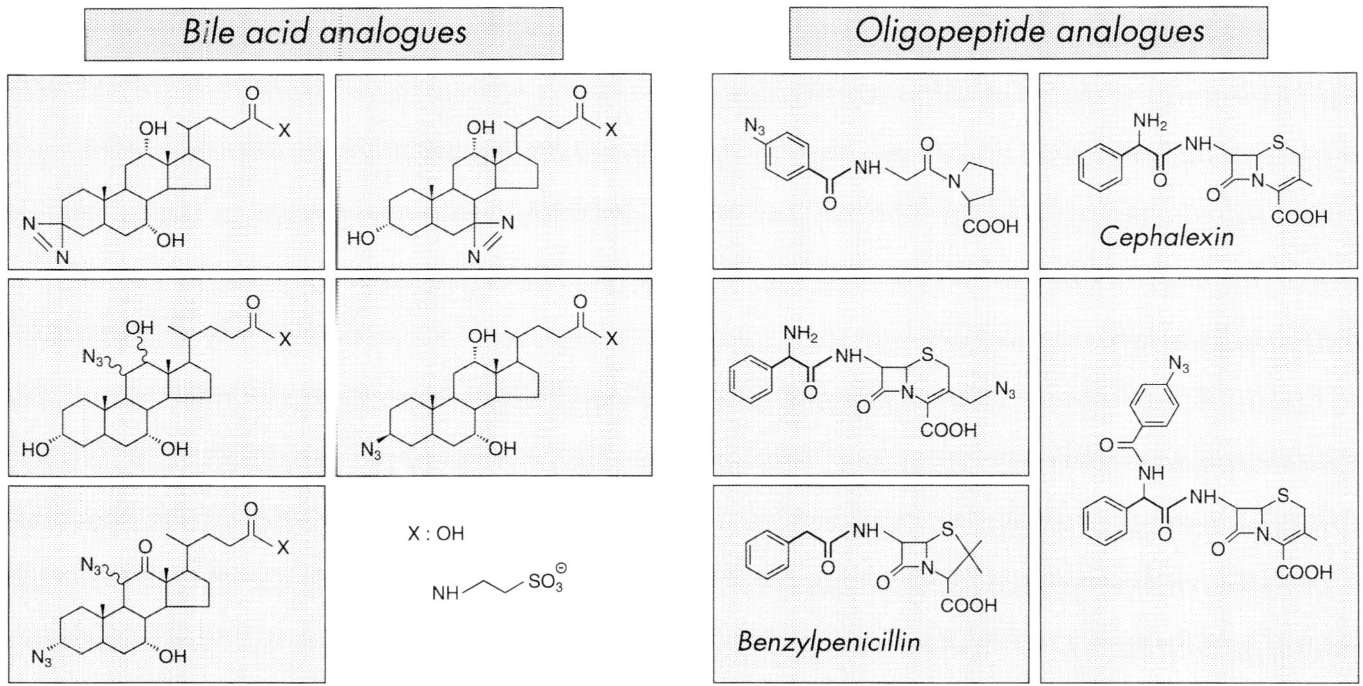

Fig. 3 Photoaffinity probes for the bile acid and oligopeptide/β-lactam antibiotic transport systems

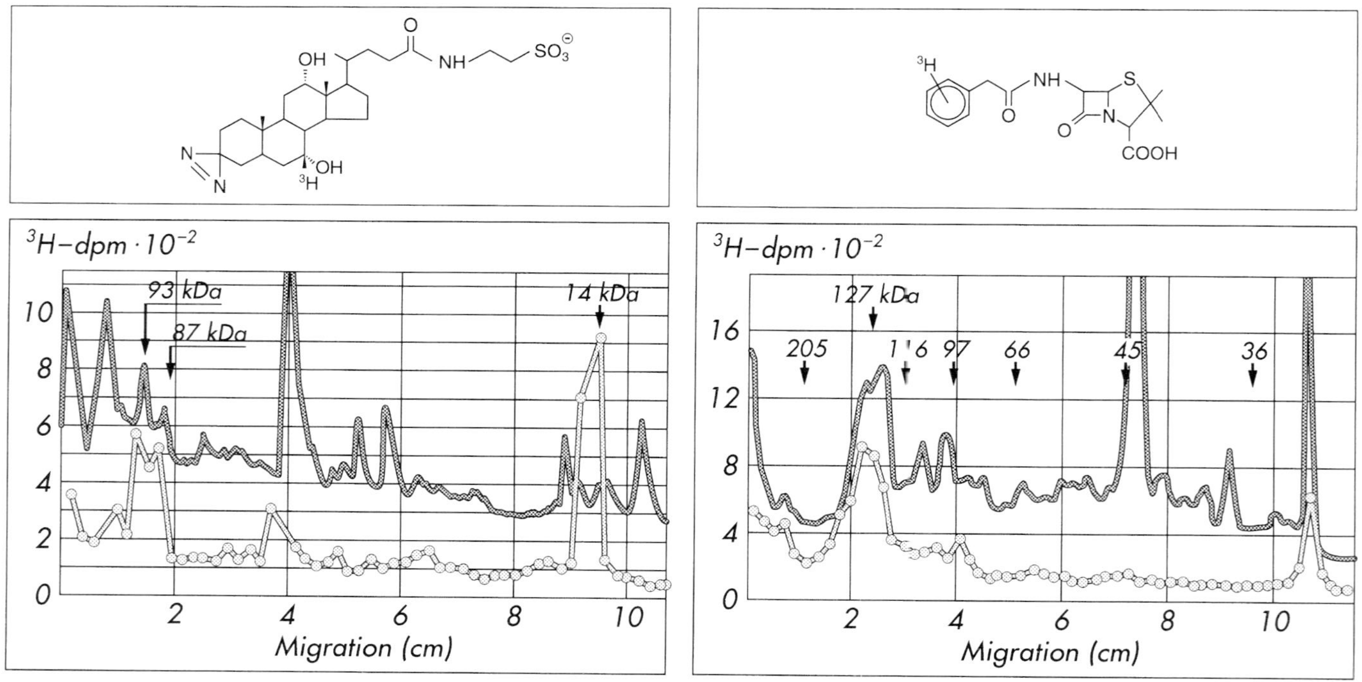

Fig. 4 Photoaffinity labelling of rabbit ileal brush-border membrane vesicles with (3,3-azo-7α,12α-dihydroxy-5β[7β-^{3}H]cholan-24-oyl)-2-aminoethanesulphonic acid (left panel) or [^{3}H]benzylpenicillin (right panel). Rabbit ileal brush-border membrane vesicles (150 μg of protein) were incubated at 30°C for 5 min in the dark either with (3,3-azo-7α,12α-dihydroxy-5β[7β-^{3}H]cholan-24-oyl)-2-aminoethanesulphonic acid or [^{3}H]benzylpenicillin (1 μmol/l) and subsequently irradiated for 10 min at 350 nm (bile acid derivative) or 2 min at 254 nm (benzylpenicillin). After washing, membrane proteins were separated by SDS-PAGE on 12% (left panel) or 7.5% gels (right panel). After slicing into 2 mm pieces the distribution of radioactivity was measured by liquid scintillation counting (lower curve)

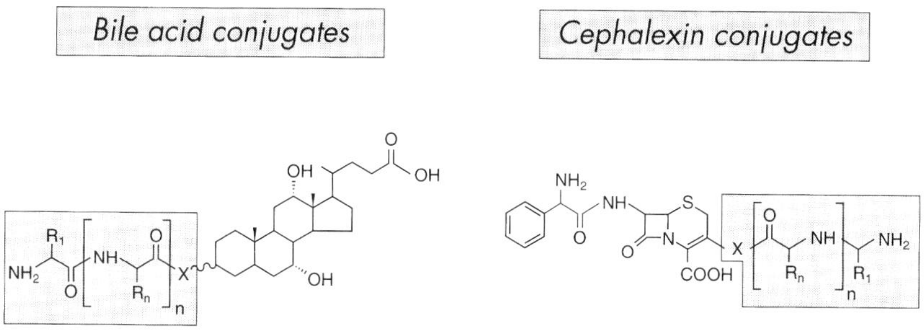

Fig. 5 Design of peptide–bile acid and peptide–cephalexin conjugates

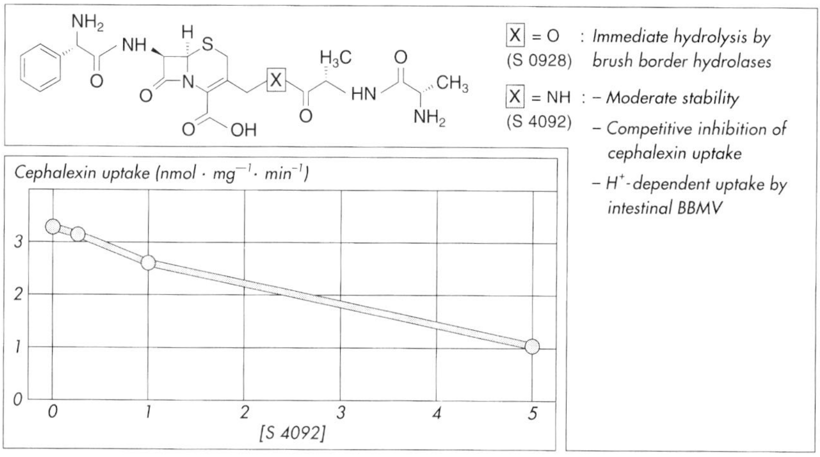

Fig. 6 Effect of peptide–cephalexin conjugates on the H^+-dependent uptake of cephalexin into rabbit small intestinal brush-border membrane vesicles. The uptake of 2 mmol/l D-cephalexin into rabbit small intestinal brush-border membrane vesicles (100 μg of protein) was measured for 1 min at 30°C in the presence of an inwardly directed H^+-gradient ($pH_{out} = 6.0$, $pH_{in} = 7.4$) in the absence and presence of the indicated concentrations of the dialanyl–cephalexin derivative

taurocholate uptake decreased with increasing chain length of the peptide radical in the bile acid conjugate, indicating a shift of the molecular characteristics of these peptide–bile acid conjugates away from bile acids. The inhibitory effect of these compounds on the H^+-dependent uptake of cephalexin was considerably lower as compared with the Na^+/bile acid co-transport system.

Photoaffinity labelling revealed a very strong inhibition of the labelling of the 93 and 14 kDa subunits of the ileal bile acid transporter by peptide–bile acid conjugates in contrast to peptides or amino acids, which did not interact with the ileal bile acid transporter and did not affect photoaffinity labelling of its protein components[17]. Labelling of the 127 kDa oligopeptide transporter was inhibited only slightly by peptide–bile acid conjugates, indicating that the peptide–bile

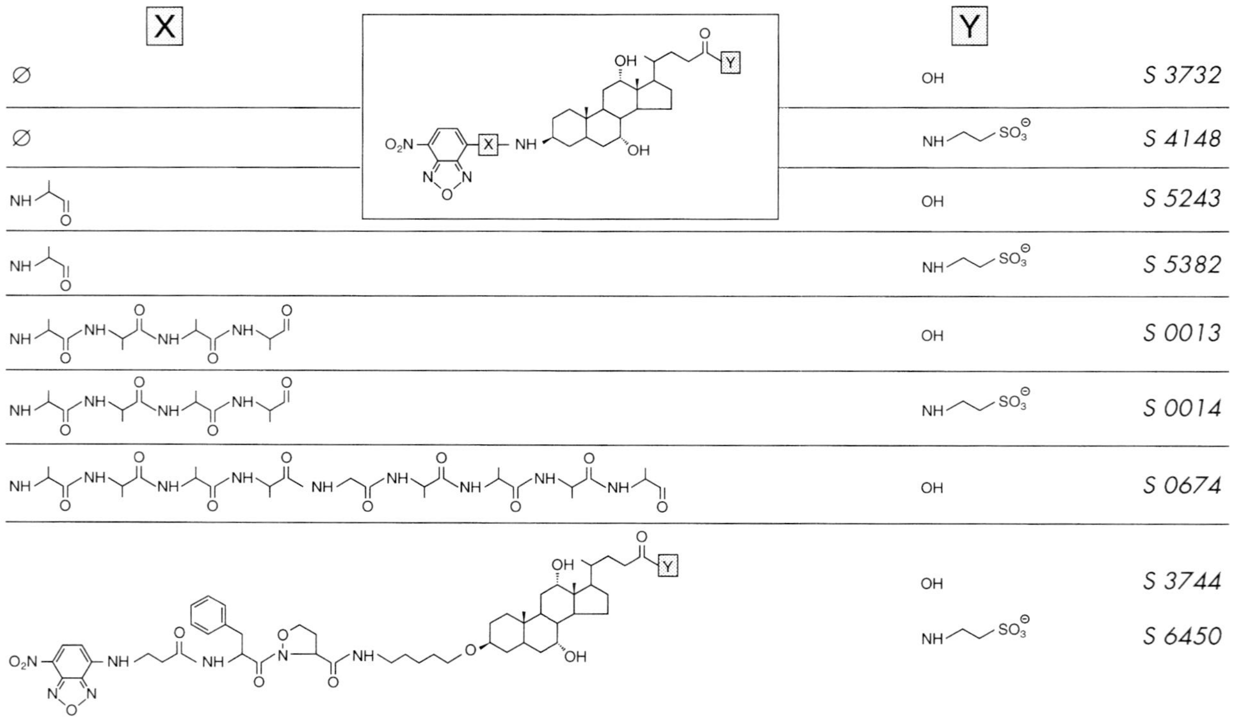

Fig. 7 Fluorescently labelled peptide–bile acid conjugates

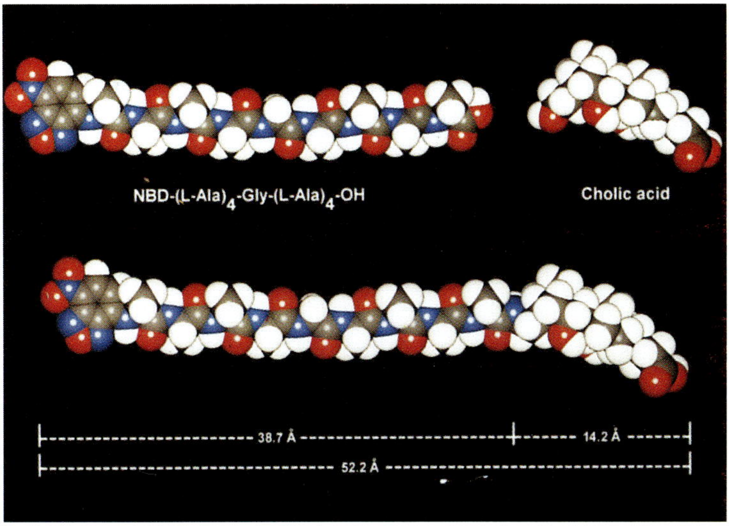

Fig. 8 Space-filling molecular modelling of cholate, the nonapeptide NBD(L-Ala)$_4$-Gly-(L-Ala)$_4$ and its bile acid conjugate S0674

acid conjugates are preferably recognized by the ileal bile acid transporter (Fig. 10).

The therapeutic use of peptides as drugs is greatly limited by their low permeability to biological membranes. Since oligopeptides do not enter hepatocytes in intact form, due to hydrolysis by membrane-bound peptidases[27], we investigated whether a peptide can be targeted to the hepatocyte after covalent linkage to a modified bile acid. For this, *in-situ* liver perfusion experiments with NBD-labelled fluorescent peptides, or their bile acid conjugates, were performed. Conjugated bile acids with a fluorescent NBD-reporter group at position 3 of the steroid nucleus were handled by the liver like natural bile acids. The taurine conjugates were transported completely unchanged from blood into bile, whereas the C-24-unconjugated acids were conjugated with taurine and secreted as taurine conjugates into bile (Fig. 11). In contrast, however, oligopeptides exerted a completely different secretion profile. Oligopeptides composed of natural L-amino acids were completely hydrolysed within seconds by liver or intestinal cells. The tetrapeptide NBD-(L-Ala)$_4$ was not transported in intact form from blood into bile, but was completely hydrolysed to amino acids during liver passage (Fig. 12). If these oligopeptides were covalently linked to modified bile acids the secretion pattern changed completely. The taurine-conjugated bile acid derivative of NBD-tetra-alanine was now transported nearly unchanged from blood into bile with only a minor hydrolysis of the attached peptide radical in contrast to the parent peptide (Fig. 13, lower panel). The C-24-unconjugated bile acid derivative was recognized within the hepatocyte by the conjugating enzymes hydroxycholanoic acid: CoA ligase (EC 6.2.1.7) and hydroxycholanoyl-SCoA: amino acid *N*-hydroxycholanoyltransferase (EC 2.3.1.?) and secreted predominantly as the corresponding taurine conjugate (Fig. 13, upper

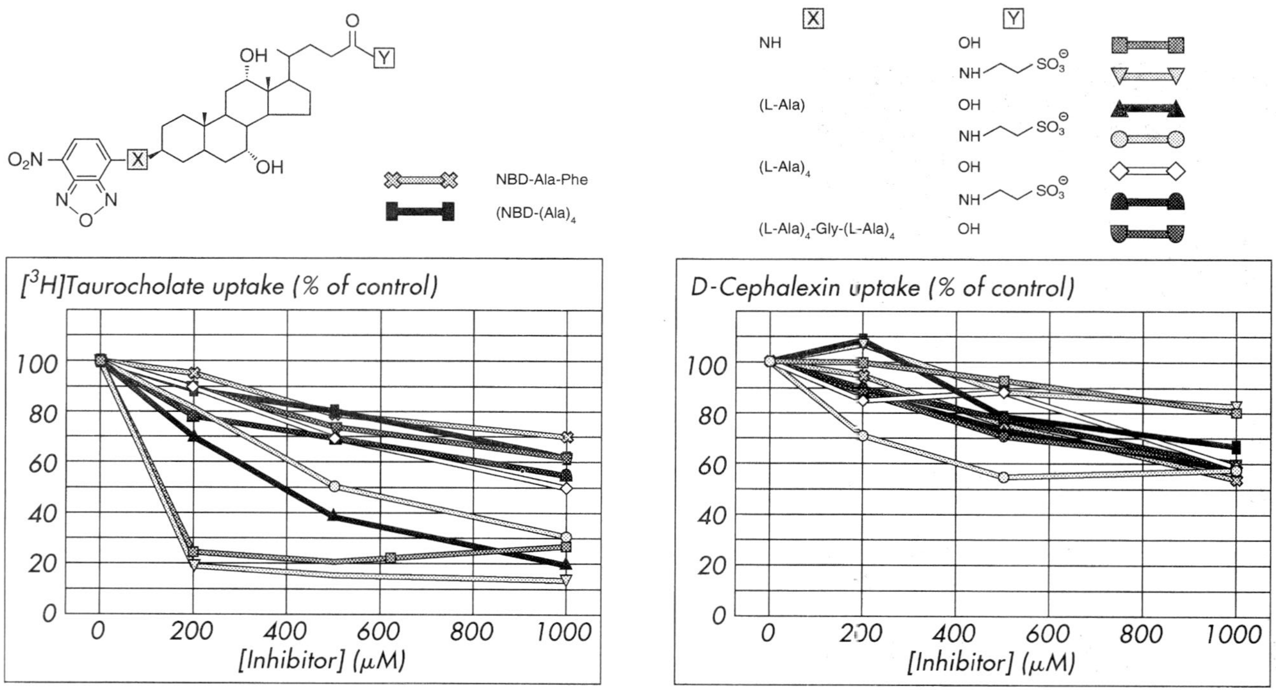

Fig. 9 Effect of NBD–peptide–bile acid conjugates on Na^+-dependent taurocholate and H^+-dependent cephalexin uptake by rabbit ileal brush-border membrane vesicles. The 60 s uptake of 50 μmol/l [^{3}H]taurocholate or 500 μmol/l D-cephalexin into rabbit ileal brush-border membrane vesicles (100 μg of protein) was measured in the presence of an inwardly-directed Na^+-gradient (taurocholate) or a H^+-gradient (cephalexin) in the absence or presence of the indicated concentrations of peptides or peptide–bile acid conjugates

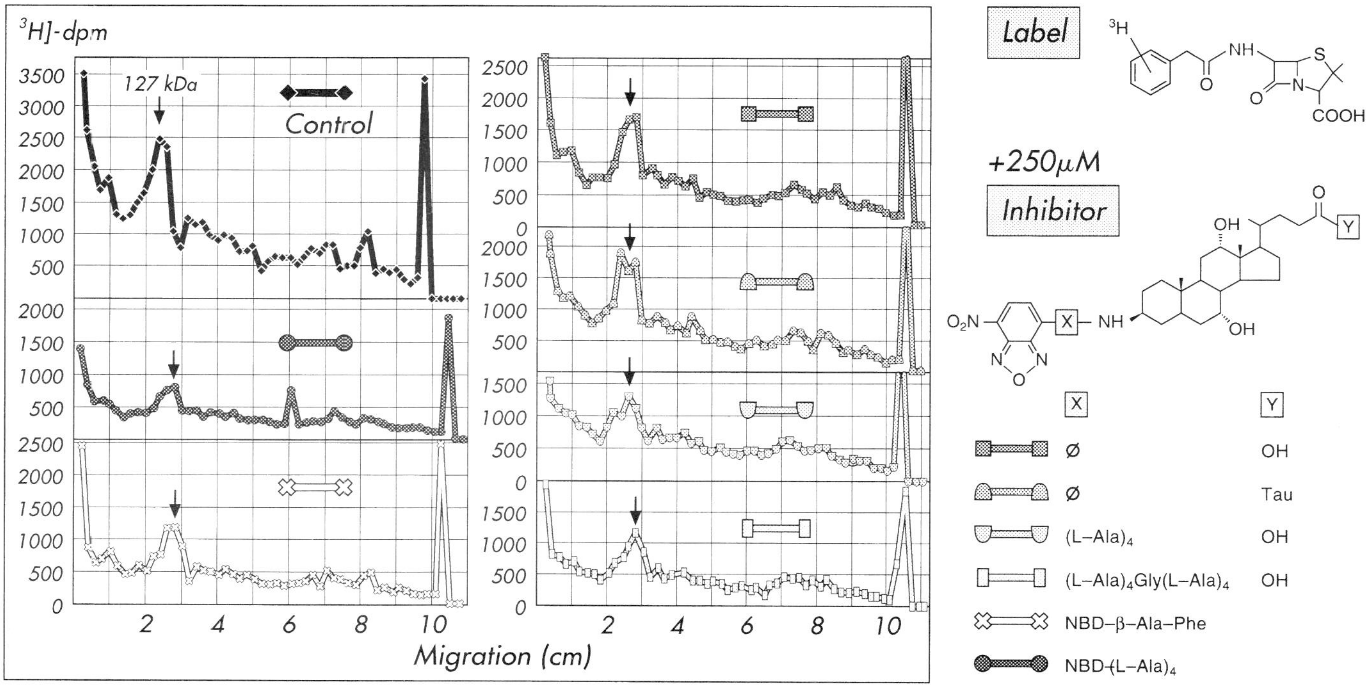

Fig. 10 Effect of NBD–peptide–bile acid conjugates on photoaffinity labelling of the rabbit intestinal H^+/oligopeptide transporter. Rabbit jejunal brush-border membrane vesicles (150 μg of protein) were incubated at 20°C for 5 min in the dark with 1.5 μmol/l of [^{3}H]benzylpenicillin in the absence or presence of 250 μmol/l of the indicated compounds, and subsequently irradiated for 2 min at 254 nm. After washing membrane proteins were separated by SDS-PAGE on 7.5% gels, and the distribution of radioactivity was determined by liquid scintillation counting as described in the legend to Fig. 4

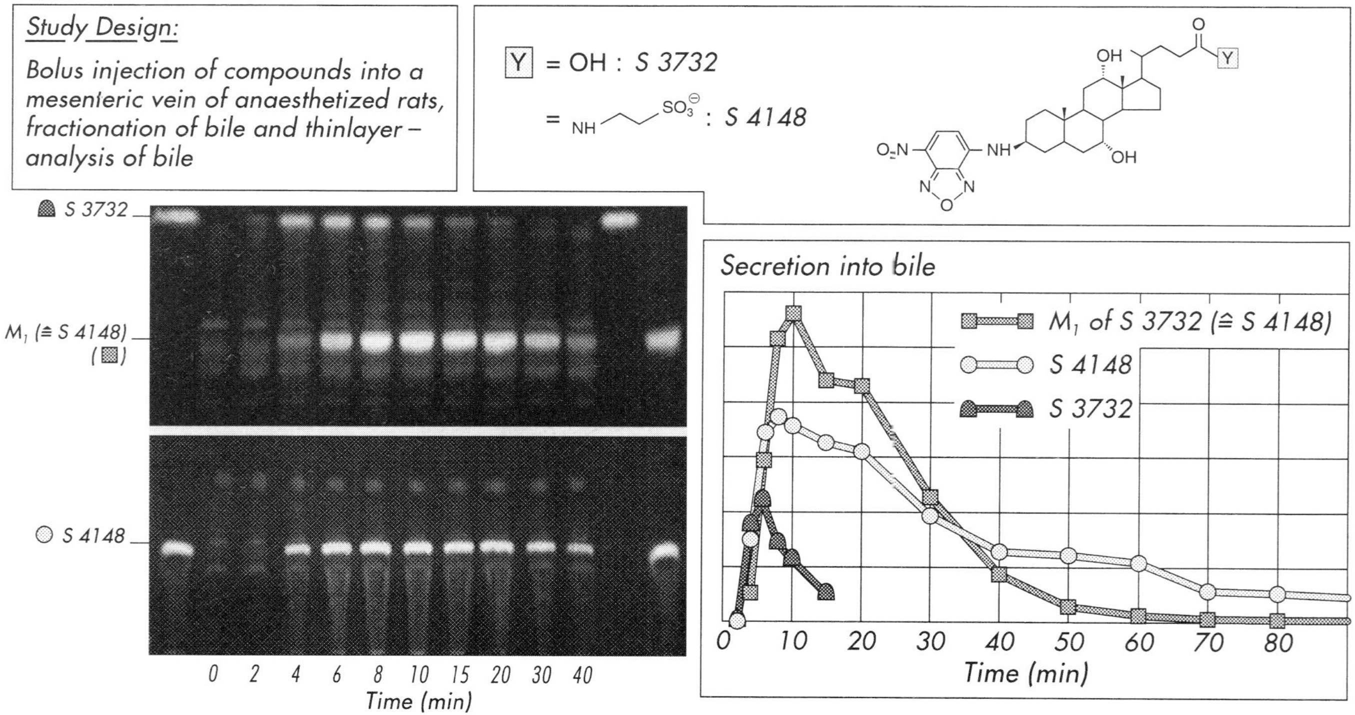

Fig. 11 Biliary secretion of NBD–bile acid derivatives. A 500 μmol/l solution of the indicated NBD–bile acid derivatives was injected as a bolus into the mesenteric vein of an anaesthetized rat after cannulation of the common bile duct. Bile was fractionated according to the indicated time periods, and 10 μl aliquots were submitted to thin-layer chromatography using *n*-butanol/acetic acid/water (5/2/3 v/v/v) as solvent system. After chromatography the NBD-labelled compounds were visualized by UV light (left panels) and the relative concentrations of the compounds and their metabolites were determined by fluorometry of the thin-layer plates

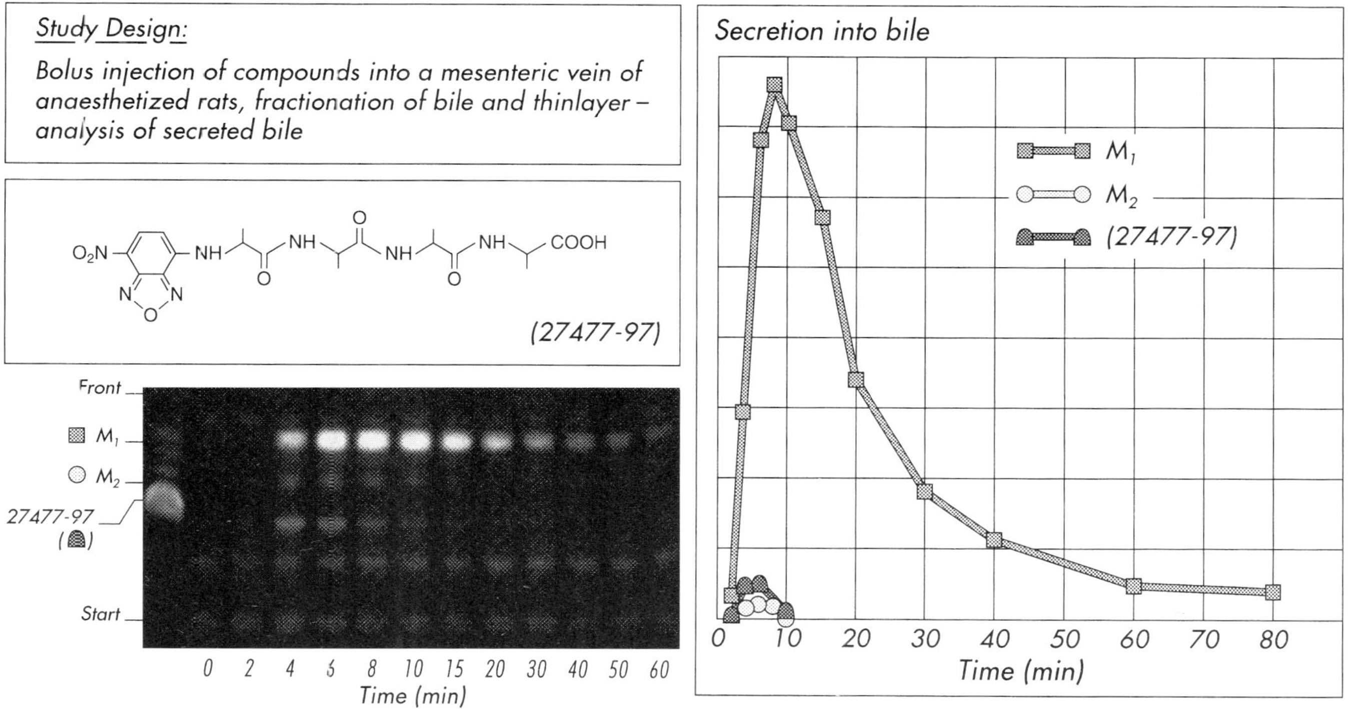

Fig. 12 Biliary secretion of NBD–tetra-alanine. A 500 μmol/l solution of NBD–tetra-alanine was injected as a bolus into the mesenteric vein of an anaesthetized rat and secreted bile was analysed as described in the legend to Fig. 11

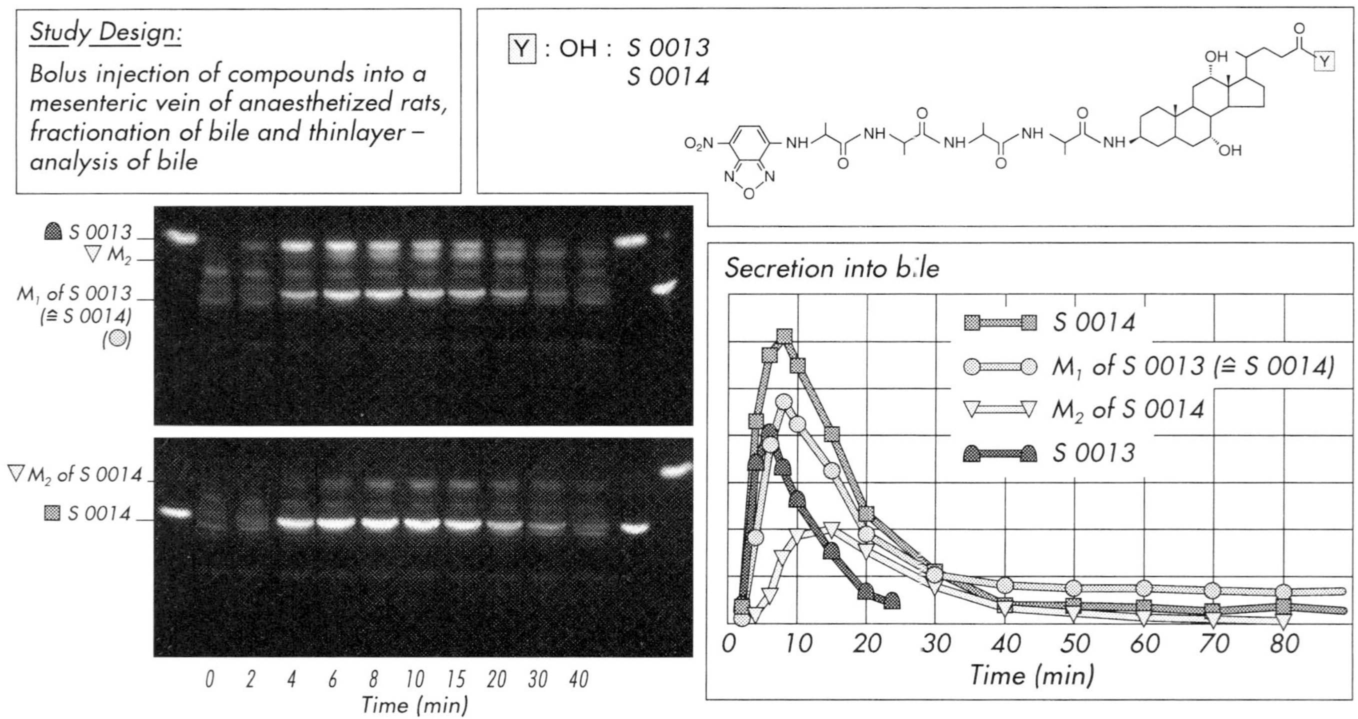

Fig. 13 Biliary secretion of NBD–tetra-alanyl–bile acid conjugates. 500 μmol/l solutions of the indicated NBD–tetra-alanyl–bile acid conjugates were injected as a bolus into the mesenteric vein of anaesthetized rats and the secreted biles were analysed as described in the legend to Fig. 11

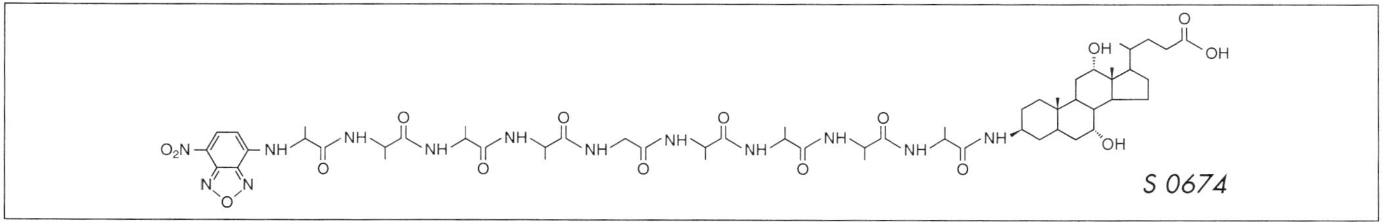

Study Design:

Bolus injection of compounds into a mesenteric vein of anaesthetized rats, fractionation of bile and thinlayer – analysis of secreted bile

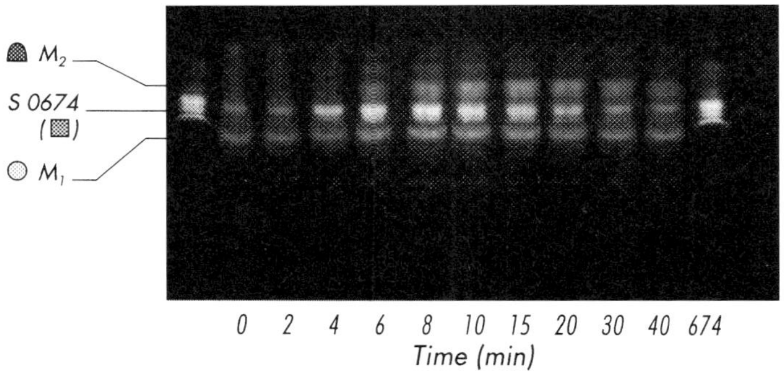

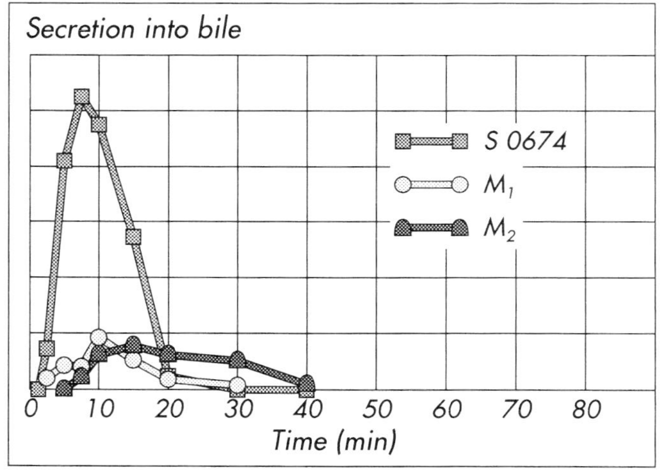

Fig. 14 Biliary secretion of the bile acid conjugate of NBD-(L-Ala)$_4$-Gly-(L-Ala)$_4$. A 500 μmol/l solution of the NBD-(L-Ala)$_4$-Gly-(L-Ala)$_4$–bile acid conjugate S0674 was injected as a bolus into the mesenteric vein of an anaesthetized rat and secreted bile was analysed as described in the legend to Fig. 11

panel). As with the taurine conjugates only a very low degree of hydrolysis of the peptide backbone occurred during liver passage. Even if the peptide chain length was increased to a nonapeptide the intact NBD–nonapeptide derivative was transported from blood into bile with a low degree of hydrolysis (Fig. 14). The metabolite M_1 formed during liver passage is presumably the corresponding taurine conjugate of S0674.

These studies clearly indicate that in the liver, as well as in the small intestine, peptides coupled to bile acids do not enter the usual transport and metabolic pathways of peptides, but are instead withdrawn from these hydrolytic events by interaction with bile acid transport systems.

In conclusion, these studies demonstrate that, by coupling of peptides to modified bile acids, peptide–bile acid conjugates are obtained which:

1. specifically interact with bile acid transport systems in the liver and the small intestine;
2. are transported in intact form into and across hepatocytes;
3. are handled like natural bile acids by the hepatocyte – the taurine conjugates are transported transcellularly unchanged whereas the C-24-bile acid derivatives are conjugated with taurine;
4. are absorbed by the ileum to a significant extent in contrast to parent peptides.

Acknowledgements

The authors are greatly indebted to F. Girbig, U. Gutjahr, C. Weyland, K. Bock, H. Kleine, K. Benstein, H. J. Dumke, W. Gerlach, C. Kremer, M. Bauer and S. Granata for their help in synthesis and biological experiments. We thank Mrs Susanne Winkler for excellent secretarial assistance.

References

1. Holmes CP, Adams CL, Fodor SPA, Yu-Yang P. New techniques in random screening: the use of light-directed spatially addressable chemical synthesis. In: Testa B, Kyburz E, Fuhrer W, Geiger R, editors. Perspectives in medicinal chemistry. Basel: Verlag Helvetica Chimica Acta: 1993:489–500.
2. Smith PL, Wall DA, Gochoco CH, Wilson G. Routes of delivery: case studies (5). Oral absorption of peptides and proteins. Adv Drug Delivery Rev. 1992;8:253–90.
3. Ganapathy V, Brandsch M, Leibach FH. Intestinal transport of amino acids and peptides. In: Johnson LR., editor. Physiology of the gastrointestinal tract, 3rd edn. New York: Raven Press; 1994:1773–93.
4. Sawyer TK. Peptidomimetic design and chemistry approaches to peptide metabolism. In: Taylor MD, Amidon GL, editors. Peptide-based drug design: controlling transport and metabolism. ACS Professional Reference Book American Chemical Society; 1995:387–422.
5. Saffran M, Kumar GS, Savariar C, Burnham JC, Williams F, Neckers DC. A new approach to the oral administration of insulin and other peptide drugs. Science. 1986;233:1081–4.
6. Lee VHL, Yamamoto A. Penetration and enzymatic barriers to peptide and protein absorption. Adv Drug Delivery Rev. 1990;4:171–207.
7. Ziv E, Lior O, Kidron M. Absorption of protein via the intestinal wall. A quantitative model. Biochem Pharmacol. 1987;36:1035–9.
8. Fujii S, Yokoyama T, Ikegaya K, Sato F, Yokoo N. Promoting effect of the new chymotrypsin inhibitor FK-448 on the intestinal absorption of insulin in rats and dogs. J Pharm Pharmacol. 1985;37:545–9.

9. Russell-Jones GJ. Oral delivery of therapeutic proteins and peptides by the vitamin B_{12} uptake system. In: Taylor MD, Amidon GL, editors. Peptide-based drug design: controlling transport and metabolism. ACS Professional Reference Book. American Chemical Society; 1995:181–98.
10. Kramer W, Dechent C, Girbig F, Gutjahr U, Neubauer H. Intestinal uptake of dipeptides and β-lactam antibiotics. I. The intestinal uptake system for dipeptides and β-lactam antibiotics is not part of a brush border membrane peptidase. Biochim Biophys Acta. 1990;1030:41–9.
11. Nakashima E, Tsuji A, Mizuo H, Yamana T. Kinetics and mechanism of in vitro uptake of amino-β-lactam antibiotics by rat small intestine and relation to the intact-peptide transport system. Biochem Pharmacol. 1984;33:3345–52.
12. Okano T, Inui K, Maegawa H, Takano M, Hori, R. H^+-gradient-dependent transport of aminocephalosporins via the dipeptide transport system in rabbit intestinal brush-border membranes. J Biol Chem. 1986;261:14130–4.
13. Kramer W. Identification of identical binding polypeptides for cephalosporins and dipeptides in intestinal brush-border membrane vesicles by photoaffinity labeling. Biochim Biophys Acta. 1987;905:65–74.
14. Kramer W, Girbig F, Leipe I, Petzoldt E. Direct photoaffinity labeling of binding proteins for β-lactam antibiotics in rabbit intestinal brush border membranes with [^{3}H]benzylpenicillin. Biochem Pharmacol. 1988;37:2427–35.
15. Kramer W, Girbig F, Gutjahr U, Kowalewski S, Adam F, Schiebler W. Intestinal absorption of β-lactam antibiotics and oligopeptides. Functional and stereospecific reconstitution of the oligopeptide transport system from rabbit small intestine. Eur J Biochem. 1992;204:923–30.
16. Kramer W, Girbig F. Gutjahr U, Kowalewski S. The intestinal oligopeptide transporter. Molecular characterization and substrate specificity. In: Taylor MD, Amidon GL, editors. Peptide-based drug design: controlling transport and metabolism. ACS Professional Book. American Chemical Society; 1995;149–79.
17. Tsuji A. Intestinal absorption of β-lactam antibiotics. In: Taylor MD, Amidon GL, editors. Peptide-based drug design: controlling transport and metabolism. ACS Professional Reference Book. American Chemical Society; 1995:101–34.
18. Kramer W, Wess G, Neckermann G *et al.* Intestinal absorption of peptides by coupling to bile acids. J Biol Chem. 1994;269:10621–7.
19. Kramer W, Kurz G. Photolabile derivatives of bile acids. Synthesis and suitability for photoaffinity labeling. J Lipid Res. 1983;24:910–23.
20. Kramer W, Schneider S. 3-Diazirine-derivatives of bile salts for photoaffinity labeling. J Lipid Res. 1989;30:1281–8.
21. Kramer W. Die Identifizierung Gallensäure-bindender Polypeptide durch Photoaffinitäts-markierung. Synthese und Anwendung photolabiler Derivate der Gallensäuren. Inaugural Dissertation (PhD thesis), Universität Freiburg; 1981:1–316.
22. Kramer W, Wess G, Schubert G *et al.* Bile acids as carrier for drugs. In: Paumgartner G, Stiehl A, Gerok W, editors. Bile acids and the hepatobiliary system. Dordrecht: Kluwer; 1993:161–76.
23. Kramer W, Wess G, European Patent Application EP 0417725 A2.
24. Wess G, Kramer W, Bartmann W *et al.* Modified bile acids: Preparation of $7\alpha,12\alpha$-dihydroxy-3β- and $7\alpha,12\alpha$-dihydroxy-3α(1-hydroxyethoxy)-5β-cholanic acid and their biological activity. Tetrahedron Lett. 1992;33:195–8.
25. Wess G, Kramer W, Enhsen A, Glombik H, Baringhaus K-H, Bock K. Dihydroxy-5β-cholanoic acid esters: versatile shuttles for drug targeting. Tetrahedron Lett. 1992;34:817–18.
26. Wess, G, Kramer W, Schubert G *et al.* Synthesis of bile acid drug conjugates: potential drug-shuttles for liver-specific targeting. Tetrahedron Lett. 1992;34:819–22.
27. Lochs H, Morse EL, Adibi SA. Mechanism of hepatic assimilation of dipeptides. Transport versus hydrolysis. J Biol Chem. 1986;261:14976–81.

8
Regulation by bile salts of the excretion of conjugated and unconjugated bilirubin in bile

J. D. OSTROW, H. OHKUBO, J. R. ASHKIN, C. WEBSTER and L. CELIC

INTRODUCTION

The excretion of bilirubins in bile is of clinical importance. Jaundice occurs when secretion of bilirubin conjugates (CB) is impaired by hepatocellular disease or cholestasis, or when hepatic uptake or conjugation of unconjugated bilirubin (UCB) is deficient[1]. Severe deficiency of UCB conjugation may lead to accumulation of neurotoxic UCB in the brain[2]. Calcium salts of UCB may precipitate in bile, leading to formation of pigment gallstones, when hydrolysis of CB and/or bilirubin loads[3] are increased. Thus, it would seem desirable to therapeutically ameliorate jaundice[4], or the supersaturation of bile with calcium bilirubinates[3,5], by modifying the excretion of bilirubins in bile. Phototherapy for severe unconjugated hyperbilirubinaemia is an established treatment based on this principle, in which UCB is converted to polar photoisomers which can be secreted in the bile of subjects with marked deficiency of bilirubin-UDPGA transferase[6–8].

Therapy with ursodeoxycholic acid (UDCA) has become popular for the amelioration of jaundice and other liver function abnormalities in cholestatic liver diseases[9]. Although UDCA does enhance excretion of CB in bile[10], this is probably not its main mechanism of action. Though UDCA and its conjugates bind Ca^{2+} more avidly than the cholate conjugates that predominate in normal bile[5,11,12], oral UDCA therapy does not dissolve pigment gallstones[13]. This is probably due to the increased secretion of ionized calcium[5,14], and increases in the pH and carbonate concentrations of bile[14], engendered by administration of UDCA or its conjugates.

This chapter explores the possibility that other bile salts, principally taurocholate (TC), might favourably alter excretion of CB and/or UCB in bile for the treatment of jaundice and/or pigment gallstones. After reviewing work by others regarding the effects of bile salts on biliary excretion of CB, we present new data regarding the effects of bile salts on UCB excretion.

EFFECTS OF BILE SALTS ON BILIARY SECRETION OF CB

Studies in rats, rabbits, dogs and ponies have shown that the endogenous biliary secretion rate of CB[15,16], as well as CB secretion at low[17] and saturating (T_{max})[10,18] CB infusion rates, are enhanced up to one-third by infusions of micelle-forming bile salts. By contrast CB secretion is not enhanced by infusion of the triketo-bile salts, dehydrocholate (DHC)[19–21] or its taurine amidate (TDHC)[16], which do not form micelles[22]. Taurocholate enhances organic anion excretion in part by stimulation of colchicine-sensitive pathways of vesicular exocytosis, but this plays a role only when the endogenous bile salt pool has been depleted by overnight external biliary drainage[17].

Mechanism of effects of bile salts on biliary secretion of CB

In vitro, bile salt micelles are known to form complexes with CB[23], suggesting that the enhanced secretion of CB might be due to bilary secretion of organic anion–bile salt complexes. Bile salts in the hepatocyte are at submicellar concentrations[24], however, and are apparently secreted into bile as monomers[25] by canalicular membrane transporters that differ from those for CB[26,27]. That massive biliary secretion of CB, engendered by intravenous boluses or infusions of large doses of UCB or bilirubin ditaurate, does not alter bile salt output[25,28], attests further to the essential independence of the canalicular membrane transporters for bile salts and CB.

It has been proposed that organic anions, including conjugated bilirubin, associate with simple and/or mixed micelles after secretion into canalicular bile, effectively removing the secreted organic anion from the gradient of unbound organic anion across the canalicular membrane[29]. Strong support for the canalicular location of this 'micellar sink' effect has been provided by the GY mutant rat, in which the deficient cMOAT canalicular transporter drastically reduces the biliary secretion of organic anions[30]. Evidence against this mechanism, however, comes from reports that infusions of TDHC and DHC both increase the maximum rate of excretion (T_{max}) of sulphobromophthalein into bile[31,32], despite the absence of micelles. Doubt regarding the association of organic anions with bile salt mixed micelles has also been engendered by studies of the co-elution of CB and bile salts during equilibrium column chromatography of bile over a wide range of dilutions[33].

Relationship to pigment gallstone formation

It has been demonstrated that there are excess UCB and bilirubin monoconjugates in the bile of most patients with pigment gallstones[34,35], whereas total bilirubin concentrations are normal[34–36]. Therefore, excess UCB in bile is important for the development of pigment gallstones, and possibly also for cholesterol gallstones, most of which have a pigmented centre[37]. This excess UCB in the bile of gallstone patients arises mainly from excessive hydrolysis of UCB conjugates after excretion into bile[34,38,39] and/or from augmented biliary excretion of hydrolysable bilirubin conjugates due to increased bilirubin production (e. g. haemolysis)[40].

Bile salt infusions increase both secretion of CB available for hydrolysis to UCB in bile[3] and the activity of free calcium ion in bile[5]. Thus, one might expect such infusions to increase the degree of saturation of calcium bilirubinates in bile, favouring pigment precipitation and pigment stone formation[3]. Nonetheless, depletion of bile salts by biliary diversion rapidly leads to precipitation of calcium bilirubinates in bile[41]; this process is prevented or reversed by intravenous infusion, or *in vitro* addition to depleted bile, of micelle-forming bile salts such as TC, but not by poor micelle-formers such as TDHC[41]. It is felt that this phenomenon results from the low ratio of bile salts to UCB in the bile-diverted animal, limiting solubilization of UCB by bile salts[3,42].

EFFECTS OF BILE SALTS ON BILIARY SECRETION OF UCB

Neither the possibility of direct biliary excretion of UCB, nor the *in vivo* effects of bile salt infusions on this process, have been studied using an assay that specifically measures UCB in bile under conditions which exclude appearance of UCB in bile due to photoisomerization of UCB[6–8] and hydrolysis of excreted CB[34,38,39]. We now report the effects of intravenous infusions of micellar TC and non-micellar TDHC on the outputs of UCB in the bile of homozygous, jaundiced Gunn rats maintained in the dark. These animals form no CB for hydrolysis to UCB[43], and the exclusion of light precludes photoisomerization of UCB[44]. To specifically measure excretion of UCB, this pigment was measured after separation from other diazo-reactive compounds in Gunn rat bile[43,45,46] by preliminary solvent partition[47] and thin-layer chromatography prior to diazo assay[48].

Materials and methods

Materials

Sodium salts of TDHC and TC, grade A, were obtained from Calbiochem, San Diego, CA and used without further purification. By thin-layer chromatography (TLC)[49] the TDHC contained no other bile salts, but the TC contained 1.5% taurochenodeoxycholate. Unconjugated bilirubin, obtained from British Drug Houses, Poole, Dorset, UK, was purified by the method of McDonagh and Assisi[50]. All solvents were HPLC grade. Pure standards of DHC and its methyl ester were a generous gift of Dr Alan F. Hofmann. Other pure bile acid standards were purchased from Applied Science or from Supelco (Bellefonte, PA),

Preparation of animals

Male albino Gunn rats, weighing 350–450 g, were anaesthetized with intraperitonal pentobarbital (5 mg/100 g body weight) and the common bile duct was cannulated with a polyethylene catheter (Intramedic PE-50, Clay Adams, New York, NY). The femoral vein was cannulated with a PE-10 catheter for continuous infusion of 2.5% dextrose–0.45% sodium chloride (w/v), with or without added bile salt, delivered by a calibrated syringe pump (Model 600–930V, Harvard Apparatus, Dover, MA) at 1.6–1.8 ml/h. Each animal was allowed to awaken in a Bollman-type restraining cage and maintained in darkness, except for a brief periods of dim indirect light (0.05 mW/cm^2) when samples were obtained or infusions changed.

Bile salt and UCB infusions

For the first 15 h after cannulation, the dextrose–saline solution without bile salts was infused while the bile salt pool was depleted by external biliary drainage. This is known to produce a stable baseline output of bile salts and phospholipids (PL) that persists until 33 h after cannulation[51–53].

Series I (10 rats) – variable bile salt infusions, with and without UCB infusions. From 15 to 33 h, each animal received two infusions each of TC and two of TDHC. The bile salts were administered in the glucose–saline solution at two different rates, ranging from 0 to 450 nmol/min per 100 g body weight, with the sequence and rates randomized among different rats. After four periods of bile salt infusion, UCB was administered at a rate of approximately 120 μg/h, dissolved in one of the TC infusion solutions used earlier in the same animal. Each bile salt or UCB solution was infused for 3.5 h, with a 30 min interval between. The bile collected during the first 30 min of each infusion period was discarded to allow a new steady state to be attained, and the bile collected on ice during the last 3 h was taken for analysis. At several intervals before and after the administration of the bilirubin load, blood from a tail vein incision was collected into a heparinized capillary tube for plasma bilirubin determination.

Series II (four rats) – variable bilirubin infusions at constant TC infusion rates. Following the 15-h period of bile salt depletion, two Gunn rats were infused with TC at a constant rate of 100 nmol/min per 100 g body weight and two at a rate of 300 nmol/min per 100 g body weight. During successive 3-h periods, following an initial period of infusion of TC alone, UCB was added to the infusate and administered at rates of 80, 160, 240 and 320 μg/h. Bile and tail vein blood were collected as above.

Analytical methods

Immediately after each infusion period, the bile volume was measured, and aliquots taken as follows: 1.5 ml was added to 10 ml of 2:1 (v/v) chloroform–methanol (Folch solvent) for separation of UCB[47]; duplicate 0.2 ml samples were taken for measurement of total diazo-reactivity; duplicate 0.1 ml samples were placed in methanol and frozen for later bile salt determination; and 0.5 ml was added to 5.0 ml of Folch solvent for PL assay.

For UCB determination the bile in Folch solvent was shaken thoroughly, 1.0 ml of 1.0 mmol/l disodium EDTA in 0.1 mol/l sodium phosphate buffer, pH 7.4 was added, and the mixture again shaken and then centrifuged at 400 *g* for 5 min. The upper phase was discarded and the lower phase washed twice with 4.0 ml distilled water. The washed lower phase was evaporated at 45°C under nitrogen in the dark and the residue dissolved in chloroform. The UCB band was separated by TLC and quantitated by diazotization with *p*-iodoaniline, as described by Boonyapisit *et al.*[48]. Internal standards of

[^{14}C]UCB were processed simultaneously to correct for losses, which averaged approximately 20%.

Total diazo-reactivity in bile (0.2 ml) and plasma (0.025 ml) was determined by the Michaelsson method[54]. Bile salts in bile and infusion solutions were measured enzymatically with 3α-hydroxysteroid dehydrogenase (Worthington Biochemicals, Freehold, NJ)[55]. Phospholipids were determined in the lower phase of the Folch partition of bile by the method of Fiske and SubbaRow[56].

Series III: Bile salt composition and phospholipid excretion after bile salt infusions

In a parallel series of experiments, rats were given infusions of TDHC exactly as above, and the bile analysed for bile acid composition by coupled gas–liquid chromatography–mass spectrometry (GLC-MS) of their methyl ester acetates[57,58].

In preparing methyl ester acetates of the bile salts, the customary time for each step was prolonged, since this was found necessary to completely derivatize the keto-bile acids, without reduction of the keto groups. Bile salts were deamidated with cholylglycine hydrolase for 30 min at 37°C according to Nair *et al.*[59]. The free bile acids were extracted (90–95% recovery) with chloroform, since keto-bile acids were poorly recovered with the customary ether extraction. The dried extracts were redissolved in chloroform–methanol (2:1 v/v) and methylated by repeated additions of diazomethane until the solution remained yellow for 1 h. The methyl esters were recovered by evaporation; and acetylated for 30 min by the method of Roovers *et al.*[60]. The methyl ester acetates were stored under vacuum over Drierite-KOH for 48–72 h to completely remove excess acetic acid prior to GLC.

For GLC-MS, a 183 cm × 1 mm glass column was packed with 1% Poly-S-179 on 100/120 mesh Gas Chrom Q (Applied Science, State College, PA), and run at 275°C, using a Hewlett-Packard 5750 instrument (King of Prussia, PA). The eluted peaks were analysed on a Biospect-GC chemical ionization mass spectrometer (Scientific Research Instruments Corp., Baltimore, MD) using isobutane as the reagent gas. 3β-Cholestanol was added as an internal standard, and retention times and mass spectra were determined with pure bile acid standards derivatized in the same manner as the bile samples. To separate and measure derivatized hyodeoxycholate and cholate, which both had a relative retention time of 1.31 min, a duplicate sample was run on an OV-17 column[57,58], on which their relative retention times were 1.22 and 1.31 respectively.

Statistical analyses

Linear regressions were performed by the method of least squares. Hyperbolic curves were fitted by linear regressions of the double reciprocal plots. Regression lines were compared by residual variances, slopes and elevations.

Results

Biliary excretion of bile salts

Total bile salt outputs, entirely as taurine conjugates, were related linearly to TC (Fig. 1) and TDHC (Fig. 2) infusion rates up to 300 nmol/min per 100 g body weight ($r = 0.89$ and 0.93, $p<0.005$), with no differences among Series I,

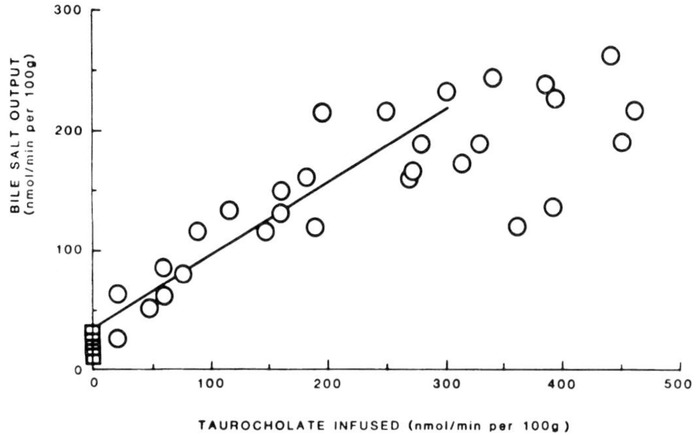

Fig. 1 Effect of intravenous taurocholate infusions (x) on bile salt outputs (y) in Gunn rat bile. At infusion rates up to 300 nmol/min per 100 g, $y = 0.612x + 33.0$, $r = 0.93$, $p<0.005$. At higher infusion rates no further increment in bile salt output occurred

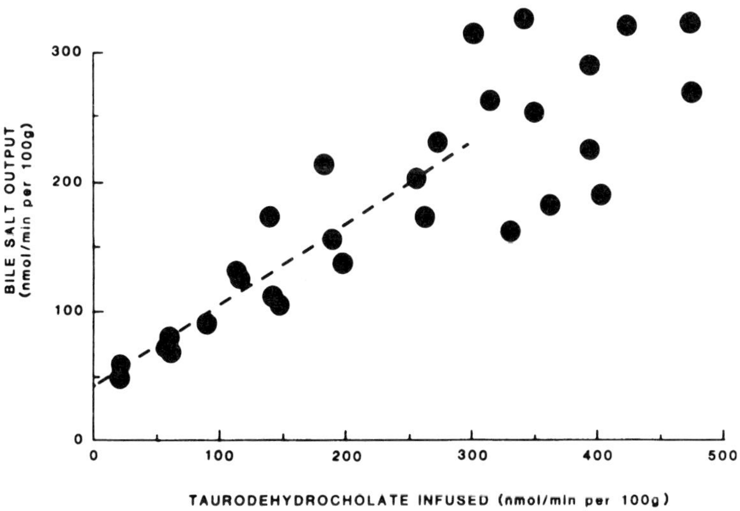

Fig. 2 Effect of intravenous taurodehydrocholate infusions (x) on bile salt outputs (y) in Gunn rat bile. $y = 0.635x + 40.5$, $r = 0.89$, $p<0.005$, with no significant plateau at bile salt outputs above 300 nmol/min per 100 g

II and III. At higher infusion rates this linear relationship persisted with TDHC, whereas the output of bile salts with TC infusion plateaued. In both cases about 60% of the infused bile salts were excreted above extrapolated baseline outputs of 33–40 nmol/min per 100 g body weight. Bile salts excreted in the baseline periods before bile salt infusions consisted almost entirely of non-keto, tri- and di-hydroxy bile salts, but included about 10% of 7-keto-deoxycholate (3α,12α-di-OH,7-keto-cholanoate) (Table 1).

Infused TC was excreted entirely as TC or tauro-β-muricholate. During TDHC infusions the output of non-keto bile acids was essentially unchanged from baseline (mean of 23 nmol/min per 100 g body weight). The exogenous bile salts emanating from the TDHC infusions consisted of 58% 3α-OH,7,12-diketo-cholanoate and 38% 7-keto-deoxycholate, each excreted in direct proportion to the TDHC infusion rate; there was no conversion to TC or 3α,7α-di-OH, 12-keto-cholanoate. When superimposed on the constant low baseline excretion rates of hydroxy-bile salts, the proportion of non-micellar bile salts in the bile rose hyperbolically with increasing TDHC infusion rates (Fig. 3). At all TDHC infusion rates above 150 nmol/min per 100 g body weight, over 80% of the total excreted bile salts was non-micellar.

Biliary excretion of phospholipids

There were no differences between Series I and III studies. As shown in Fig. 4, with both TC and TDHC infusions, phospholipid excretion increased linearly with total bile salt output during infusions of either bile salt, but was about 6.5-fold greater with TC than with TDHC (p<0.01).

Table 1 Gas–liquid chromatography of bile acids as methyl ester acetates on poly S-179 column

Bile acids (5β-Cholanoate Derivatives)		*Relative retention times*	*Major mass ions detected (m/e)*	*Percentage in pre-infusion bile samples*[d]
Trivial name (-cholate)	*Steroid groups*[a]			
Litho-	3α-OH	0.55	373	0.0–1.0
Deoxy-	3α,12α-di-OH	0.74	371, 431	2.7–3.3
Chenodeoxy-	3α,7α-di-OH	1.00[b]	371, 431	9.5–12.7
Hyodeoxy-	3α,6α-di-OH	1.31	371, 431	11.9–13.2[e]
Cholate	3α,7α,12α-tri-OH	1.31	369, 429	45.7–50.6[e]
Hyo-	3α,6α,12α-tri-OH	1.70	369, 429	6.9–8.2
7-Ketodeoxy-	3α,12α-di-OH, 7K	2.21	385, 445	8.0–10.5
β-Muri-	3α,6β,7β-tri-OH	2.43	369, 429	7.6–8.5
12-Keto-chenodeoxy-	3α,7α-di-OH, 12K	2.63	385, 445[c]	0
Dehydro-	3,7,12-tri-K	3.70	417[c]	0
7,12-di-Keto-litho-	3α-OH,7,12-di-K	4.49	401, 461	0.0–0.8

[a] -OH denotes (acetylated) hydroxyl- group, K denotes keto- group.
[b] Relative retention times taken with chenodeoxycholate as 1.00, since lithocholate and deoxycholate were undetectable in all bile samples after 15 h interruption of EHC.
[c] These peaks were absent from all bile samples, so that mass spectral analysis was obtained only with standard compounds.
[d] Miscellaneous minor peaks, with relative retention times more than 4.5, constituting collectively less than 2.5% of total bile acids, were detected but not identified.
[e] Distinguished by parallel gas–liquid chromatography on OV-17 columns.

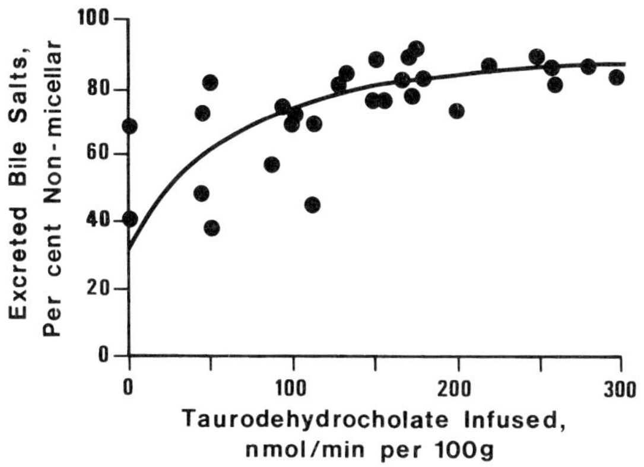

Fig. 3 Percentage of 'non-micellar' bile salts (y) in Gunn rat bile during intravenous infusion of taurodehydrocholate at various rates (x). $y/100 = (x + 18.75)/(x + 59.64)$, $p<0.001$

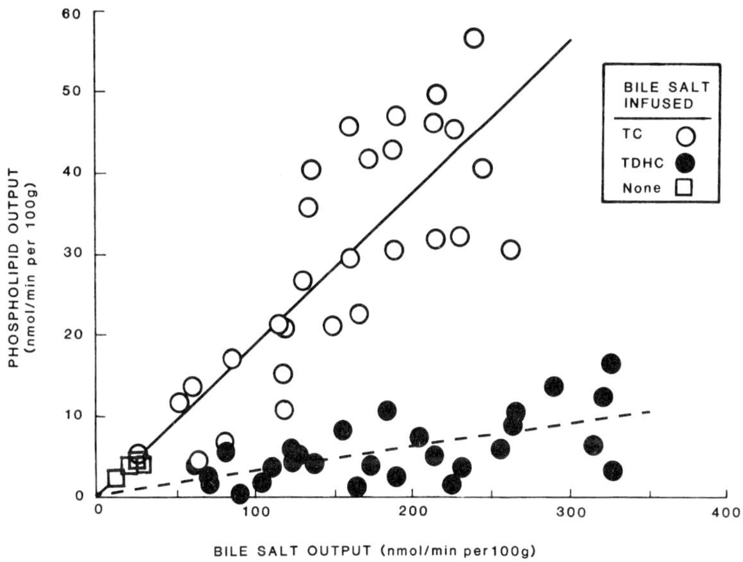

Fig. 4 Effects of intravenous bile salt infusions (x) on phospholipid outputs (y) in Gunn rat bile. For taurocholate (TC) infusions, $y = 0.188x - 0.02$, $r = 0.86$, $p<0.005$. For taurodehydrocholate (TDHC) infusions, $y = 0.029x + 0.22$, $r = 0.60$, $p<0.01$. PL excretion is 6.5 times greater with TC infusion ($p<0.01$)

Biliary excretion of bile pigments

Excretion of total diazo-reactive pigments (Fig. 5) exhibited saturable, hyperbolic relationships to bile salt outputs that did not differ significantly between TC and TDHC infusions. By contrast, outputs of endogenous UCB *per se*

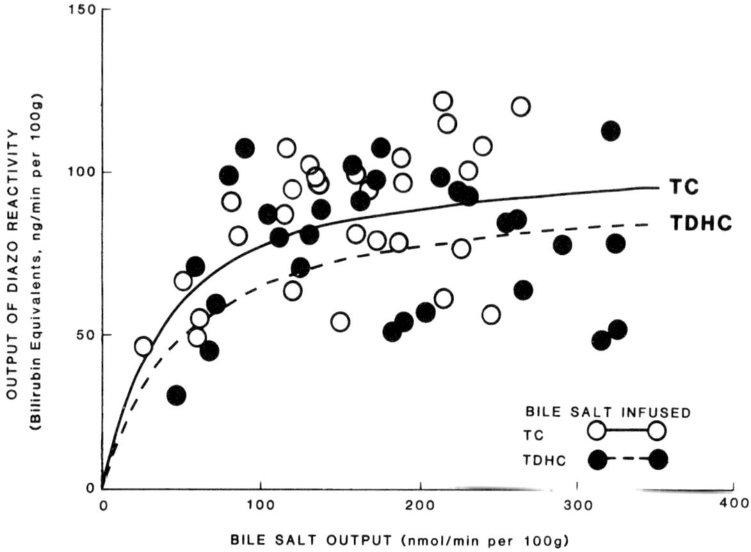

Fig. 5 Effects of bile salt infusions (x) on outputs of diazo-reactivity (y) in Gunn rat bile, expressed as the amount of bilirubin, in ng/min per 100 g, that would yield the same diazo-reactivity. For TC infusions, $1/y = (0.3404/x) + 0.0096$, $r = 0.62$. For TDHC infusions, $1/y = (0.4977/x) + 0.0104$, $r = 0.45$ ($p<0.02$ for each). There is no significant difference between the effects of the two bile salts

(Figs 6 and 7) were related linearly to bile salt outputs, but were 60% greater with TC than with TDHC infusions ($p<0.05$) (Fig. 7). In each case the ratio of UCB to diazo-reactivity increased with increasing bile salt output ($p<0.01$, not

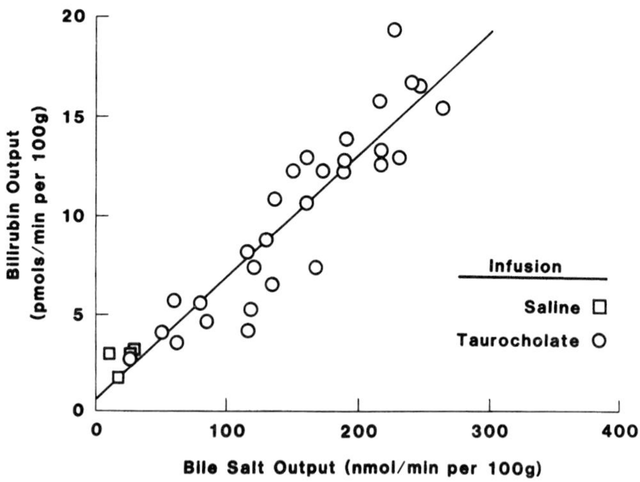

Fig. 6 Effects of infusions of TC (x) on endogenous outputs (y) of unconjugated bilirubin (UCB) in Gunn rat bile. Note the different units on the two axes. $y = 0.0629x + 0.648$, $r = 0.93$, $p<0.005$. Square symbols represent saline infusions without TC

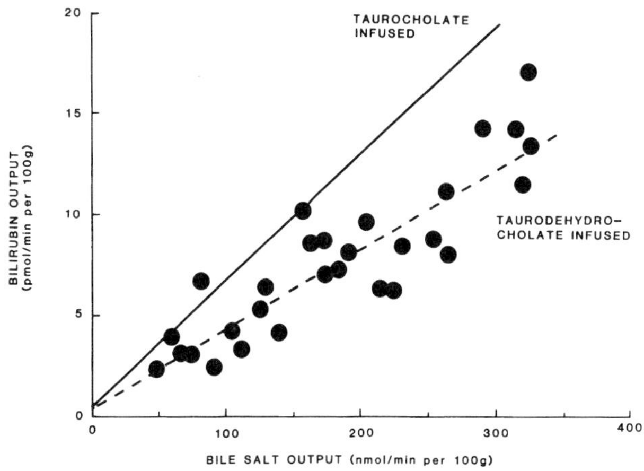

Fig. 7 Effects of infusions of TDHC (x) on outputs of UCB (y) in Gunn rat bile, represented by broken line ($y = 0.0395x + 0.472$, $r = 0.89$, $p<0.005$). Slope of the linear regression for TC infusions from Fig. 6 (solid line), is 60% greater than that for TDHC

shown). Less than 18%, and usually less than 10% of the total diazo-reactivity in the bile represented UCB.

With either bile salt infusion, endogenous UCB output showed a weak linear correlation with bile flow ($r = 0.55$, $p<0.02$, not shown). By contrast there were excellent linear correlations ($r = 0.70$ and 0.87, $p<0.005$) between UCB outputs and phospholipid outputs (Fig. 8); with TC infusions the increment in the output of UCB per increment in phospholipid output was 2.4 times that with TDHC

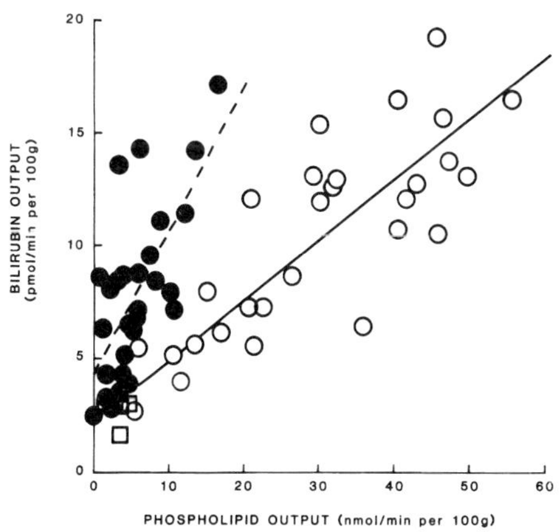

Fig. 8 Relationships of UCB outputs (y) to phospholipid outputs (x) in Gunn rat bile during infusions of TC (○) and TDHC (●) at various rates. For TC infused, $y = 0.268x + 2.25$, $r = 0.87$, $p<0.005$. For TDHC infused, $y = 0.632x + 4.39$, $r = 0.68$, $p<0.01$. Square symbols represent saline infusions without bile acids

infusions ($p<0.05$). There was, however, a small but significant excretion of UCB (2–4 pmol/min per 100 g body weight) at essentially zero phospholipid output.

Effects of added bilirubin loads during TC infusions

Among the 10 rats in Series I that received a single UCB infusion at a rate that increased by 3-fold the estimated normal bilirubin load, plasma UCB increased by 2.1 ± 0.7 mg/dl in five rats, but did not change in the remaining five rats. In the four rats in Series II that received added UCB loads varying from 2 to 8 times the normal UCB production rate in these animals, plasma UCB levels did not increase significantly until the UCB infusion rate exceeded 160 μg/h (4× baseline), irrespective of the TC infusion rate. As shown in Fig. 9, for both series of rats the biliary output of UCB during these added UCB loads bore the same relationship to total bile acid output as during infusions of TC without added UCB, with about 1 nmol of UCB secreted per 16 000 nmol of bile salt. The output of total diazo-reactive compounds in bile likewise did not increase as a result of the UCB loads (not shown).

DISCUSSION

Normally, UCB appears in bile mainly by hydrolysis of excreted CB[34,38,39]. In subjects with unconjugated hyperbilirubinaemia undergoing phototherapy[6,46,61]

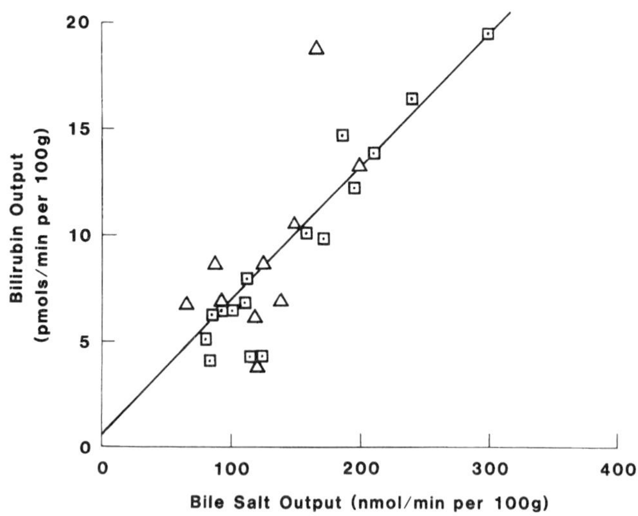

Fig. 9 Effects of intravenous infusions of unconjugated bilirubin in Gunn rats receiving intravenous infusions of taurocholate. Series I (10 rats, △) received varied TC infusion rates + UCB infused at 120 μg/h, Series II (four rats, ⊡) each received TC at 100 or 300 nmol/min per 100 g body weight, and UCB infusions ranging from 80 to 120 μg/h. The regression of UCB output on bile salt output is not significantly different from that obtained with infusions of TC alone (——, from Fig. 6)

(and, to a lesser extent, under normal lighting conditions[44]), more UCB-IXα-Z,Z appears in bile. This is due to formation of more polar E,Z photoisomers that can be excreted into bile, where some revert spontaneously to the poorly-soluble, parent Z,Z isomer of UCB[6–8]. This chapter considers a third possibility: that some UCB *per se* is passed into bile directly from the hepatocytes and/or across the biliary epithelium, and that this excretory process is mediated by bile salt secretion. Evidence cited in favour of this possibility is the presence of low concentrations of UCB in the bile of patients with Crigler–Najjar syndrome[62] and Gunn rats[43–45,61], neither of which can form bilirubin conjugates that could be hydrolysed to UCB after excretion.

Methodological considerations: bilirubin

The above studies, however, were not performed in total darkness, so that photoreactions were not excluded[44]. We therefore studied the output of UCB by Gunn rats maintained in the dark, thus excluding both hydrolysis of bilirubin conjugates and excretion of UCB photoisomers as sources of UCB in the bile. The absence of bilirubin conjugates also eliminated possible interference of these normally predominant pigments with accurate measurement of UCB. The bile of Gunn rats, however, contains other diazo-positive pigments[43,45] that preclude equating diazo-reactivity with UCB content, as had been done by others[63]. We therefore employed an assay for UCB in which these non-bilirubin bile pigments were separated from UCB by Folch solvent partition[47] and TLC[34,48], and the pure UCB band was quantitated accurately by diazotization[48].

Methodological considerations: bile salt infusions

Another refinement in our studies was the use of TDHC infusions to study whether micelle formation was essential to the mechanism of UCB excretion. Unlike the significant formation of non-keto bile salts, principally cholate conjugates, during infusions of unconjugated DHC, or its glycine amidate, reported by most other investigators[64–68], we observed that none of the infused TDHC was converted to trihydroxy bile salts. Rather the TDHC was completely metabolized to two keto-hydroxy bile salts which form micelles only at quite high concentrations[22,52,69], but the 7-keto-, rather than the 12-keto-dihydroxy-cholanoate[64] was the major metabolite. By performing the TDHC infusions only during the prolonged nadir of endogenous bile salt output that occurs from 15 to 33 h after biliary diversion in the rat[46,51,53] at least 80% of the excreted bile salts was 'non-micellar' at TDHC infusion rates greater than 150 nmol/min per 100 g body weight. The very low output of phospholipids supports the concept that, at the concentrations achieved in bile in these studies, both the diketo and diol metabolites of infused TDHC formed micelles poorly, as reported by others[22,52,64,65,69].

Mechanism of bile salt-induced biliary secretion of UCB

Using these methods we were able to document that non-micellar bile salts secreted during TDHC infusions were about 60% as effective as micellar bile salts secreted during TC infusions in promoting the direct excretion of UCB into bile. This contrasts with the lack of effect of DHC or TDHC infusions on CB secretion by various animal species[16,19–21] and the striking decrease in CB excretion during infusions of unconjugated DHC in human subjects[70]. In confirmation of observations of Billing *et al.*[63], the output of diazo-reactive pigments was related hyperbolically to bile salt output during TC infusions. By contrast the output of UCB, measured specifically, was related linearly to the output of bile salts. This bile salt-related mechanism for excretion of UCB was, however, extremely inefficient, with only one molecule of UCB secreted per 16 000 molecules of bile salt (UCB/TC ratio = 6.3×10^{-5}). This is quite similar to the maximum ratio of UCB bound to TC at pH 7.4 during solvent partition of UCB into 50 mmol/l TC solution[42], a bile salt concentration similar to that found in normal rat bile[51]. In addition, the 40% lower excretion of UCB during TDHC as compared with TC infusions is similar to the 40% lower *in vitro* solubilization of UCB in 50 mmol/l TDHC as compared with 50 mmol/l TC[42].

UCB is known also to interact with phospholipids[42], and we found a linear relationship of UCB excretion to phospholipid output. This relationship differed, however, for TC and TDHC infusions, indicating that the bile salts, and not the phospholipids, were the determining factor. These results suggested that bile salts directly mediate the excretion of UCB into bile. Since bile salts enter bile primarily via canalicular secretion after passage across the hepatocyte[25], it seems likely that the excreted UCB also entered the bile via the hepatocyte and canaliculus.

These results indicate that interaction of UCB with bile acid micelles is not essential for biliary excretion of UCB. This is in keeping with studies, by solvent partition, of UCB solubilization by various bile salts, which suggest that UCB interacts serially with bile salt monomers, rather than with preformed bile salt micelles[42]. Together these findings suggest that biliary secretion of UCB is not mediated by a 'micellar sink' phenomenon[25,29].

Relevance to severe unconjugated hyperbilirubinaemia

Whatever the mechanism by which bile salts mediated the direct excretion of UCB into bile, it was apparently saturated at the normal rates of UCB production in the Gunn rat (about 1 mg/day for a 350 g rat)[44]. Our prior studies in Gunn rats maintained in the dark[44] have shown that only about 2–4% of total [^{14}C]bilirubin turnover can be accounted for by this bile salt-related mechanism which, in the present studies, showed no compensatory increase in response to acute UCB loads up to 8 times normal UCB production rates. Neither was there an increase in biliary excretion of diazo-positive UCB derivatives, suggesting that alternative, oxidative pathways of UCB catabolism[4,43,45,71,72] likewise did not compensate for the acutely increased UCB load. These findings do not exclude the possibilities that one or both of these mechanisms for removal of UCB would not increase adaptively to chronic bilirubin overloads, or that the photoisomerization mechanism, not studied here, would not increase in response to the higher levels of UCB in the skin that would occur in response to increased UCB formation[73]. In this regard it is noteworthy that, despite the lack of compensatory increases in biliary excretion of UCB or its diazo-positive derivatives, no significant increase in plasma UCB concentration occurred in these Gunn rats until the bilirubin load was more than 5 times normal. This suggests that the tissues of the jaundiced Gunn rat possess considerable reserve capacity for uptake and storage of UCB, and that this may be one mechanism for protection of these animals against kernicterus in the face of haemolysis.

In humans, biliary excretion of UCB extrapolates to zero at zero bile salt output[40]. By contrast, extrapolation of our data suggested that, in the Gunn rat, approximately 0.5 pmol/min of UCB per 100 g body weight was excreted independently of bile salt output or photoisomerization of UCB. Possibly, geometric isomerization of UCB can occur to a limited degree in the absence of light[6] and account for the bile-salt-independent excretion of UCB in the dark. Alternatively, as occurs in the intestine[72], there might be some diffusion of UCB from the hyperbilirubinaemic plasma across either the intrahepatocytic tight junctions or the biliary epithelium.

Relevance to pigment gallstone formation

Calcium bilirubinates precipitate in the bile after biliary diversion, both in normal rats[41] and during phototherapy of Gunn rats[46]. In both cases, as in our animals at baseline, the excretion of bile salts is markedly depleted, so that the bile salt-related excretion of UCB should be comparably reduced. Nonetheless, in both models the biliary concentration of UCB remains high or increases. In the normal rats this is due to the relative independence of excretion of bilirubin conjugates on bile salt output, so that significant concentrations of bilirubin conjugates remain available in bile for hydrolysis to UCB. In the Gunn rats this is due to enhanced excretion of UCB via the photoisomerization mechanism.

CONCLUSIONS

These results indicate that some UCB is excreted directly into rat bile in the absence of hydrolysis of bilirubin conjugates or photoisomerization of UCB. This process is mediated mainly by association of UCB with bile salts, rather than phospholipids, and involves principally non-micellar interactions, akin to those seen *in vitro*. This bile-salt-mediated excretion of UCB is apparently saturated even at normal rates of bilirubin formation in the Gunn rats, and cannot accommodate increased bilirubin loads, so that it can play no role in protecting glucuronosyl transferase-deficient subjects against the consequences of haemolysis. Though TC infusions may enhance UCB excretion by as much as 20-fold, the very low ratio of UCB to bile salt output, the haemolytic effects of high bile salt loads, and the increases in both UCB and ionized calcium concentrations, preclude a clinically-useful enhancement of UCB excretion by infusion of bile salts into patients with severe unconjugated hyperbilirubinaemia. Compared with the hydrolysis of excreted CB, this bile-acid-mediated excretion of UCB contributes minimally to UCB concentrations in bile, and thus plays little role in the pathogenesis of pigment gallstones.

Acknowledgements

This work was supported by Medical Investigator and Merit Review Research Awards to Dr Ostrow from the US Department of Veterans Affairs. We are grateful to Dr Patricia Szczepanik for her performance of the gas–liquid chromatographic/mass spectrometric analyses of the biliary bile salts in the Series III experiments, which were performed while Dr Ostrow and Dr Ashkin were at the University of Pennsylvania and Philadelphia Veterans Administration Hospital.

Dr Ostrow's current address is: M.D.L., Room CZ-111, Academic Medical Center, Meibergdreef 9, 1105 AZ Amsterdam Zuidoost, The Netherlands.

References

1. Ostrow JD. Jaundice and disorders of bilirubin metabolism. In: Stein JH, editor. Internal medicine, 4th edn. St Louis, MO: Mosby-Year book; 1994:556–70.
2. Cashore WJ. The neurotoxicity of bilirubin. Clin Perinatol. 1990;17:437–47.
3. Ostrow JD. Unconjugated bilirubin and cholesterol gallstone formation. Hepatology. 1990;12:219S–26S.
4. Ostrow JD. Therapeutic amelioration of jaundice. Hepatology. 1988;8:683–9.
5. Moore EW. Biliary calcium and gallstone formation. Hepatology. 1990;12:206S–18S.
6. McDonagh AF, Lightner DA. Phototherapy and photobiology of bilirubin. Semin Liver Dis. 1988;8:272–81.
7. Stoll MS, Zenone EA, Ostrow JD. Excretion of administered and endogenous photobilirubins in the bile of the jaundiced Gunn rat. J Clin Invest. 1981;68:134–41.
8. Onishi S, Kawade N, Itoh S, Isobe K, Sugiyama S. High pressure liquid chromatographic analysis of anerobic photoproducts of bilirubin IX *in vitro*, and its comparison with photoproducts *in vivo*. Biochem J. 1980;190:527–32.
9. Poupon RE, Poupon R. Ursodeoxycholic acid for the treatment of cholestatic diseases. In: Boyer JL, Ockner RK, editors. Progress in liver diseases, 10th edn. Philadelphia: Saunders; 1992:219–38.
10. Galan AI, Jimenez R, Munoz ME, Gonzalez J. Effects of ursodeoxycholate on maximal biliary secretion of bilirubin in the rat. Biochem Pharmacol. 1990;39:1175–80.
11. Marteau C, Portugaal H, Pauli A-M, Gerolami A. Effect of glycoursodeoxycholate on precipitation of calcium carbonate. Hepatology. 1985;5:1209–12.
12. Donovan JM, Leonard MR, Batta AK, Carey MC. Calcium affinity for biliary lipid aggregates in model biles: complementary importance of bile salts and lecithin. Gastroenterology. 1994;107: 831–46.
13. Salen G, Tint GS, Shefer S. Oral dissolution treatment of gallstones with bile acids. Semin Liver Dis. 1990;10:181–6.
14. Knyrim K, Vakil N, Pfab R, Classen M. The effects of intraduodenal bile acid administration on biliary secretion of ionized calcium and carbonate in man. Hepatology. 1989;10:134–42.
15. Mesa VA, Fevery J. Heirwegh KPM, DeGroote J. Effects of ioglycamide on the hepatic transport of bilirubin and its mono- and di-conjugates in the rat. Hepatology. 1985;5:600–6.
16. Gonzalez J, Hidalgo F, Lopez MA, Esteller A. Influence of bile salts on the endogenous excretion of bile pigments. Rev Esp Fisiol. 1983;39:69–76.
17. Crawford JM, Gollan JL. Hepatocyte cotransport of taurocholate and bilirubin glucuronides: role of microtubules. Am J Physiol. 1988;255:G121–31.
18. Goresky CA, Haddad HH, Kluger WS, Nadeau BE, Bach GG. The enhancement of maximal bilirubin excretion with taurocholate-induced increments in bile flow. Can J Physiol Pharmacol. 1974;52:389–403.
19. Engelking LR, Gronwall R, Anwer MS. Effect of dehydrocholic, chenodeoxycholic and taurocholic acids on the excretion of bilirubin. Am J Vet Res. 1980;41:355–61.
20. Esteller A, Gonzalez J, Hidalgo F, Lopez MA. Enhancement of maximal bilirubin excretion by bile salts in the anesthetized rabbit. Q J Exp Physiol. 1984;69:217–25.
21. Garcia-Marin JJ, Gonzalez J, Esteller A. Influence of dehydrocholate on bilirubin transport into bile in the rat. Digestion. 1986;33:80–8.
22. Roda A, Hofmann AF, Mysels KJ. The influence of bile salt structure on self-association in aqueous solutions. J Biol Chem. 1983;258:6362–70.

23. Carey MC, Spivak W. Physical chemistry of bile pigments and porphyrins with particular reference to bile. In: Ostrow JD, editor. Bile pigments and jaundice; molecular, metabolic and medical aspects. New York: Marcel Dekker; 1986:81–132.
24. Ostrow JD. Metabolism of bile salts in cholestasis in humans. In: Tavaloni N, Berk PD, editors. Hepatic transport and bile secretion; physiology and pathophysiology. New York: Raven Press; 1993:673–712.
25. Verkade HJ, Havinga R, Gerding A, Vonk RJ, Kuipers F. The mechanism of bile acid-induced biliary lipid secretion in the rat. Effect of conjugated bilirubin. Am J Physiol. 1993;264:G462–9.
26. Jansen PLM, Groothuis MM, Peters HM, Meijer FM. Selective hepatobiliary transport defect for organic anions and neutral steroids in mutant rats with hereditary conjugated hyperbilirubinemia. Hepatology. 1987;7:71–6.
27. Takikawa H, Sano N, Narita T *et al.* Biliary excretion of bile acid conjugates in a hyperbilirubinemic mutant Sprague-Dawley rat. Hepatology. 1991;14:352–60.
28. Usui R, Ise H, Kitayama O *et al.* Bilirubin conjugation and biliary bilirubin excretion after intravenous bilirubin injection in dogs. Tohoku J Exp Med. 1991;165:67–77.
29. Scharschmidt BF, Schmid R. The micellar sink. A quantitative assessment of the association of organic anions with mixed micelles and other macromolecular aggregates in bile. J Clin Invest. 1978;62:1122–31.
30. Verkade HJ, Wolbers MJ, Havinga R, Uges DRA, Vonk RJ, Kuipers F. The uncoupling of biliary lipid from bile acid secretion by organic anions in the rat. Gastroenterology. 1990;99:1485–92.
31. Binet S, Delage Y, Erlinger S. Influence of taurocholate, taurochenodeoxycholate, and taurodehydrocholate on sulfobromophthalein transport into bile. Am J Physiol. 1979;236:E10–14.
32. Ritt DJ, Combes B. Enhancement of apparent excretory maximum of BSP by taurocholate and dehydrocholate. J Clin Invest. 1967;46:1108–9.
33. Reuben A, Howell KE, Boyer JL. Effects of taurocholate on the size of mixed lipid micelles and their associations with pigment and proteins in rat bile. J Lipid Res. 1982;23:1039–52.
34. Boonyapisit ST, Trotman BW, Ostrow JD. Unconjugated bilirubin and the hydrolysis of conjugated bilirubin in gallbladder bile of patients with cholelithiasis. Gastroenterology. 1978;74:70–4.
35. Masuda H, Nakayama F. Composition of bile pigment in gallstones and bile and their etiological significance. J Lab Clin Med. 1979;93:353–60.
36. Trotman BW, Ostrow JD, Soloway RD. Pigment vs cholesterol cholelithiasis: comparison of stone and bile composition. Am J Dig Dis. 1974;19:585–90.
37. Been JM, Bills PM, Lewis D. Microstructure of gallstones. Gastroenterology. 1979;76:548–55.
38. Maki T. Pathogenesis of calcium bilirubinate gallstones: Role of *E. coli*, β-glucuronidase and coagulation by inorganic ions, polyelectrolytes and agitation. Ann Surg. 1966;164:90–100.
39. Ho K-J, Hsu SC, Chen JS *et al.* Human biliary β-glucuronidase: correlation of its activity with deconjugation of bilirubin in the bile. Eur J Clin Invest. 1986;16:361–7.
40. Shull SD, Wagner CI, Trotman BW, Soloway RD. Factors affecting bilrubin excretion in patients with cholesterol or pigment gallstones. Gastroenterology. 1977;72:625–9.
41. Angelico M, De Sanctis SC, Gandin C, Alvaro D. Spontaneous formation of pigmentary precipitates in bile salt-depleted rat bile and its prevention by micelle-forming bile salts. Gastroenterology. 1990;98:444–53.
42. Ostrow JD, Mukerjee P, Tiribelli C. Structure and binding of unconjugated bilirubin: relevance for physiological and pathophysiological function. J Lipid Res. 1994;35:1715–37.
43. Blanckaert N, Fevery J, Heirwegh KPM, Compernolle F. Characterization of the major diazo-positive pigments in bile of homozygous Gunn rats. Biochem J. 1977;164:229–36.
44. Zenone EA, Stoll MS, Ostrow JD. The effect of elimination of environmental light on the metabolism of unconjugated bilirubin in the Gunn rat. Dig Dis Sci. 1982;27:1117–20.
45. Berry CS, Zarembo JE, Ostrow JD. Evidence for conversion of bilirubin to dihydroxyl derivatives in the Gunn rat. Biochem Biophys Res Commun. 1972;49:1366–75.
46. Ostrow JD, Berry CS, Zarembo JE. Studies on the mechanism of phototherapy in the congenitally jaundiced rat. In: Odell GB, Schaffer R, Simoupoulis AP, editors. Phototherapy in the newborn: an overview. Washington, DC: National Academy of Sciences, USA; 1974:74–92.
47. Ostrow JD, Murphy NH. Isolation and properties of conjugated bilirubin from bile. Biochem J. 1970;120:311–27.

48. Boonyapisit ST, Trotman BW, Ostrow JD, Olivieri PJ, Gallo D. Measurement of conjugated and unconjugated bilirubin in bile: II. A new thin-layer chromatographic method. J Lab Clin Med. 1976;88:857–63.
49. Chavez MN, Krone CI. Silicic acid thin-layer chromatography of conjugated and free bile acids. J Lipid Res. 1976;17:545–7.
50. McDonagh AF, Assisi F. The ready isomerization of bilirubin-IXα in aqueous solution. Biochem J. 1972;129:797–800.
51. Balint JA, Beeler DA, Kyriakides EC, Treble DH. The effect of bile salts upon lecithin synthesis. J Lab Clin Med. 1971;77:122–33.
52. Sewell RB, Hoffman NE, Smallwood RA, Cockbain S. Bile acid structure and bile formation: a comparison of hydroxy and keto bile acids. Am J Physiol. 1980;238:G10–17.
53. Kuipers F, Havinga R, Bosschieter H, Toorop GP, Hindriks FR, Vonk RJ. Enterohepatic circulation in the rat. Gastroenterology. 1985;88:403–11.
54. Michaelsson M. Bilirubin determination in serum and urine. Studies on diazo methods and a new copper–azopigment method. Scand J Clin Lab Invest. 1961;13(Suppl. 56):1–80.
55. Mashige F, Kazuhiro I, Osuga T. A simple and sensitive assay of total serum bile acids. Clin Chim Acta. 1976;70:79–86.
56. Fiske CH, SubbaRow Y. The colorimetric determination of phosphorus. J Biol Chem. 1925;66:375–400.
57. Szczepanik PA, Hachey DL, Klein PD. Evaluation of Poly S-179 as a stationary phase for the gas-liquid chromatography-mass spectrometry of bile acid methyl ester acetates. J Lipid Res. 1978;19:280–3.
58. Szczepanik PA, Hachey DL, Klein PD. Characterization of bile acid methyl ester acetate derivatives using gas-liquid chromatography, electron impact, and chemical ionization mass spectrometry. J Lipid Res. 1976 17:314–34.
59. Nair PP, Gordon M, Reback J. The enzymatic cleavage of the carbon-nitrogen bond in 3-alpha, 7-alpha, 12-alpha trihydroxy-5-beta-cholan-24-oylglycine. J Biol Chem. 1967;242:7–11.
60. Roovers J, Evrard E, Vanderhaeghe H. An improved method for measuring human blood bile acids. Clin Chim Acta. 1968;19:449–57.
61. Ostrow JD. Photocatabolism of labeled bilirubin in the congenitally jaundiced (Gunn) rat. J Clin Invest. 1971;50:707–18.
62. Fevery J, Blanckaert N, Heirwegh KPM *et al.* Unconjugated bilirubin and an increased proportion of bilirubin monoconjugates in the bile of patients with Gilbert's syndrome and Criglar-Najjar disease. J Clin Invest. 1977;60:970–9.
63. Billing BH, Jansen FH, Bilton E. The effect of bile depletion on the biliary excretion of unconjugated bilirubin and bilirubin conjugates. In: Preisig R, Paumgartner G, editors. The liver; quantitative aspects of structure and function. Basel: Karger; 1973:386–91.
64. Soloway RD, Hofmann AF, Thomas PJ, Schoenfield LJ, Klein PD. Triketocholanoic (dehydrocholic) acid: hepatic metabolism and effect on bile flow and biliary lipid secretion in man. J Clin Invest. 1973;52:715–24.
65. Hardison WG. Metabolism of sodium dehydrocholate by rat liver: its effect on micelle formation in bile. J Lab Clin Med. 1971;77:811–20.
66. Parkhill BJ, Jr, Barnhart JL, Combes B. Hepatic metabolism of glyco-dehydrocholic acid in the dog and rat. Proc Soc Exp Biol Med (NY). 1979;162:495–502.
67. Ogura M, Wakutani T, Yamasaki K. The fate of 14C-dehydrocholate administered to the bile-fistula rabbit. Yonaga Acta Med. 1960;4:179–86.
68. Ogura M, Yamasaki K. The fate of C14-labelled dehydrocholic acid in the guinea pig. J Biochem (Tokyo). 1961;49:649–59.
69. Hoffman NE, Sewell RB, Smallwood RA. Bile acid structure and biliary lipid secretion II: a comparison of three hydroxy and two keto bile acids. Am J Physiol. 1978;234:G637–41.
70. Bloomer JR, Boyer JL, Klatskin G. Inhibition of bilirubin excretion in man during dehydrocholate choleresis. Gastroenterology. 1973;65:929–35.
71. Kapitulnik J, Ostrow JD. Stimulation of bilirubin catabolism in jaundiced Gunn rats by an inducer of microsomal mixed-function monooxygenases. Proc Natl Acad Sci (USA). 1977;75:682–5.
72. Schmid R, Hammaker L. Metabolism and disposition of C14-bilirubin in congenital nonhemolytic jaundice. J Clin Invest. 1963;42:1720–34.
73. Kapoor CL, Krishna Murti CR, Bajpai P. Uptake and release of bilirubin by skin. Biochem J. 1973;136:35–43.

Section III
Bile Acids and Lipoproteins

9
Plasma lipoprotein metabolism

A. D. COOPER

INTRODUCTION

An overview of lipoprotein metabolism is presented in Fig. 1. Endogenous and exogenous pathways are generally held to be separate, but in fact are quite similar and are interactive. The state of the enterohepatic circulation of bile salts and cholesterol plays a major role in determining the rate of flux through their pathways. The apoproteins play a major role in directing lipoprotein metabolism. Accordingly, each major apoprotein will be described, followed by discussion of the metabolism of each class of lipoproteins.

THE LIPOPROTEIN CLASSES

Since lipids are relatively insoluble in water, a carrier system must exist to transport them from sites of synthesis or absorption through the circulation to sites of their utilization. The first evidence of such a transport system was described in 1929[1] and the existence of discrete lipid–protein complexes was subsequently demonstrated[2]. The initial descriptions of lipoprotein subclasses made in the 1950s and 1960s were based on chemical precipitation procedures and electrophoretic mobilities. These studies were extended using ultracentrifugation techniques, resulting in the delineation of four lipoprotein classes based on their buoyant densities[3] (Table 1). *Chylomicrons* are triglyceride-rich lipoproteins synthesized by the intestine. *Very low-density lipoproteins* or VLDL are triglyceride-rich lipoproteins synthesized by the intestine, and have pre-beta mobility on electrophoresis. *Low-density lipoproteins* or LDL are the major carriers of cholesterol in serum, and on electrophoresis have beta mobility. They are produced largely by the catabolism of VLDL. *High-density lipoproteins* or HDL are derived from several different tissue sources including the liver and intestine, as well as other lipoproteins. On electrophoresis they have primarily alpha mobility.

One of the major determinants of the physical properties of a lipoprotein is its protein and lipid composition. The more triglyceride a lipoprotein contains, the larger and more buoyant it is. Chylomicrons are exceedingly rich in triglyceride

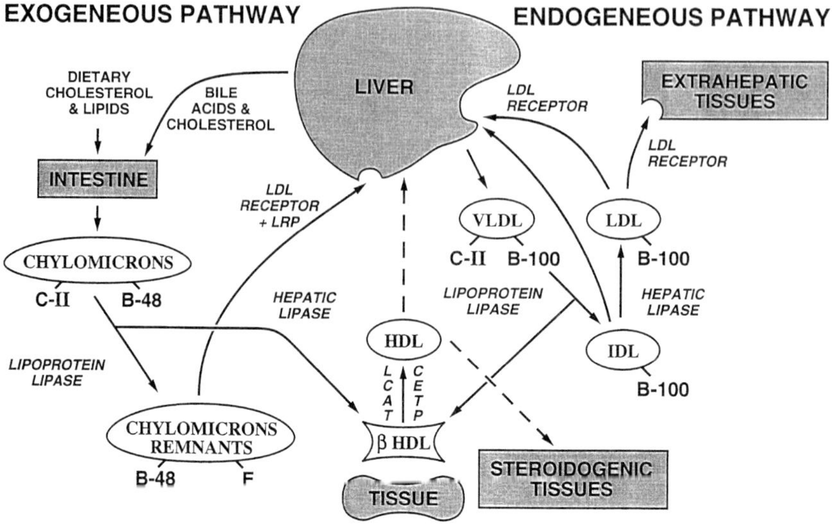

Fig. 1 An overview of lipoprotein metabolism. The process is divided into endogenous and exogenous pathways. These proceed by generally similar mechanisms, with triglyceride-rich lipoproteins formed by intestine and liver. Large chylomicrons and very low-density lipoprotein (VLDL) are depleted of triglycerides and form remnants and high-density lipoproteins (HDL) under the influence of the enzyme lipoprotein lipase. Chylomicron remnants are removed rapidly and specifically by the liver, while VLDL remnants can become low-density lipoproteins (LDL) and deliver cholesterol to peripheral tissues by interaction with LDL receptors. Remnants are removed by the hepatic LDL receptor as well as by the LDL receptor-like protein (LRP). Together liver-derived hepatic lipase, lecithin cholesterol acyl transferase (LCAT) and cholesterol ester transfer protein (CETP) facilitate the transport of cholesterol from peripheral tissues to the liver via HDL. Apoproteins, B_{100}, B_{48}, C_{II} and E are referred to as B-100, B-48, C-II and E, respectively. From Cooper A. D. In: Zakim D., Boyer T., editors. Hepatology: a textbook of liver disease, 2nd edn, vol. 1. Philadelphia: WB Saunders; 1989:96–123

Table 1 Characteristics of the lipoprotein classes

	Chylomicrons	*VLDL*	*LDL*	*HDL*
Density (g/ml)	<0.95	0.95–1.006	1.006	1.063
SF°[a]	>400	20–400	0–20	—
Size (Å)	750–3000	300–700	180–300	50–120
Composition (%)				
Triglyceride	80–95	45–65	4–8	2–7
Cholesterol, free	1–3	4–8	6–8	3–5
Cholesterol, ester	2–4	16–22	45–50	15–20
Phospholipid	3–6	15–20	18–24	26–32
Protein	1–2	6–10	18–22	45–35
Apoproteins				
Major	B, C[b], A[b]	B, C, E	B	A
Minor	E[b]	A		C, E

a SF° = corrected flotation at $d = 1.063$, expressed as Svedberg units = 10^{-3}cm/(s dyne^{-1} g^{-1})
b Chylomicron composition changes with duration of exposure to serums. Initially chylomicrons contain apoproteins B and A. With time they lose A and acquire C and E.
From: Cooper A.D In: Zakim D, Boyer T, editors. Hepatology: a textbook of liver disease, 2nd edn, vol. 1. Philadelphia: WB Saunders; 1989:96–123.

and are thus the largest lipoproteins. They contain variable amounts of cholesteryl ester and relatively small amounts of protein, phospholipid, and unesterified cholesterol. At the other end of the spectrum, HDL, the smallest class of lipoproteins, contain virtually no triglyceride and are relatively richer in protein, cholesterol and phospholipid than are other types of lipoproteins.

The protein constituents of the lipoproteins are referred to as apolipoproteins or apoproteins. A particular lipoprotein class may contain several different apoproteins, and certain apoproteins are found in more than one lipoprotein class (Table 1). Five major families of apoproteins have been described and are named A, (a) or apoprotein little a, B, C, and E. At least four of these contain several different proteins, designated A-I, A-II, A-IV; B-48, B-100; C-I, C-II, C-III; E2, E-3 and E-4. Several apoproteins of lower abundance have also been described. The amount of a particular apoprotein in a lipoprotein class is variable, and often changes as the lipoproteins circulate in plasma.

THE APOPROTEINS

Individual apoproteins play a critical role in determining the structure and metabolism of the lipoprotein particle. The amino acid sequences of the apoproteins were either derived by direct protein sequencing of the purified proteins or deduced from the cDNAs. The primary structure of the exchangeable apoproteins, apo A-I, A-II, AIV, C-I, C-II, C-III, and E, revealed that these proteins are characterized by the presence of amphipathic helixes[4]. In this formulation the polar and non-polar amino acids reside on opposite sides of the helix. Most important in terms of lipid metabolism is the 'Type A' helix in which there is a clustering of positive charged amino acids at the polar–non-polar interfaces and negative amino acid residues located at the centre of the polar face[4]. Lipid affinity resides in this motif, and thus may be responsible for ordering the apoprotein on the lipoprotein surface (see below). A brief description of each apoprotein is given below; see ref. 4 for a more comprehensive review of the apoprotein structure and function.

Apoprotein A-I is a 28 kDa protein that is the most abundant protein of the HDL subclasses. It is synthesized by liver and intestine and is secreted into the blood as a constituent of newly formed HDL and chylomicrons[5,6]. The same is true for the 17 kDa apoprotein A-II; in this case, however, the liver is the main site of synthesis. In humans, but not in other non-human primates, apo A-II consists of two identical chains of M_r = 8707 linked together by a Cys 6–Cys 6 disulphide bridge[7]. Human apo A-I and apo A-II are synthesized as preproproteins containing 18 or 17 amino acid prepeptides, respectively, and six amino acid propeptides[5,6]. Cleavage of the pre-segment occurs within the cell for both A-I and A-II. Proteolytic cleavage of the apo A-I hexapeptide prosegment occurs in the serum[8], while most of the apo A-II pro-segment is cleaved within the cell. Apoproteins A-I and A-II bind phospholipids avidly. In the presence of phospholipids they form complexes that have many of the characteristics of HDL.

Recent evidence from studies in mice transgenic for human apo A-I, apo A-II or both[9–11] and humans with apo A-I and apo A-II gene mutations[12] and gene targeting in apo A-I 'knock-out' mice[13] demonstrated that expression of apo A-I is a major contributing factor in determining HDL cholesterol levels, the distribution of HDL subclasses, and conferring resistance to diet-induced atherosclerosis. Apoprotein A-II, on the other hand, appears to play a more limited structural role in HDL formation and may, in fact be pro-atherogenic. This notion is supported by the recent observation that transgenic mice over-expressing mouse apo A-II have increased HDL cholesterol levels and increased atherosclerotic lesion development[11]. The role that apo A-II plays in HDL metabolism is thus not entirely clear. Apoprotein A-I is also a co-factor for the enzyme that is responsible for the esterification of serum cholesterol, namely, lecithin : cholesterol acyltransferase (LCAT).

Apoprotein A-IV is a 46 kDa protein synthesized in the intestine. The apoprotein A-IV gene is localized on chromosome 11q23 in humans in a multigene cluster with the apoprotein A-I and C-III genes, suggesting a common evolutionary origin[14]. Like the other apo A's, it is synthesized as a larger precursor prepeptide that undergoes proteolytic cleavage prior to secretion[15]. However, it does not contain a prepeptide and does not undergo a second proteolytic cleavage. Several electrophoretic variants of apo-IV have been described, and the molecular bases for these variants have been determined[16]. The distribution of apo A-IV in serum is not established and, depending on the fractionation method used, it may exist free or totally associated with lipoproteins. Apo A-IV in humans can, however, be found as a component of both chylomicrons and HDL[6]. Although it is a relatively abundant protein in human serum its physiological function is unknown. Recent studies have linked apo A-IV to hydrolysis of triglyceride-rich lipoproteins, the interconversion of HDL subclasses, and it may participate in reverse cholesterol transport (see below). The increased concentration of serum apo A-IV after a fat meal, interestingly, might act as a satiation signal[17].

Apoprotein (a) is a glycoprotein component of a lipoprotein called Lp(a) that resembles normal human LDL in lipid composition and content of apoprotein B-100. Lp(a) differs from normal LDL, however, by the presence of apoprotein (a), a polypeptide chain that varies in size from 300 to 800 kDa[18,19]. Apoprotein (a) is disulphide bonded to apoprotein B-100 in the LDL particle. The highly polymorphic apoprotein (a) gene resides on the long arm of chromosome 6 in humans in the vicinity of the plasminogen gene. Studies of apoprotein (a) cDNA clones demonstrated that apoprotein (a) is structurally similar to plasminogen. It has the same protease region and similar 'kringle 4' and 'kringle 5' domains; however, in apoprotein (a), the kringle 4 domain occurs in multiple tandem copies whose number is inversely related to the plasma levels of Lp(a). The liver appears to be a major, if not the sole, site of apoprotein (a) synthesis. Apoprotein (a) is synthesized as a lower molecular weight precursor in hepatocytes and is glycosylated within the Golgi compartment to a mature form of higher apparent molecular weight. The major site of covalent linkage to apoprotein B-100 is not known; however, recent work in mice transgenic for human apoprotein (a) suggests that at least a portion of this may occur within the plasma compartment[20]. The plasma concentration of Lp(a) varies widely between individuals in spite of rather limited intra-individual variation[21]. The level of Lp(a) in the blood is an independent risk factor for the risk of cardiovascular disease; however, the precise mechanism for this is not clear. It may involve stimulation of smooth muscle cell proliferation[22], interference of plasmin generation and clot lysis, oxidation and modification of the Lp(a) particle and uptake by macrophages and accumulation in the arterial intima[18,19].

Apoprotein B is the principal protein of LDL and is the integral protein of the triglyceride-rich lipoproteins VLDL and chylomicrons[23]. Because of its large size (about 512 kDa) and insolubility, it has been difficult to study. Using molecular cloning procedures its amino acid sequence has been derived[24,25]. There are two different but related B apoproteins. In humans, apo B-48 (241 kDa) is synthesized and secreted by the small intestine and the other, apo B-100 (512 kDa), is made in the liver[26]. The entire sequence of the intestine form is contained within hepatic apo B-100, but lacks the carboxy terminal region that mediates binding to the LDL receptor. There is one gene for apo B. The message is edited post-transcriptionally in intestinal enterocytes by a specific cytidine deaminase that converts codon 2153 (CAA, glutamine) to a stop translation codon (UAA) by a process known as mRNA editing[27]. This editing process for the apoprotein B gene is under tisue-specific, developmental, hormonal, and nutritional control[28]. The amount of apoprotein B per lipoprotein particle is the same regardless of the particle size. This is true both within a single class, such as VLDL, and between lipoprotein classes. Synthesis of apoprotein B appears to be necessary for the release of triglyceride-rich lipoprotein particles from both the intestine and liver. This apoprotein, moreover, is one of the ligands recognized by the LDL receptor[29].

The C apoproteins are low molecular weight proteins found in HDL, VLDL and chylomicrons. There are three distinct proteins in humans: CI (5.8 kDa), CII (9.1 kDa) and CIII (8.75 kDa). All three C apoproteins are synthesized in the liver. The C apoproteins are important in the metabolism of triglyceride-rich lipoproteins. Apoprotein CII is an activator of lipoprotein lipase, the enzyme responsible for hydrolysing the triglyceride of lipoproteins. The congenital absence of this protein results in profound hypertriglyceridaemia[30]. Apo CIII plasma levels are often elevated in hypertriglyceridaemic individuals, and over-expression of CIII in transgenic mice results in hypertriglyceridaemia[31,32]. This may be due to delayed clearance of triglyceride-rich lipoproteins by the liver[33]. Deficiency of apoprotein AI and CIII occurs owing to a major rearrangement of the apoprotein AI gene. Absence of these apoproteins results in low levels of HDL, and premature atherosclerosis.

Apoprotein E was also called the arginine-rich protein because arginine comprises about 10% of its amino acids. It has a molecular weight of about 33 000 and is polymorphic when studied by isoelectric focusing. This is due to differences in glycosylation and to variation in amino acid sequence. As noted below, apoprotein E is a ligand for the LDL receptor. Interestingly, it has been mapped to the same chromosome on which the LDL receptor resides. There are three common alleles for the apoprotein E gene, apo E2, E3, and E4[34]. The gene products differ by one charge unit each. E4 is the most acidic and E2 is the most basic. E4 differs from E3 because of a substitution of arginine for cysteine at residue 112; E2 differs from E3 by the substitution of cysteine for arginine at residue 158. Apoprotein E is present in most mammalian species and can be found in all the lipoprotein fractions except human LDL[35]. It is produced by the liver, and the rate of its production is related to the rate of secretion of cholesteryl ester. It is the protein responsible for determining whether a lipoprotein will be removed by the liver[35,36] or bind to its membranes[37]. This conclusion is strongly supported by the changes in lipoprotein metabolism observed in mice transgenic for human apoprotein E[38,39] and in apoprotein E 'knock-out' mice[40]. Overproduction of human apoprotein E in transgenic mice reduced the plasma levels of cholesterol, triglyceride, and apoprotein B in VLDL and LDL. These animals were also resistant to dietary-induced hyperlipoproteinaemia. In contrast, the apoprotein E-deficient mice had elevated levels of VLDL and IDL and developed marked hyperlipoproteinaemia and atherosclerosis[40]. These studies unequivocally demonstrate that apoprotein E is a major regulator of lipoprotein clearance from the circulation. Although most apoprotein E comes from liver, it is also synthesized by a number of extrahepatic tissues including macrophages and glial cells of the nervous system[41,42]. In this regard, it may play a role in diseases of the central nervous system, since apoprotein E binds with high affinity to the β-amyloid protein of senile plaque and the apoprotein E type 4 allele is linked genetically to late onset Alzheimer's disease[43,44].

CHYLOMICRON METABOLISM

Chylomicrons are formed in intestinal epithelial cells and are secreted into the mesenteric lymph, from which they ultimately reach the systemic circulation (Fig. 2). Their precise size and composition depend on the lipid constituents of

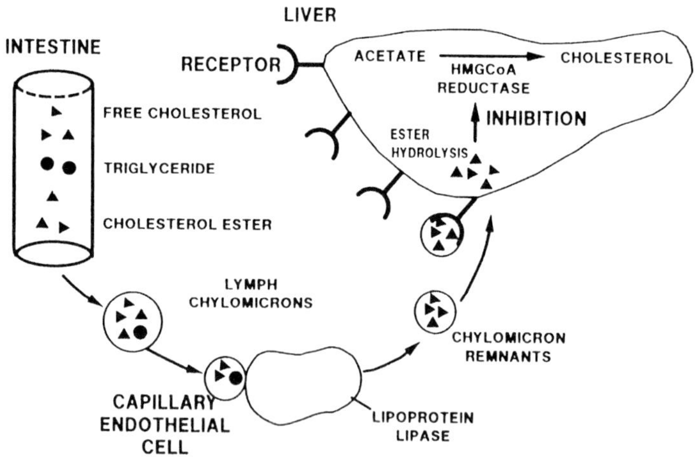

Fig. 2 An outline of chylomicron metabolism. After chylomicrons are formed in the intestine from dietary lipids, they are secreted into the lymph. They then reach the general circulation and attach to the capillary endothelium, where the enzyme lipoprotein lipase catalyzes the hydrolysis of triglycerides. A new particle called a chylomicron remnant is eventually produced. This particle is then removed by the liver and catabolized, with several metabolic effects on hepatic lipid homeostasis. From: Cooper A. D. In: Zakim D., Boyer T., editors. Hepatology: a textbook of liver disease, 2nd edn, vol. 1. Philadelphia: WB Saunders; 1989: 96–123

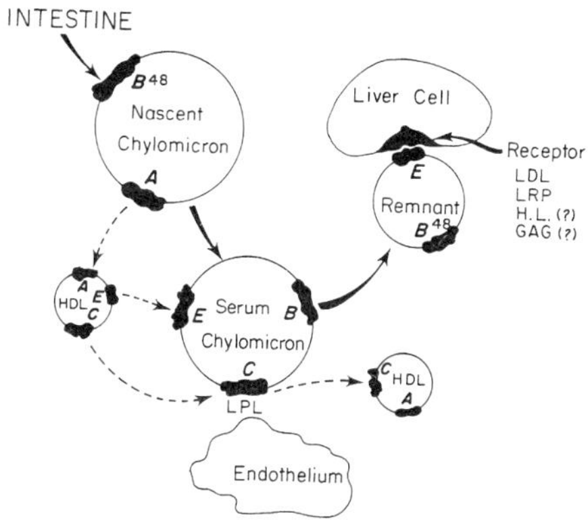

Fig. 3 Apoprotein transfers during chylomicron metabolism. When formed, chylomicrons contain primarily B and A apoproteins. As the result of contact with high-density lipoproteins (HDL), they lose the A apoproteins and gain C and E apoproteins. During the process of hydrolysis the C apoproteins are lost. The remnant contains primarily B and E apoproteins. Proposed receptors include the LDL receptor, the LDL receptor-related protein (LRP), hepatic lipase (HL), and glycosaminoglycans (GAG). From: Cooper A. D. In: Zakim D., Boyer T., editors. Hepatology: a textbook of liver disease, 2nd edn, vol. 1. Philadelphia: WB Saunders; 1989: 96–123

the diet. Their cores are always extremely rich in triglyceride and contain varying amounts of esterified cholesterol. When initially synthesized, these particles contain apoproteins B-48, AI, AII, and AIV[5,6]. Before reaching the systemic circulation, however, chylomicrons undergo significant alterations in their composition. The amount of apoprotein A decreases substantially, and apoproteins E and C are acquired. These changes are thought to occur as the result of interaction between chylomicrons and HDL that have filtered through the intestinal capillaries into the lymph (Fig. 3)

Normally, chylomicrons have a very short residence in the circulation. Their time in the circulation is likely to be less than 30 min under most circumstances. They bind to the endothelial cells that line the surfaces of a number of tissues, including adipose tissue, mammary gland, and smooth and striated muscle. While bound, they are substrates for the enzyme lipoprotein lipase[45]. This enzyme hydrolyses most of the triglyceride in the core region of the chylomicron. The resultant fatty acids enter nearby cells by diffusion and are immediately metabolized or converted to triglycerides and stored[46].

Concomitant with the removal of core lipid from the chylomicron, other major changes in lipoprotein structure take place. The depletion of the core of the particle creates an excess of surface material. Phospholipid, free cholesterol, and apoproteins separate from the particle surface in some unknown way to form new lipoproteins that have the characteristics of HDL[47,48]. This may constitute a major pathway for HDL formation. Since apoprotein CII is an activator of LPL, its transfer out of the chylomicron particle causes the lipolytic reaction to slow and ultimately stop. The altered chylomicron separates from the endothelium and re-enters the circulation. It is now referred to as a chylomicron remnant[49]. Remnants are smaller than their chylomicron precursors, are markedly depleted of triglyceride and C apoproteins, and are at least relatively enriched in esterified cholesterol. They retain apoprotein B-48 and E of the precursor chylomicron[50].

A number of investigators have shown that the isolated liver can take up remnant particles avidly under circumstances in which chylomicrons are not removed from the liver's perfusate. Further work indicated that the particles are removed as a unit by a process that is saturable and specific, and has a high affinity[51,52]. Once removed, the particles are metabolized and have physiological effects on the liver consistent with their composition[52].

The cell responsible for remnant removal appears to be the hepatocyte[53]. Although Kupffer cells can also remove these particles with a high affinity, because of their small number, they make a small overall contribution. Remnant removal is dependent on apoprotein E[36,54], independent of apoprotein B[55], and inhibited by the C-apoprotein[35,41]. The LDL receptor can recognize chylomicron remnants[56] and plays an important role in their removal from the circulation[57,58]. Moreover, the rate of remnant removal can be altered by physiological manipulations that change the number of LDL receptors expressed in the liver[59]. However, patients and animals lacking LDL receptors remove remnants relatively normally, suggesting that there is also a separate, non-LDL receptor-dependent mechanism for removal of remnants[60].

Recent information suggests that a candidate for this remnant removal pathway is another member of the LDL receptor gene family, the LDL receptor-related protein or LRP[61]. This protein, whose cDNA was cloned by homology with the complement repeat region of the LDL receptor sequence, is much larger than the LDL receptor and shares many of the same domains. Although LRP is present on a variety of cells and tissues, its function in the body is expressed primarily in the liver. This protein can initiate the uptake of cholesterol from apoprotein E-rich lipoproteins in cells lacking the LDL receptor, providing they are supplemented with apoprotein E or lipoprotein lipase (LpL)[62–65]. The LRP undergoes endocytosis and is identical to the receptor that mediates the removal of activated α_2-macroglobulin–protease complexes from the blood[66,67]. It also binds vitellogenin, *Pseudomonas* exotoxin A, lactoferrin, and fibrinolytic–anti-fibrinolytic complexes[68,69]. It also appears to be the interspecies homologue of gp330, the protein responsible for the induction of the rat autoimmune disease Heymann nephritis[70,71]. LRP co-purifies with a 39 kDa protein called receptor-associated protein (RAP) that may control the availability of the receptor sites for the various ligands[70,72,73]. The RAP has been identified as the interspecies homologue of heparin-binding protein 44. Recent evidence suggests that the LRP-mediated clearance of remnant lipoproteins may involve a complex formed between cell surface proteoglycans and lipoprotein lipase bound to the lipoproteins[63–65]. These are summarized in Fig. 4.

Recent studies from our laboratory[57,58,74] estimate that the LDL receptor and the LRP are required for remnant removal. In the normal mouse (Fig. 5) a minimum of 50% is removed by the LDL receptor and 10% by the LRP. The distribution of the remaining 40% between these receptors is not yet resolved.

Because of the high affinity and large capacity of the remnant removal system, it is likely that under normal circumstances the concentration of remnants in the blood of the rat is low. Whether this is true in other species is

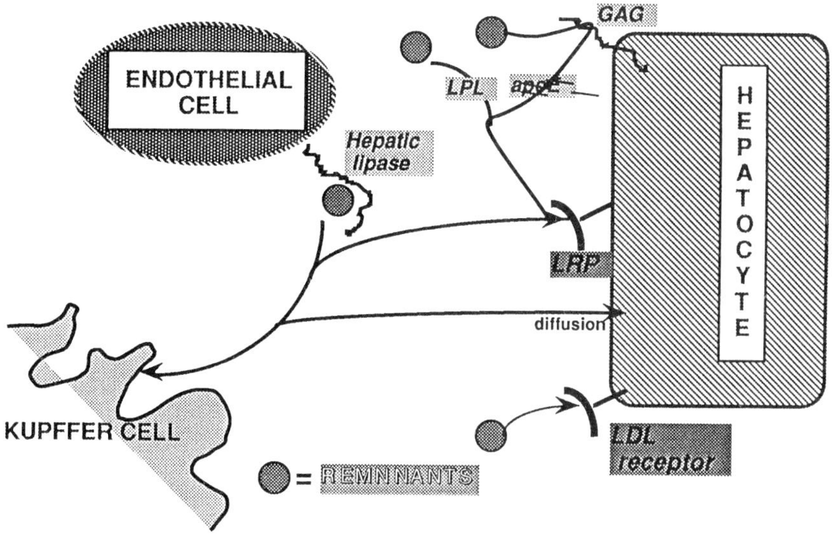

Fig. 4 Possible mechanisms of uptake of chylomicron remnants by the liver. There are several mechanisms by which chylomicron remnants have been shown to enter the liver. First, remnants are good substrates for the LDL receptor. Second, remnants can bind to the LDL receptor-like protein (LRP), especially in the presence of additional apo E. It has also been proposed that glycosamino-glycans may serve as an anchoring site for remnants before they are removed by the LRP. Similar proposals have been made for hepatic lipase. In addition, in the absence of both receptors it is conceivable that remnants are completely metabolized on the surface of endothelial cells and their lipids enter the cell

unknown. It has been established that type III hyperlipoproteinaemia in humans represents a remnant removal disorder brought about by the presence of an abnormal apoprotein E.

Following its removal by liver, the remnant is degraded. Studies with inhibitors of lysosomal function suggest that the lysosome is the site of this process[75]. The degradation process appears to involve the catabolism of each of the constituents of the remnants. The cholesteryl esters are hydrolysed to free cholesterol and fatty acids, the triglycerides to free fatty acids and glycerol, and the apoproteins to small peptides and amino acids. Once released from the remnant, these constituents have their expected metabolic effects. The free cholesterol suppresses cholesterol synthesis[52], and the fatty acids cause the stimulation of VLDL secretion[76]. Little is known about the regulation of the degradation process, nor have acquired defects in this process been found. In congenital lysosomal dysfunction, however, there is massive lipid accumulation in liver[77].

Because chylomicron formation requires HDL constituents such as apoproteins C and E, and remnant formation results in HDL formation, there is likely to be an important relationship between dietary composition and HDL metabolism. This relationship, which is not yet completely understood, may be important in a number of disease processes, including alcohol-induced hyperlipidaemia and atherosclerosis.

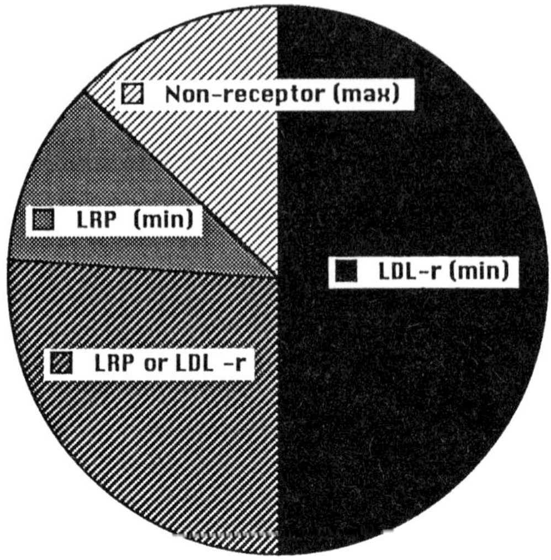

Fig. 5 Estimates of the amount of remnant uptake by various mechanisms. Based on studies discussed in the text, our laboratory has concluded that, in the normal mouse, a minimum of 50% of remnant uptake is by the LDL receptor (LDLR). A minimum of 10% is by the LDL receptor-like protein (LRP). A maximum of 20% of remnant uptake is non-receptor-mediated. This would include the plasma space unless there is an overestimate. The remaining uptake may be the LDL receptor or the LRP

VERY LOW-DENSITY LIPOPROTEIN METABOLISM

Very low-density lipoproteins appear to be metabolized by a pathway generally similar to that for chylomicrons, but with several important differences. As defined by density and size, VLDL are formed both by liver and intestine[78,79], but it is not yet known whether the VLDL of intestinal origin and the VLDL of hepatic origin are identical in composition or in metabolism. It is likely that there are significant differences between them.

The principal lipoprotein secreted by the liver is VLDL. The early work of Steinberg and co-workers[80], and Marsh[81], using liver slices and perfused livers, demonstrated that radiolabelled amino acids were incorporated into plasma lipoprotein-like products, and that the liver secreted particles that were immunologically similar to plasma lipoproteins. Initially, investigators focused their attention on the secretion of LDL, because these are quantitatively the principal lipoproteins in human serum. When rat livers were perfused, using techniques that minimize changes in lipoprotein composition after secretion[81], most of the lipid and apoprotein isolated, however, had a density of less than 1.006; that is, it was VLDL. Any material that was isolated in the LDL density range had a lipid composition intermediate between that of serum VLDL and LDL. In other species also, substantial evidence suggests that VLDL, not LDL, is the most abundant lipoprotein product secreted by the liver.

The intracellular formation and secretion of the VLDL have been examined in detail by electron microscopy. The synthesis of apoproteins begins in the rough endoplasmic recticulum. However, lipoprotein particles are not seen in this region of the endoplasmic reticulum. Lipid-containing particles are present throughout the smooth endoplasmic reticulum where triglyceride synthesis occurs. It has been proposed that assembly of the lipoprotein particle occurs at the junction of the smooth and rough endoplasmic reticulum, and that the lipid and protein constituents flow separately to this region[82]. The precise steps in the assembly are still not understood. One perplexing problem is that the enzymes of triglyceride and phospholipid synthesis are located on the outer, cytosolic side of the endoplasmic reticulum, whereas the lipoprotein particle is formed on the inner side of the organelle[83]. Accordingly, the lipids must cross the membrane before they can be incorporated into the particle. This process may be facilitated by a microsomal triglyceride transfer protein that has been suggested to be required for triglyceride-rich lipoprotein secretion[84]. Absence of this protein results in the disease abetalipoproteinaemia[85].

The newly formed VLDL particles appear to move through specialized tubules, ultimately reaching the area of the Golgi apparatus. Clusters of particles are seen in the Golgi region, where it is likely that the apoproteins are glycosylated. The clustering of particles in this region represents the first step in the formation of secretory vesicles. These vesicles bud off the Golgi apparatus, and the secretory vesicles migrate to the plasma membrane. The newly formed VLDL is then discharged into Disse's space by reverse endocytosis, which involves fusion of the vesicle membrane with the plasma membrane.

Protein synthesis is required for lipoprotein formation. Inhibitors of protein synthesis almost invariably cause a decrease in VLDL secretion. Compounds acting by this mechanism include not only classic inhibitors of protein synthesis such as cycloheximide and puromycin, but also agents such as orotic acid and the tetracyclines. Since these agents do not affect triglyceride formation, triglycerides accumulate in the liver. The lipid that accumulates under these conditions takes the form of lipid droplets located outside the endoplasmic reticulum–Golgi complex. Histologically, the pattern induced by these agents is indistinguishable from the nutritional or alcoholic fatty liver. This leads to the speculation that an imbalance between triglyceride accumulation and apoprotein synthesis is a general mechanism for the development of fatty liver[86].

The details of how apoprotein synthesis and triglyceride synthesis are coordinated is slowly becoming established[87]. The major advance in this area was the cloning and sequencing of the apoprotein B gene and the determination of its amino acid sequence. This information has been used by a number of workers to delineate the protein sequences important for lipid binding and lipoprotein assembly in liver cells. This information has recently been reviewed[88]. The transport of apoprotein B across the endoplasmic reticulum membrane is believed to proceed by a mechanism similar to that of other secretory proteins. Translocation of apoprotein B across the membrane may be controlled by a 33 amino acid 'pause–transfer' sequence which causes the newly synthesized B protein to pause in the membrane allowing for lipid binding and post-translational modification of the protein[89]. Pause–transfer sequences would allow the proper folding of apoprotein B around a requisite amount of lipid during translocation. In this way lipids may integrate into the growing lipoprotein particle without apoprotein B integrating into endoplasmic reticulum membrane[87]. Transfer of neutral lipids from the cytoplasm to apoprotein B, probably facilitated by the microsomal triglyceride transfer protein, results in growth of a neutral lipid core. The rate-limiting step appears to be assembly of these apoprotein B/lipid complexes in the endoplasmic reticulum membrane. Once enough core components are assembled the lipoprotein can be released into the endoplasmic reticulum lumen.

The composition of the VLDL particle, when isolated from the Golgi apparatus or immediately following secretion, differs from the composition of plasma VLDL. Especially in humans the nascent particles are relatively poor in cholesteryl esters. In addition, nascent VLDL contains more apoprotein E and less C apoproteins than does VLDL in serum. Newly synthesized lipoproteins thus may serve as a source of apoprotein E for HDL and, ultimately, chylomicrons. They are also an important acceptor for the cholesteryl ester generated by the combined action of LCAT and the CETP on HDL.

Through standard molecular manipulation of the gene and transfection of liver cells with plamids containing the mutated apoprotein B cDNAs, carboxyterminal deletions of apoprotein B-100 were prepared. These revealed that a linear relationship exists between the size of the apoprotein B fragment produced in the cell and the radii of the lipoproteins on which it resides. About 1 kDa of protein corresponds to about 1.1 Å of core circumference[90,91]. These data predict a model in which the apoprotein B-100 forms a 'belt' around a growing triglyceride nucleus within the bilayer of the endoplasmic reticulum membrane. Apoprotein B would then direct the droplet to bulge into the lumen where it pinches off to form a lipoprotein particle. By this mechanism large apoprotein B peptides direct the synthesis of large lipoproteins, whereas short peptides direct the synthesis of small lipoproteins. Carboxyterminal deletion of 75% of apoprotein B, however, abolishes the ability of the protein to form buoyant lipoproteins. These data are consistent with observations of humans with genetic disorder familial hypobetalipoproteinaemia, in which a variety of small apoprotein B peptides are found in the serum in a variety of lipoprotein density classes[92].

It is not yet known how apoprotein and triglyceride synthesis are coordinated. In cultured hepatocytes and hepatoma cells only a small portion of the apoprotein B-100 synthesized in the liver cell is actually secreted; the majority is degraded within the endoplasmic reticulum[93]. Many factors affecting VLDL output by the liver have been identified (see ref. 94 for review). Hepatic VLDL secretion is increased in experimental animals by conditions that promote lipogenesis, such as sucrose feeding and glucocorticoid treatment. Conversely, conditions that depress lipogenesis, such as starvation and glucagon treatment, decrease VLDL secretion. One of the factors that most clearly regulates VLDL secretion is the amount of free fatty acid reaching the liver[95]. Fatty acid flux across the liver increases the apoprotein B-100 synthesized that is actually secreted in the media. This occurs in the absence of changes in the level of apoprotein B-100 mRNA, or in its rate of translation. Fatty acids apparently shift newly synthesized apoprotein B-100 from a degradatory to the secretory pool in the endoplasmic reticulum[96]. As the amount of free fatty acid entering the liver increases, there is a concomitant increase in the rate of secretion of VLDL. The relationship between free fatty acid input and VLDL output is not linear, but

VLDL production is saturable. Free fatty acids increase the number of VLDL particles secreted, as well as increasing the size of each particle.

Cholesterol is necessary for VLDL secretion, and inhibitors of cholesterol synthesis reduced hepatic VLDL secretion from rat liver[97]. In cell culture studies these agents appear to have either no effects or to stimulate apoprotein B-100 secretion[87]. The lipid content of lipoproteins entering the liver cell also appears to regulate both apoprotein B-100 secretion and the lipid content of the secreted lipoproteins[98,99]. In these studies, when triglyceride was the major lipid entering the cell (chylomicron remnants), they were also the major lipid component of the particles leaving the cell. When cholesterol was the major lipid entering the cell (cholesterol-rich βVLDL) secretion of an apoprotein B-100 particle with a higher cholesterol content was observed.

Phospholipid availability is also required for VLDL secretion[100]. The secreted phospholipids appear to be newly synthesized, and are present in the endoplasmic reticulum in amounts that are probably not rate-limiting for secretion[101]. It is thus unlikely that phospholipid availability regulates VLDL secretion in the normal state.

Hormones also alter synthesis of apoproteins and lipoproteins. Oestrogens cause a marked increase in secretion of VLDL[86]. Both *in vitro* and *in vivo*, livers from females produce significantly more VLDL than do livers from males. The basis for the oestrogen effect remains controversial, but it is physiologically important. Thyroid status affects hepatic secretion of lipoprotein. Secretion of triglyceride by livers from hyperthyroid animals is decreased, whereas an increased rate of triglyceride secretion is found in hypothyroid animals.

Diet is another determinant of the rate of VLDL production and composition. A high-carbohydrate diet increases VLDL production substantially, and can cause profound hyperlipaemia in susceptible individuals[102]. High-carbohydrate diets increase the synthesis and secretion of triglyceride in humans, but apoprotein B-100 production is generally unchanged. Carbohydrate feeding appears to alter the composition of the particles produced, so that they are larger and triglyceride-enriched. Consumption of a cholesterol-rich diet results in the synthesis and secretion of markedly altered VLDL; cholesteryl esters are substituted for triglyceride in the cores of the particles, and there is a marked enrichment in the amount of apoprotein E secreted[103]. These varied observations demonstrate that secretion of VLDL by the liver is a complex process that is susceptible to regulation by a large number of factors.

Once in the serum the VLDL bind to the lipoprotein lipase 'site' in much the same manner as do chylomicrons. The affinities of the two lipoprotein classes for the site differ, since it has been shown that the affinity of the enzyme is proportional to the triglyceride content of the lipoprotein. The existence of a single common site explains how change in the amount of VLDL can affect chylomicron metabolism and vice-versa[104].

As with chylomicrons (Fig. 6), a VLDL remnant is formed following the action of lipoprotein lipase on the VLDL particle. This remnant contains less triglyceride than did the parent VLDL, and has lost its C apoproteins. VLDL remnants have a greater buoyant density than do VLDL (to 1.019 rather than 1.006)[105]. Serum lipoprotein particles isolated at densities between 1.006 and 1.019 g/ml are often referred to as intermediate density lipoproteins (IDL), and it

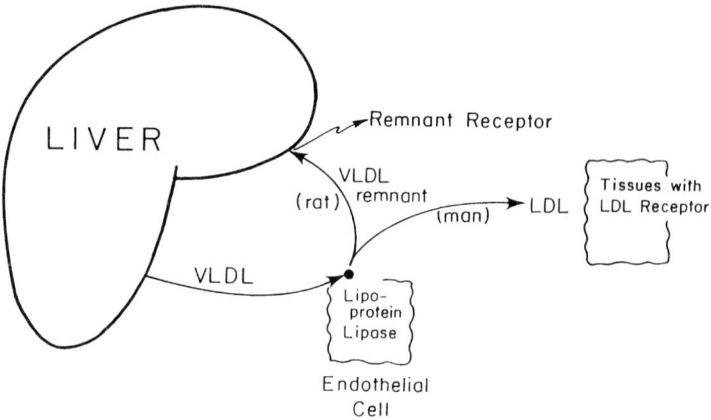

Fig. 6 Very low-density lipoprotein (VLDL) metabolism proceeds along two pathways. One, similar to the chylomicron remnant pathway, leads to the return of partially metabolized VLDL particles to the liver. This is the predominant pathway in the rat. The other pathway involves more extensive hydrolysis of the triglycerides, resulting ultimately in the formation of low-density lipoproteins (LDL). This is the predominant pathway in humans

is generally believed that they are VLDL remnants. VLDL remnants have a dual fate: they may be removed by the liver, much as chylomicron remnants are, or they may undergo further lipolysis to form LDL in a reaction possibly catalysed by hepatic lipase. This enzyme does not require apoprotein CII as a cofactor. The quantitative distribution of VLDL remnants between these pathways varies among species. In the rat virtually all of the VLDL remnants are removed by the liver. In humans, on the other hand, the majority are converted to LDL[106]. In normal humans the bulk of the circulating LDL is created in this manner[107]. The reason for the species differences in the metabolism of VLDL is not yet fully understood, but such differences have a profound effect on the concentration of circulating lipoprotein classes, and perhaps on species susceptibilities to atherosclerosis.

Remnants prepared from freshly isolated hepatic VLDL have been found to compete with chylomicron remnants for hepatic removal, implying that they share a common transport mechanism, at least in part[108]. In contrast, it has been reported that remnants prepared from serum VLDL behave differently from chylomicron remnants, and are removed by the liver in a manner strictly analogous to LDL[109]. This removal is defective in LDL receptor-defective rabbits.

A unique receptor for VLDL has recently been isolated that binds VLDL, VLDL remnants, and IDL, but not LDL[110]. The mRNA for this receptor is abundant in heart, adipose tissue, and muscle, but not in liver, suggesting that it may play a role in fatty acid metabolism but not in lipoprotein clearance by the liver. Thus, it appears that a portion of VLDL is converted to LDL, another portion becomes IDL, and behaves like LDL in terms of hepatic removal, while a third portion may behave like chylomicrons and spend only a brief time in the circulation.

LOW-DENSITY LIPOPROTEIN METABOLISM

The metabolism of LDL has received a great deal of attention because of the well-established association of the serum level of this lipoprotein class with atherosclerosis. Under normal circumstances in humans all LDLs are derived from the degradation of VLDL. A number of studies using perfused rat livers and cells in culture have failed to reveal secretion of an LDL-like particle. *In vitro*, substrate-deprived hepatocytes secrete apoprotein B-100 containing particles with a density similar to LDL[111]. Kinetic studies in humans indicate that, in normal humans, LDL formation results primarily from VLDL catabolism, and the amount of apoprotein B-100 secreted in VLDL is adequate to account for apoprotein B-100 in LDL[107]. The livers of cholesterol-fed animals, however, produce small cholesterol-enriched particles that have a density similar to LDL and humans with the disease familial hypercholesterolaemia[112] produce small cholesterol-rich apoprotein B-100-containing lipoproteins. This would be anticipated from the above discussion in that, with a greater flux of cholesterol across the cell, the liver would produce apoprotein B-100-containing particles that are cholesterol rather than triglyceride-rich. Since cholesteryl esters have a partial specific volume less than triglyceride, the lipoproteins produced are smaller, more dense particles. It therefore seems reasonable to conclude that normally there is little or no secretion of LDL by the liver, but in some diseases and conditions of fatty acid deprivation or cholesterol overloading the liver may make a significant direct contribution to the pool of circulating LDL.

Our understanding of the degradation of LDL has been expanded enormously by the Nobel-prize-winning work of Brown and Goldstein, who have described a pathway for the metabolism of these lipoproteins[113]. The essential features of the LDL receptor pathway are illustrated in Fig. 7. The first step is the binding

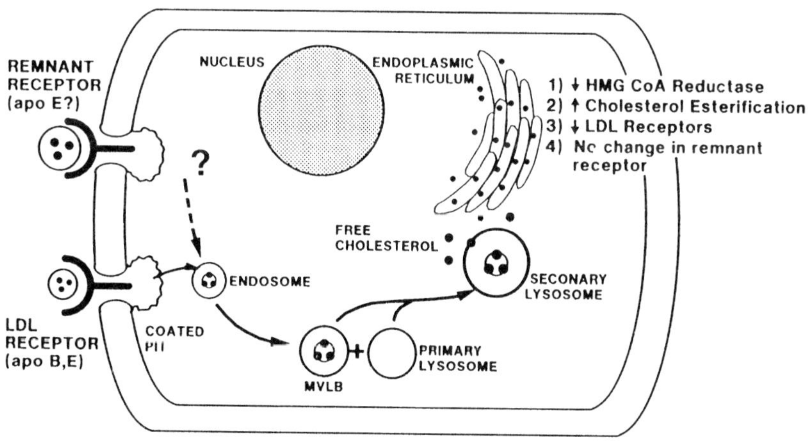

Fig. 7 Sequential steps in the low-density lipoprotein (LDL) pathway in cultured human fibroblasts. The numbers indicate the regulatory actions of LDL: (1) decrease in HMG-CoA reductase and cholesterol synthesis; (2) increase in ACAT and cholesterol esterification; (3) decrease in the number of cell surface receptors for LDL. HMG CoA reductase = 3-hydroxy-3-methylglutyrl coenzyme A reductase; ACAT = acyl coenzyme A: cholesterol acyltransferase

of LDL to a specific receptor on the plasma membrane of a cell. This receptor was originally identified in cultured human skin fibroblasts. It is most abundant in the adrenal gland, liver and intestine[114,115], but virtually any tissue can express the receptor if grown under conditions of cholesterol deprivation. Binding of LDL to its receptor is saturable, has a high affinity, requires divalent cations and is partially reversible.

The LDL receptor is synthesized as a lower molecular weight precursor of ~120 kDa and is processed within the endoplasmic reticulum and Golgi compartments to a mature glycoprotein of ~160 kDa. Based on the amino acid sequence of the receptor and the exon/intron organization of the gene, the receptor is organized into five domains. All the domains have separate functions that were deduced by site-directed mutagenesis of the receptor and from natural genetic mutations. The five domains are the ligand binding domain, the epidermal growth factor (EGF) precursor homology domain, the O-linked sugar domain, the membrane spanning domain, and the cytoplasmic domain[116]. The amino terminal ligand binding domain is an exceptionally interesting structure in that this region contains seven copies of a 40-residue repeat, the subunits of which are held together by disulphide bridges. The distal segment of each repeat element contains a conserved sequence of negatively charged amino acids that are postulated to interact with the receptor binding domains of apoprotein B-100 and apoprotein E. Electron microscopy shows that the receptors are clustered in specialized areas of the cell surface that are characterized by a thickened, indented, fuzzy segment of the membrane, referred to as a coated pit.

Following binding of LDL, the receptor–lipoprotein complex is internalized by endocytosis, with the formation of an endocytic vesicle. As the endocytic vesicle becomes acidified through the action of a proton pump, the receptor and its ligand dissociate. The receptor returns to the cell surface while the vesicles containing the lipoprotein migrate to the Golgi-rich region of the liver cell, where they are identified as multivesicular-like bodies (MLLB)[117]. These ultimately merge with primary lysosomes to form secondary lysosomes. The lipoprotein is degraded within this secondary lysosome; the cholesteryl ester is hydrolysed to free cholesterol, and the apoprotein B-100 is degraded to small peptides and amino acids. As a consequence of the availability of free cholesterol there is a decrease in the rate of *de novo* cholesterol synthesis by the cell. Sterol-mediated feedback repression is discussed later in this chapter. Any cholesterol liberated in excess of cellular needs is re-esterified by a microsomal enzyme, acyl coenzyme A : cholesterol acyltransferase (ACAT), and is stored in the form of cholesterol esters.

The role of the liver as the primary site of LDL degradation has become established during the past decade. Initially, however, it was not clear whether the liver was important in this process. Several tissues, particularly the adrenal gland, have a higher specific activity of LDL binding than liver[114]. However, LDL receptors can be identified on the liver of normal adults of most species, including humans[118] and, considering the relative mass of these tissues, the contribution of the liver to total binding, and thus to LDL removal, would be substantial. Further, it has been observed that perfused livers degrade LDL, although at a rate far slower than the rate at which they remove and degrade remnants[119]. Perhaps the best data on the importance of the liver in LDL catabolism have been provided by studies using LDL labelled with residualizing labels such as [^{14}C]sucrose or [^{125}I]tyramine cellobiose[120]. Since these molecules are not catabolized by lysosomes, it was reasoned that their accumulation would reflect cumulative LDL degradation. From these studies it was concluded that the liver is responsible for about 40–60% of LDL degradation, with no other tissue contributing more than 9%. When patients who lack LDL receptors undergo hepatic transplantations, their serum LDL levels fall dramatically but remain about 33% higher than normal. It has been suggested that this failure is due to failure to correct the non-hepatic contribution to LDL degradation[121]. Deitschy and his colleagues[122] have studied this process in detail in the rat and hamster. By using LDL that contain apoprotein B with a chemically modified binding site for receptor recognition, the amount of non-receptor-mediated LDL transport by the liver has been estimated. In normal animals about 90% of the LDL are taken up by the LDL receptor pathway, and the rest by the low-affinity (receptor-independent) pathway[122]. However, the proportion transported by the two pathways varies, depending on the metabolic state of the animal. If the serum content of cholesterol is low, the number of LDL receptors will be high. This will lead to little receptor-independent transport. When the serum concentration of cholesterol is high, this will lead to more receptor-independent transport. Consistent with this notion, in the Watanabe heritable hyperlipidaemic rabbit, which has a defective LDL receptor, it was observed that the liver was still the principal site of LDL degradation[123]. Presumably, in this case all of the transport is by the low-affinity pathway. Interestingly, the expression of hepatic LDL receptors appears to be less sensitive to sterol-mediated down-regulation than other tissues such as fibroblasts[124]. The mechanism for this is not entirely clear.

The LDL receptor pathway can be regulated by a number of hormones and serum factors[125–128], and other factors such as dietary fat content. A striking example of the sensitivity of plasma LDL cholesterol to small changes in hepatic LDL receptor expression was noted when Watanabe heritable hyperlipidaemic rabbits that lack normal LDL receptor were given autologous hepatocytes transfected with the LDL receptor gene[129]. A 30% reduction in the serum cholesterol was achieved with a 2–4% reconstitution of LDL receptor gene expression. This has led to the concept that somatic cell gene therapy might be an important intervention for familial hypercholesterolaemia. Thus, it is now established that the liver is quantitatively the major site of LDL degradation, and that most of this is mediated by the LDL receptor.

It is now clear that LDL can be divided into subclasses characterized by variations in density, size and chemical composition. Using gradient gel electrophoresis (GGE), for example, LDL can be found in two subclasses termed type A and type B[130]. LDL subclass phenotype A is characterized by the presence of large LDL particles with a peak particle diameter of about 263 Å Subclass phenotype B is characterized by smaller particles of peak particle diameter of 248 Å that are more dense, and more apoprotein B-100 enriched. It is now widely recognized that an increased coronary heart disease risk is associated with a predominance of the small LDL particles. Subclass phenotype B is common in the population, with a prevalence of about 30%.

HIGH-DENSITY LIPOPROTEIN METABOLISM

The metabolism of HDL is not understood in as much detail as the metabolism of the other lipoprotein classes. This situation has changed in the past few years with the appreciation of an inverse correlation between serum levels of HDL and atherosclerosis. HDL is thought to participate in 'reverse cholesterol transport', a process described more than 20 years ago[131] in which cholesterol in peripheral tissues is delivered to the liver, either for excretion or recycling[132,133]. Although unsubstantiated as yet, this process is widely thought to be anti-atherogenic. Studies of HDL metabolism are complicated by the fact that HDL are not a single homogeneous class of particles. At least two groups of HDL particles can be distinguished in normal individuals by ultracentrifugation, and on the basis of their compositions. These are referred to as HDL_2 (densities between 1.063 and 1.120) and HDL_3 (densities between 1.120 and 1.210). Overlapping these classes, it is now clear that human HDL can also be divided into two major subpopulations on the basis of apoprotein composition: those that contain apoprotein A-I but no apoprotein A-II (called LpA-I) and those containing apoproteins A-I and A-II (called LpA-I, A-II)[132]. In addition, the composition of HDL *in vivo* is constantly changing because of the extensive exchange and transfer of both lipid and proteins between HDL particles and other lipoprotein classes.

It now seems that HDL are formed by more than one mechanism, and originate in more than one tissue (Fig. 8). HDL production by the liver was enigmatic for many years. It was clear that the liver was capable of synthesizing and secreting the important apoproteins of HDL (AI, AII, AIV, and Cs), but HDL particles were not visualized in the Golgi complexes of the liver. This problem

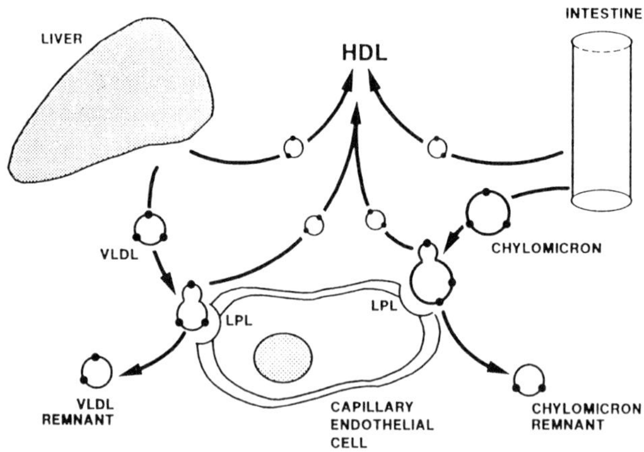

Fig. 8 HDL formation. There are several mechanisms whereby HDL can be formed. First, they appear to be formed following the *de novo* synthesis of apo A-I from either the liver or the intestine. The Apo A-I is probably secreted as a pre-β HDL with very little associated lipid. It acquires phospholipid and cholesterol while in the circulation, probably from contact with cells. In addition, HDL can be formed by budding off of the surface of the larger lipoproteins, chylomicrons, or VLDL during the process of remnant formation

was probably resolved by the observation that newly synthesized HDLs are disc-shaped rather than spheroidal, and undergo a transformation catalysed by LCAT and CETP following secretion into the serum[134]. It remains unclear whether the discs are formed in the Golgi apparatus or whether free apoproteins are secreted into the plasma and then HDL are formed from the association of apoprotein with phospholipid and cholesterol. HDL do not appear to be formed as a consequence of VLDL secretion, since blockade of VLDL secretion does not prevent HDL secretion. When the serum cholesterol-esterifying enzyme, LCAT, is inhibited during liver perfusion experiments, the HDL particles accumulating in the perfusate are not spherical but biconcave discs. When analysed chemically, these discs are virtually devoid of cholesteryl ester; thus they lack a core. These particles undergo, however, a rapid transformation to a spherical shape in the serum of intact animals. This occurs because free cholesterol on the surface of the particle is esterified in serum by the enzyme LCAT. This enzymatic reaction is central to HDL metabolism. The details of this reaction were elucidated, initially, by Glomset[131]. He and his associates first established that the esterification of serum cholesterol was catalysed by LCAT. It was subsequently discovered that this process was important not only in cholesterol transport but also in determining lipoprotein metabolism and structure[135], (see refs 136 and 137 for review).

In humans, significant expression is found only in hepatocytes. The enzyme LCAT catalyses the formation of cholesteryl esters and lysolecithin by combining phospholipase A2 and acyltransferase activities and translocating unsaturated sn-2 fatty acids from phosphatidylcholine to the 3β-hydroxyl group of cholesterol (Fig. 9). LCAT can also catalyse the reverse reaction; however, the significance of this *in vivo* is unknown. Unesterified cholesterol that is a substrate for the LCAT reaction is derived from cell membranes, HDL, or to a limited extent, from LDL[138]. Prior to esterification, cell membrane cholesterol is taken up by nascent, predominantly apoprotein AI-containing HDL particles

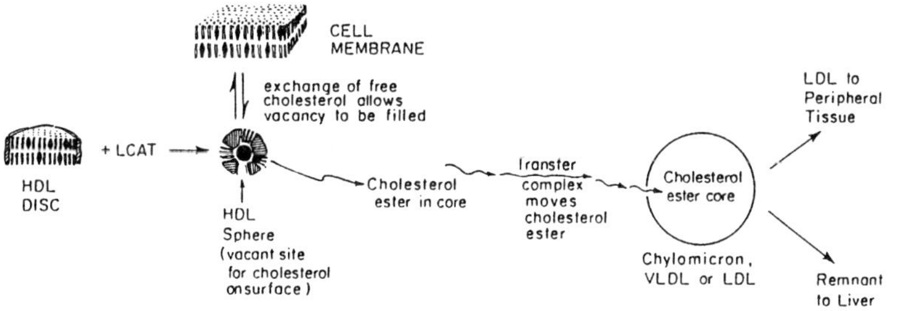

Fig. 9 The lecithin–cholesterol acyltransferase (LCAT) reaction. A proposed mechanism whereby LCAT regulates movement of cholesterol from tissues in which it is in excess of those in which it can be utilized. The LCAT causes transformation of an HDL disc into an HDL sphere. During this process a free cholesterol molecule moves from the surface of the lipoprotein to the core of the particle. This shifts the equilibrium of cholesterol exchange between cell membranes and lipoproteins so that there can be net movement of free sterol from a cell to the lipoprotein. The cholesterol ester is ultimately transferred to a lower-density particle, which carries it to a tissue with a metabolic requirement for cholesterol. From: Cooper A. D. In: Zakim D., Boyer T., editors. Hepatology: a textbook of liver disease, 2nd edn, vol. 1. Philadelphia: WB Saunders; 1989:96–123

called preβ-HDL because of their mobility on agarose gel electrophoresis[139]. The small preβ-HDL appear to the initial acceptor of cholesterol from cell membranes in the reverse cholesterol transport pathway, and are a major substrate for LCAT. Through the LCAT reaction these small HDL are converted to larger, more complex HDL. The rate of the reaction is accelerated by the presence of apoprotein AI.

Any cholesteryl esters that are formed by the LCAT reaction are packed within the core of the particle, making them spherical. During the process, preβ-HDL may acquire apoprotein D, CETP and possibly apoprotein AIV. The CETP transfers cholesterol ester from the HDL core to LDL or VLDL, allowing continual packing of the HDL core with cholesterol ester.

When a molecule of free cholesterol has been esterified and transferred from the surface of HDL to its core, the lipoprotein surface membrane has a vacancy for another molecule of free cholesterol. This cholesterol molecule may be provided by the plasma membrane of any cell with which the lipoprotein comes into contact. Thus, the LCAT reaction and the CETP may be the driving forces in the transport of cholesterol from cells to the liver, with HDL serving primarily as the site of the esterification reaction.

It is not surprising that diseases affecting the quantity of LCAT in blood have profound effects on the metabolism of serum lipoproteins. Patients who have congenital deficiencies of LCAT have numerous abnormalities of lipoprotein composition, structure and function. These are manifested by low concentrations of cholesteryl ester in serum, the persistence of HDL discs in serum, and the failure of reverse cholesterol transport[140,141]. Patients with liver disease also have varying degrees of LCAT deficiency, and hence similar abnormalities of lipoprotein metabolism.

Several factors including gender and feeding of fat alter the apparent activity of LCAT in serum. It is not known whether this is the result of a change in the rate of LCAT secretion, a change in the rate of activation of the enzyme, or alteration of the amount of substrate available to the enzyme. Several liver diseases are associated with changes in LCAT activity, presumably owing to changes in the rate of LCAT secretion, although this has not been proven.

The movement of cholesterol esters from HDL to VLDL and LDL is catalysed by the CETP. The liver also synthesizes and secretes the cholesteryl ester transfer protein or CETP. This protein is thought to play a role in the speciation of HDL subclasses and in reverse cholesterol transport[142]. It mediates the transfer of cholesteryl ester, triglyceride, retinyl ester and phospholipids between the various lipoprotein classes. The mechanism of lipid transfer is not known with certainty. Kinetic data support the hypotheses that CETP may act as a free carrier of lipids, or may form a ternary complex between the donor and acceptor lipoproteins. The CETP accounts for all of the neutral lipid transfer activity in human serum and about 50% of the phospholipid transfer activity. Another phospholipid transfer protein has been purified from human serum that appears to be responsible for the remainder of the serum phospholipid transfer activity. The human CETP is a glycoprotein of approximately 74 kDa. CETP mRNA can be found in a variety of tissues with a species-specific distribution. In humans the liver, spleen and adipose tissue have the highest levels. The cell type producing CETP in the different tissues is not entirely clear; however, in the liver both parenchymal and non-parenchymal cells produce CETP mRNA. Human plasma CETP concentrations of 1.50 ± 0.26 and 1.92 ± 0.52 μg/ml have been noted in normolipidaemic males and females, respectively. Recent studies have shown that CETP gene expression is regulated by hormones, cholesterol, drugs and, apparently, the apo E genotype. Regulation is primarily at the level of transcription with the liver-enriched transcription factor C/EBP positively regulating the CETP gene promoter[143]. CETP plasma activity is increased by high-cholesterol, high-fat diets and by probucol therapy, and is inversely related to plasma post-heparin lipoprotein lipase activity and parameters of insulin activity. Furthermore, dietary cholesterol increases transcription of the CETP gene in transgenic mice[144]. Corticosteroid therapy and exercise conditioning, in contrast, decrease plasma CETP activity. Studies of mice transgenic for human CETP or CETP and human apoprotein AI, and humans with CETP genetic deficiency, have revealed that high levels of CETP in plasma are associated with low HDL cholesterol and elevated VLDL plus LDL and apoprotein B-100 concentrations. Low levels of CETP, in contrast, are associated with elevated levels of HDL cholesterol and reduced concentrations of VLDL and LDL cholesterol. In dysbetalipoproteinaemia, the nephrotic syndrome, familial hypercholesterolaemia, insulin-dependent diabetes mellitus and peripheral vascular disease (conditions that are associated with accelerated atherosclerosis) the levels of CETP plasma activity are elevated. Alcoholism, in contrast, is associated with elevated HDL cholesterol concentrations and plasma CETP activity is decreased. Despite its importance, virtually nothing is known about the regulation of the process of HDL secretion. Few, if any, quantitatively meaningful studies of the regulation of HDL secretion by the liver have been reported, because of the complexity of controlling the LCAT reaction and because production of HDL is slower than that of VLDL. Protein is secreted in HDL at roughly one-tenth the rate of its secretion in VLDL. Accordingly, isolated liver perfusion, which has been the basic tool for studying VLDL secretion is less likely to be used in studying HDL secretion.

Concomitant with the conversion of the discoidal HDL to a sphere there is an alteration in the apoprotein composition of the particle. The discs, which initially contain a significant amount of apoprotein E, lose the apoprotein E and become enriched in the A and C apoproteins[120]. These changes do not occur in the absence of LCAT[135], and appear to be influenced by the ratio of apoproteins AI and AII in the particles, hepatic lipase activity, and by the activity of the cholesteryl ester transfer protein (CETP, discussed below).

Disc-like structures similar to nascent hepatic HDL have been found in mesenteric lymph[145]. Because the intestine is a site of synthesis of apoprotein AI and AII it is plausible that these also represent nascent HDL particles that subsequently undergo a structural conversion to spherical HDL.

As already mentioned, an alternative pathway for the formation of HDL exists. HDL can be produced in the serum as a product of the metabolism of chylomicrons and VLDL. In this scheme HDL is formed from the excess surface material of the triglyceride-rich lipoproteins during the process of lipolysis and remnant formation. This has been demonstrated *in vitro* and in hepatectomized rats. The quantitative aspects of HDL formation have not yet been elucidated in any detail; hence the relative contribution of these two pathways and of liver and intestine to the circulating pool of HDL is not known.

The fate of circulating HDL is not entirely clear. The surface apoproteins of both A and C groups are able to transfer back and forth among HDL and VLDL and chylomicrons (see Fig. 5). The half-life in serum of the A apoproteins (4–5 days) is substantially longer than that of the C apoproteins (10–18 h)[146]. The free cholesterol of HDL can exchange with plasma membranes and other lipoproteins, and has a half-life that is different from that of HDL cholesteryl esters. The latter cannot exchange readily but are transferred by the CETP[142] from small HDL particles, possibly a subclass called pre β-HDL [139,147], to larger HDL particles, LDL or VLDL[132].

Although it seems logical that the liver should be a major site of HDL catabolism, definitive proof of this is lacking. The half-life of the HDL particle is thus difficult to determine precisely, because it has no fixed constituent. Evidence from liver perfusion studies suggests that the liver can account for only a limited amount of direct HDL catabolism[148]. At physiological concentrations of HDL the rate of HDL degradation by the isolated perfused liver is only 7% of the rate *in vivo*. Additional recent evidence suggests that, at least in some species, HDL may serve as a source of cholesterol for extrahepatic tissues[149]. Since many HDL constituents are transferred to other lipoprotein classes that undergo direct hepatic catabolism, the liver may in this way become the eventual site of catabolism of lipids and proteins that originated in HDL. Support for the concept that HDL is not metabolized as a unit is provided by studies of Pittman and his colleagues[150] using non-metabolizable markers, as was done for LDL. As compared with the ratio in the HDL particle, twice as much cholesterol ether (a non-metabolizable analogue of cholesteryl ester) as labelled apoprotein AI accumulated in the liver. The amount was seven-fold higher in the adrenal. The ratio was 1 : 1 in most other tissues, except the kidney, in which labelled apoprotein AI accumulated in excess of the labelled cholesterol. Moreover, free cholesterol in HDL rapidly equilibrates with liver plasma membranes and bile, whereas cholesterol ester in HDL enters the organ much more slowly[151]. The possibility of separate mechanisms for removal of HDL constituents by the liver then seems likely. Although receptors for HDL and apo AI in the liver have been described[152], the physiological relevance of these receptors has not been established. They are not analogous to the LDL receptors, but may facilitate transfer of HDL constituents by mechanisms other than endocytosis.

SUMMARY

Lipoproteins are produced in the liver and the intestine. Thus, production requires the synthesis of several apolipoproteins by these organs. The rates of this formation are regulated by the flux of fatty acids through these organs. The rate of bile salt formation and secretion is a key determinant of lipid absorption, and thus plays a major regulatory role. The rate of lipoprotein catabolism is regulated largely by the level LDL receptors expressed on the liver. This is also determined by the cholesterol balance in this organ which, in turn, is regulated by the rate of conversion of cholesterol to bile salt and the rate of bile salt secretion. These regulatory interactions are depicted in Fig. 10.

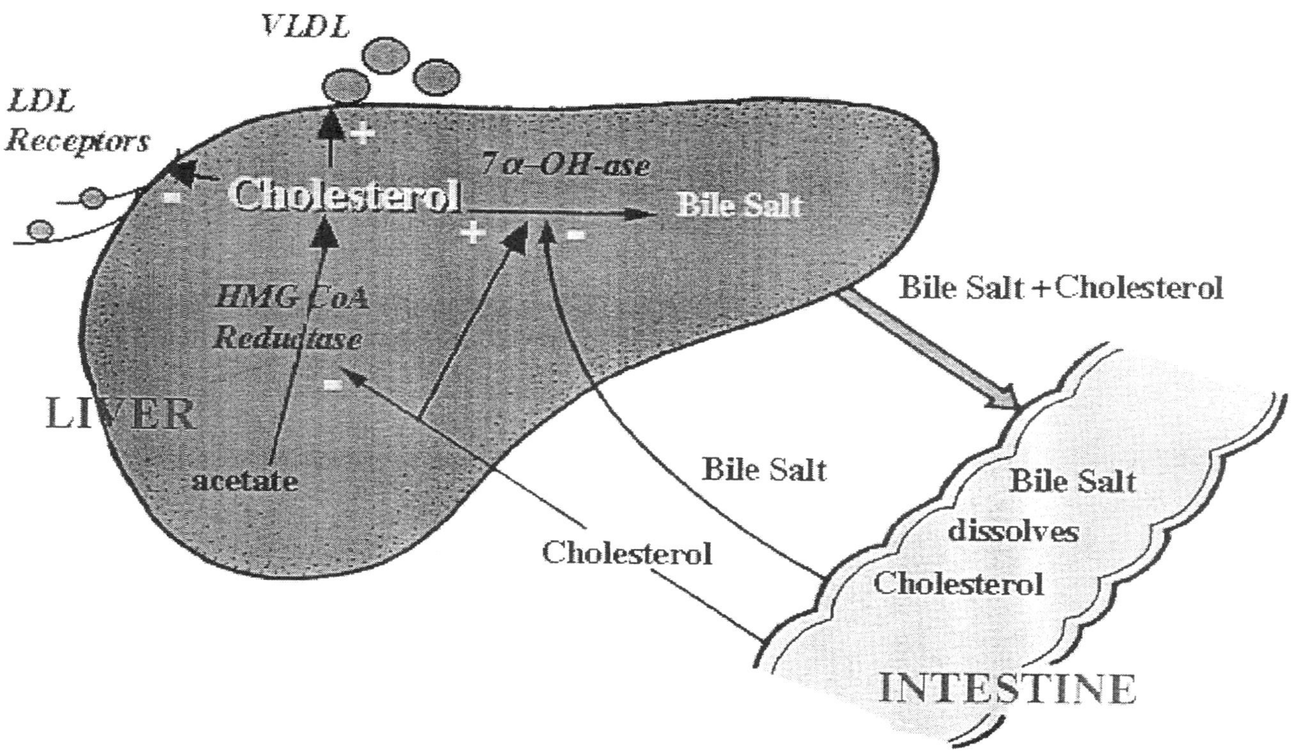

Fig. 10 The enterohepatic circulation in the control of lipoprotein metabolism. Various interactions that determine hepatic cholesterol homeostasis are outlined. Those functions inhibited by cholesterol or bile salts are indicated with a minus sign, and those which are stimulated are indicated with a plus sign

Acknowledgements

I thank Ms Kathe O'Hearn for preparing the manuscript. Original studies cited were supported by Grant DK38318 from the National Institutes of Health and the Stanford University Digestive Diseases Core Center, DK38707.

References

1. Machebouef M. Recherches sur les phosphoaminolipides et les sterides du serum et du plasma sanguine: entrainement des phospholipides, des sterides par les diverses fractions au cours du fractionnement des proteides du serum. Bull Soc Chem Biol. 1929;11:268.
2. Gofman JW, Lindgren FT, Elliott H. Ultracentrifugal studies of lipoproteins of human serum. J Biol Chem. 1949;179:973–9.
3. Havel RJ, Eder HA, Bragdon HJ. Distribution and chemical composition of ultracentrifugally separated lipoproteins in human serum. J Lipid Res. 1955;21:436–42.
4. Segrest JP, Jones MK, De Loof H, Brouillette CG, Venkatachalapathi YV. The amphipathic helix in the exchangeable apolipoproteins: a review of secondary structure and function. J Lipid Res. 1992;33:141–66.
5. Windmueller HG, Wu A-L. Biosynthesis of plasma apolipoproteins by rat small intestine without dietary or biliary fat. J Biol Chem. 1981;256:3012–16.
6. Green PH, Glickman RM, Saudek CD, Blum LB, Tall AR. Human intestinal lipoproteins. J Clin Invest. 1979;64:233–42.
7. Brewer HB, Jr, Lux SE, Ronan R, John KM. Amino acid sequence of human apoLp-Gln-II (apo A-II), an apolipoprotein isolated from the high-density lipoprotein complex. Proc Natl Acad Sci USA. 1972;69:1304–8.
8. Sliwkowski MB, Windmueller HG. Rat liver and small intestine produce proapolipoprotein A-I which is slowly processed to apolipoprotein A-I in the circulation. J Biol Chem. 1984;259:6459–65.
9. Schultz JR, Gong EL, McCall MR, Nichols AV, Clift SM, Rubin EM. Expression of human apolipoprotein A-II and its effect on high density lipoproteins in transgenic mice. J Biol Chem. 1992;267:21630–6.
10. Rubin EM, Ishida BY, Clift SM, Krauss RM. Expression of human apolipoprotein A-I in transgenic mice results in reduced plasma levels of murine apolipoprotein A-I and the appearance of two new high density lipoprotein size subclasses. Proc Natl Acad Sci USA. 1991;88:434–8.
11. Warden CH, Hedrick CC, Qiao J-H, Castellani LW, Lusis AJ. Atherosclerosis in transgenic mice overexpressing apolipoprotein A-II. Science. 1993;261:469–72.
12. Schmitz G, Lackner KJ. High-density lipoproteins and atherosclerosis. Curr Opin Lipidol. 1993;4:392–400.
13. Williamson R, Lee D, Hagaman J, Maeda N. Marked reduction of high density lipoprotein cholesterol in mice genetically modified to lack apolipoprotein A-I. Proc Natl Acad Sci USA. 1992;89:7134–8.
14. Karathanasis SK. Apolipoprotein multigene family: tandem organization of human apolipoprotein AI, CIII, and AIV genes. Proc Natl Acad Sci USA. 1985:82:6374–8.
15. Gordon JI, Bisgaier CL, Sims HF, Sachdev OP, Glickman RM, and Strauss AW. Biosynthesis of human preapolipoprotein A-IV. J Biol Chem. 1984;259:468–74.
16. Tenkanen H, Ehnholm C. Molecular biology of apolipoprotein A-IV. Curr Opin Lipidol. 1993;4:95–9.
17. Tso P, Cardelli JA, Fujimoto K. Increased apolipoprotein A-IV in rat mesenteric lymph after lipid meal acts as a physiological signal for satiation. FASEB J. 1992;6:A1205.
18. Scanu, AM. Lipoprotein (a): a genetic risk factor for premature coronary heart disease. JAMA. 1992;267:3326–9.
19. Lawn RM. Lipoprotein (a) in heart disease: a remarkable protein that transports cholesterol and binds with blood clots can raise the risk of a heart attack. Comparisons between it and other blood proteins may explain why. Sci Am. 1992;June:54–60.
20. Chiesa G, Hobbs HH, Koschinsky ML, Lawn RM, Maika SD, Hammer RE. Reconstitution of lipoprotein (a) by infusion of human low density lipoprotein into transgenic mice expressing human apolipoprotein (a). J Biol Chem. 1992;267:24369–74.

21. Boerwinkle E, Leffert CC, Lin J, Lackner C, Chiesa G, Hobbs HH. Apolipoprotein (a) gene accounts for greater than 90% of the variation in plasma lipoprotein (a) concentrations. J Clin Invest. 1992;90:52–60.
22. Grainger DJ, Kirschenlohr HL, Metcalfe JC, Weissberg PL, Wade DP, Lawn RM. Proliferation of human smooth muscle cells promoted by lipoprotein (a). Science. 1993;260:1655–8.
23. Young SG. Recent progress in understanding apolipoprotein B. Circulation. 1990;82:1574–94.
24. Law SW, Lackner KJ, Hospattankar AV *et al.* Human apolipoprotein B-100: cloning, analysis of liver mRNA, and assignment of the gene to chromosome 2. Proc Natl Acad Sci USA. 1985;82:8340–4.
25. Chen SH, Yang CY, Chen PF *et al.* The complete cDNA and amino acid sequence of human apolipoprotein B-100. J Biol Chem. 1986;261:12918.
26. Kane JP, Hardman DA, Paulus HE. Heterogeneity of apolipoprotein B: isolation of a new species from human chylomicrons. Proc Natl Acad Sci USA. 1980;77:2465–9.
27. Hodges P, Scott J. Apolipoprotein B mRNA editing: a new tier for the control of gene expression. TIBS. 1992;17:77–81.
28. Davidson NO, Powell LM, Wallis SC, Scott J. Thyroid hormone modulates the introduction of a stop codon in rat liver apolipoprotein B messenger RNA. J Biol Chem. 1988;263:13482–5.
29. Powell LM, Wallis SC, Pease RJ, Edwards YH, Knott TJ, and Scott J. A novel form of tissue-specific RNA processing produces apolipoprotein-B48 in intestine. Cell. 1987;50:831–40.
30. Goldstein JL, Brown MS. The low-density lipoprotein pathway and its relation to atherosclerosis. Annu Rev Biochem. 1977;46:897–930.
31. Ito Y, Azrolan N, O'Connell A, Walsh A, and Breslow JL. Hypertriglyceridemia as a result of human apo CIII gene expression in transgenic mice. Science. 1990;249:790–3.
32. Aalto-Setälä K, Fisher EA, Chen X *et al.* Mechanism of hypertriglyceridemia in human apolipoprotein (apo) CIII transgenic mice. Diminished very low density lipoprotein fractional catabolic rate associated with increased apo CIII and reduced apo E on the particles. J Clin Invest. 1992;90:1889–1900.
33. Cox DW, Breckenridge WC, and Little JA. Inheritance of apolipoprotein C-II deficiency with hypertriglyceridemia and pancreatitis. N Engl J Med. 1978;299:1421–4.
34. Zannis V, Breslow JL, Utermann G *et al.* Proposed nomenclature of apoE isoproteins, apoE genotypes, and phenotypes. J Lipid Res. 1982;23:911–14.
35. Shelburne F, Hanks J, Meyers W, Quarfordt S. Effect of apoproteins on hepatic uptake of triglyceride emulsions in the rat. J Clin Invest. 1980;65:652–8.
36. Sherrill BC, Innerarity TL, Mahley RW. Rapid hepatic clearance of the canine lipoproteins containing only the E apoprotein by a high affinity receptor. Identity with the chylomicron remnant transport process. J Biol Chem. 1980;255:1804–7.
37. Cooper A, Erickson S. Evidence that apo E is the determinant of chylomicron remnant binding to liver plasma membrane. Clin Res. 1980;28:518.
38. Shimano H, Yamada N, Katsuki M *et al.* Plasma lipoprotein metabolism in transgenic mice overexpressing apolipoprotein E. Accelerated clearance of lipoproteins containing apolipoprotein B. J Clin Invest. 1992;90:2084–91.
39. Smith JD, Plump AS, Hayek T, Walsh A, Breslow JL. Accumulation of human apolipoprotein E in the plasma of transgenic mice. J Biol Chem. 1990;265:14709–12.
40. Plump AS, Smith JD, Hayek T *et al.* Severe hypercholesterolemia and atherosclerosis in apolipoprotein E-deficient mice created in homologous recombination in ES cells. Cell. 1992;71:343–53.
41. Windler E, Chao Y-S, Havel RJ. Determinants of hepatic uptake of triglyceride-rich lipoproteins and their remnants in the rat. J Biol Chem. 1980;255:5475–80.
42. Basu SK, Brown MS, Ho YK, Havel RJ, Goldstein JL. Mouse macrophages synthesize and secrete a protein resembling apolipoprotein E. Proc Natl Acad Sci USA. 1981;78:7545–9.
43. Strittmatter WJ, Weisgraber KH, Huang DY *et al.* Binding of human apolipoprotein E to synthetic amyloid B peptide: isoform-specific effects and implications for late-onset Alzheimer disease. Proc Natl Acad Sci USA. 1993;90:8098–102.
44. Strittmatter WJ, Saunders AM, Schmechel D *et al.* Apolipoprotein E: high-avidity binding to β-amyloid and increased frequency of type 4 allele in late-onset familial Alzheimer disease. Proc Natl Acad Sci USA. 1993;90:1977–81.
45. Korn E. Clearing factor, a heparin activated lipoprotein lipase. J Biol Chem. 1955;215:1.
46. Robinson D. The function of the plasma triglycerides in fatty acid transport. In: Florkin SE, editor. Comprehensive biochemistry. Amsterdam: Elsevier; 1970:51.

47. Tall AR, Green PHR, Glickman RM, Riley JW. Metabolic fate of chylomicron phospholipids and apoproteins in the rat. J Clin Invest. 1979;64:977–89.
48. Redgrave TG, Small DM. Quantitation of the transfer of surface phospholipid of chylomicrons to the high density lipoprotein fraction during the catabolism of chylomicrons in the rat. J Clin Invest. 1979;64:162–71.
49. Redgrave TG. Formation of cholesteryl ester-rich particulate lipid during metabolism of chylomicrons. J Clin Invest. 1970;49:465–71.
50. Mjos OD, Faergeman O, Hamilton RL, Havel RJ. Characterization of remnants produced during the metabolism of triglyceride-rich lipoproteins in blood plasma and intestinal lymph in the rat. J Clin Invest. 1975;56:603–15.
51. Sherrill BC, Dietschy JM. Characterization of the sinusoidal transport process responsible for uptake of chylomicrons by the liver. J Biol Chem. 1977;253:1859–67.
52. Cooper AD. The metabolism of chylomicron remnants by isolated perfused rat liver. Biochim Biophys Acta. 1977;488:464–74.
53. Nilsson A, Zilversmit DB. Distribution of chylomicron cholesteryl ester between parenchymal and Kupffer cells of rat liver. Biochim Biophys Acta. 1979;248:137.
54. Mahley RW. Alterations in plasma lipoproteins induced by cholesterol feeding in animals including man. In: Dietschy JM, Gotto AM, Ontkyo JA, editors. Disturbances in lipid and lipoprotein metabolism. Bethesda, MD: American Physiological Society; 1978:181.
55. Cooper AD, Erickson SK, Nutik R, Shrewsbury MA. Characterization of chylomicron remnant binding to rat liver membranes. J Lipid Res. 1982;23:42–52.
56. Ellsworth JL, Kraemer FB, Cooper AD. Transport of β-very low density lipoproteins and chylomicrons remnants by macrophages is mediated by the low density lipoprotein receptor pathway. J Biol Chem. 1987;262:2316–25.
57. Choi SY, Fong LG, Kirven MJ, Cooper AD. Use of an anti-LDL receptor antibody to quantify the role of the LDL receptor in the removal of chylomicron remnants in the mouse *in vivo*. J Clin Invest. 1991;88:1173–81.
58. Choi SY, Cooper AD. A comparison of the roles of the low density lipoprotein (LDL) receptor and the LDL receptor-related protein α_2-macroglobulin receptor in chylomicron remnant removal in the mouse *in vivo*. J Biol Chem. 1993;268:15804–11.
59. Szanto A, Balasubramaniam S, Roach PD, Nestel PJ. Modulation of the low-density-lipoprotein-receptor-related protein and its relevance to chylomicron-remnant metabolism. Biochem J. 1992;288:791–4.
60. Rubinsztein DC, Cohen JC, Berger GM, van der Westhuyzen DR, Coetzee GA, Gevers W. Chylomicron remnant clearance from the plasma is normal in familial hypercholesterolemic homozygotes with defined receptor defects. J Clin Invest. 1990;86:1306–12.
61. Herz J. The LDL-receptor-related protein – portrait of a multifunctional receptor. Curr Opin Lipidol. 1993;4:107–13.
62. Kowal RC, Herz J, Goldstein JL, Esser V, Brown MS. Low density lipoprotein receptor-related protein mediates uptake of cholesteryl esters derived from apoprotein E-enriched lipoproteins. Proc Natl Acad Sci USA. 1989;86:5810–14.
63. Beisiegel U, Weber W, Bengtsson-Olivecrona G. Lipoprotein lipase enhances the binding of chylomicrons to low density lipoprotein receptor-related protein. Proc Natl Acad Sci USA. 1991;88:8342–6.
64. Chappell DA, Fry GL, Waknitz MA *et al.* Lipoprotein lipase induces catabolism of normal triglyceride-rich lipoproteins via the low density lipoprotein receptor-related protein/a2-macroglobulin receptor *in vivo*. J Biol Chem. 1993;268:14168–75.
65. Nykjaer A, Bengtsson-Olivecrona G, Lookene A *et al.* The alpha2-macroglobulin receptor/low density lipoprotein receptor-related protein binds lipoprotein lipase and beta -migrating very low density lipoprotein associated with the lipase. J Biol Chem. 1993;268:15048–55.
66. Kristensen T, Moestrup SK, Gliemann J, Bendtsen L, Sand O, Sottrup-Jensen L. Evidence that the newly cloned low-density-lipoprotein receptor related protein (LRP) is the a2-macroglobulin receptor. FEBS Lett. 1990;276:151–5.
67. Strickland DK, Ashcom JD, Williams S, Burgess WH, Migliorini M, Argraves WS. Sequence identity between the α_2-macroglobulin receptor and low density lipoprotein receptor-related protein suggests that this molecule is a multifunctional receptor. J Biol Chem. 1990;265:17401–4.

68. Kounnas MZ, Morris RE, Thompson MR, FitsGerald DJ, Strickland DK, Saelinger CB. The alpha 2-macroglobulin receptor/low density lipoprotein receptor-related protein binds and internalizes *Pseudomonas* exotoxin. J Biol Chem. 1992;267:12420–3.
69. Bu G, Williams S, Strickland DK, Schwartz AL. Low density lipoprotein receptor-related protein/α_2-macroglobulin receptor is an hepatic receptor for tissue-type plasminogen activator. Proc Natl Acad Sci USA. 1992;89:7427–31.
70. Kounnas MZ, Argraves WS, Strickland DK. The 39-kDa receptor-associated protein interacts with two members of the low density lipoprotein receptor family, af2-macroglobulin receptor and glycoprotein 330. J Biol Chem. 1992;267:21162–6.
71. Willnow TE, Goldstein JL, Orth K, Brown MS, Herz J. Low density lipoprotein receptor-related protein and gp330 bind similar ligands, including plasminogen activator–inhibitor complexes and lactoferrin, an inhibitor of chylomicron remnant clearance. J Biol Chem. 1992;267:26172–80.
72. Herz J, Goldstein JL, Strickland DK, Ho YK, Brown MS. 39 kDa protein modulates binding of ligands to low density lipoprotein receptor-related protein/α_2-macroglobulin. J Biol Chem. 1991;266:21232–8.
73. Williams SE, Ashcom JD, Argraves WS, Strickland DK. A novel mechanism for controlling the activity of α_2-macroglobulin receptor/low density lipoprotein receptor-related protein. Multiple regulatory sites for 39-kDa receptor-associated protein. J Biol Chem. 1992;267:9035–40.
74. de Faria EC, Komaromy MC, Fong LG, Cooper AD. An anti-hepatic lipase antibody that does not inhibit lipolysis delays removal and reduces hepatic uptake of chylomicron remnants in mice. Circulation 1994;90:I–289.
75. Floren C-H, Nordgren H, Nilsson A. Effects of chloroquine and colchicine on the degradation of chyle cholesteryl ester and phospholipids *in vivo*. Eur J Biochem. 1977;80:331.
76. Van Zuiden PEA, Erickson SK, Cooper AD. Effect of removal of lipoproteins of different composition on hepatic 3-hydroxy-3-methylglutaryl coenzyme A reductase activity and hepatic very low density lipoprotein secretion. J Lipid Res. 1983;24:418–28.
77. Patrick AD, Luke BD. Deficiency of an acid lipase in Wolmans disease. Nature (Lond). 1969;222:1067.
78. Ockner RK, Hughes FB, Isselbacher KJ. Very low density lipoproteins in intestinal lymph: origin, composition and role in lipid transport in the fasting state. J Clin Invest. 1969;48:2079–88.
79. Jones AL, Ruderman NB, Herrera MG. Electron microscopic and biochemical study of lipoprotein synthesis in the isolated perfused rat liver. J Lipid Res. 1967;8:429.
80. Radding CM, Bragdon JH, Steinberg D. The synthesis of low and high density lipoproteins by rat liver *in vitro*. Biochim Biophys Acta. 1958;30:443.
81. Marsh JB. Lipoproteins in a nonrecirculation perfusate of rat liver. J Lipid Res. 1974;15:544.
82. Alexander CA, Hamilton RL, Havel RJ. Subcellular localization of B apoprotein of plasma lipoproteins in rat liver. J Cell Biol 1976;69:241.
83. Colman, R, and Bell, RM. Triacylglycerol synthesis in isolated fat cells. J Biol Chem. 1976;251:4537.
84. Atzel A, Wetterau JR. Mechanism of microsomal triglyceride transfer protein catalyzed lipid transport. Biochemistry. 1993;32:10444–50.
85. Wetterau JR, Aggerbeck LP, Bouma ME *et al.* Absence of microsomal triglyceride transfer protein in individuals. Science. 1992;258:999–1001.
86. Stein O, Bar-on H, Stein Y. Lipoproteins and the liver. In: Popper SF, editor. Progress in liver disease. New York: Grune & Stratton; 1972:45.
87. Dixon JL, Ginsberg HN. Regulation of hepatic secretion of apolipoprotein B-containing lipoproteins: information obtained from cultured liver cells. J Lipid Res. 1993;34:167–79.
88. Young SG. Recent progress in understanding apolipoprotein B. Circulation. 1989;80:219–33.
89. Chuck SL, Lingappa VR. Pause transfer: a topogenic sequence in apolipoprotein B mediates stopping and restarting of translocation. Cell. 1992;68:9–21.
90. Spring DJ, Chen-Liu LW, Chatterton JE, Elovson J, Schumaker VN. Lipoprotein assembly: apolipoprotein B size determines lipoprotein core circumference. J Biol Chem. 1992;267:14839–45.
91. Graham DL, Knott TJ, Jones TC, Pease RJ, Pullinger CR, Scott J. Carboxyl-terminal truncation of apolipoprotein B results in gradual loss of the ability to form buoyant lipoproteins in cultured human and rat liver cell lines. Biochemistry. 1991;30:5616–21.

92. Linton MR, Farese R, Young S. Familial hypobetalipoproteinemia. J Lipid Res. 1993;34:521–41.
93. Sato R, Imanaka T, Takatsuki A, Takano T. Degradation of newly synthesized apolipoprotein B-100 in a pre-golgi compartment. J Biol Chem. 1990;265:11880–4.
94. Sniderman AD, Cianflone K. Substrate delivery as a determinant of hepatic ApoB secretion. Arterioscler Thromb. 1993;13:629–36.
95. Heimberg M, Wilcox HG, Dunn GD, Woodside WF, Breen KJ, Soler-Argilage C. Studies on the synthesis and secretion of the very low density lipoprotein and on ketogenesis by the liver. In: Lundquist F, Tygstrup N, eds Regulation of hepatic metabolism. New York: Academic Press; 1974:119–43.
96. White AL, Graham L, LeGros J, Pease RJ, Scott J. Oleate-mediated stimulation of apolipoprotein B secretion from rat hepatoma cells. J Biol Chem. 1992;267:15657–64.
97. Khan B, Fungwe TV, Wilcox HG, Heimberg M. Cholesterol is required for the secretion of the very-low-density lipoprotein: *in vivo* studies. Biochim Biophys Acta. 1990;1044:297–304.
98. Craig WY, Cooper AD. Effects of chylomicron remnants and β-VLDL on the class and composition of newly secreted lipoproteins by HepG2 cells. J Lipid Res. 1988; 29:299–308.
99. Craig WY, Nutik R, Cooper AD. Regulation of apoprotein synthesis and secretion in the human hepatoma HepG2. The effect of exogenous lipoprotein. J Biol Chem. 1988;263:13880–90.
100. Robinson BS, Yao Z, Baisted DJ, Vance DE. Lysophosphatidylcholine metabolism and lipoprotein secretion by cultured rat hepatocytes deficient in choline. Biochem J. 1989;260:207–14.
101. Vance JE. The use of newly synthesized phospholipids for assembly into secreted hepatic lipoproteins. Biochim Biophys Acta. 1989;1006:59–69.
102. Ahrens JEH, Hirsh J, Oette K *et al.* Carbohydrate-induced and fat-induced lipemia. Trans Assoc Am Phys. 1961;74:134.
103. Kris-Etherton PM, Cooper AD. Studies on the etiology of the hyperlipemia in rats fed an atherogenic diet. J Lipid Res. 1980;21:435–42.
104. Brunzell JD, Hazzard WR, Porte Jr, D, Bierman EL. Evidence for a common, saturable, triglyceride removal mechanism for chylomicrons and very low density lipoproteins in man. J Clin Invest. 1973;52:1578–85.
105. Faergeman O, Havel RJ. Metabolism of cholesteryl esters of rat very low density lipoproteins. J Clin Invest. 1975;55:1210–18.
106. Faergeman O, Sata T, Kane JP, Havel RJ. Metabolism of apoprotein B of plasma very low density lipoproteins in the rat. J Clin Invest. 1975;56:1396–403.
107. Berman M, Hall M, Levy RI *et al.* Metabolism of apo B and apo C lipoproteins in man: kinetic studies in normal and hyperlipoproteinemic subjects. J Lipid Res. 1978;19:38.
108. Cooper AD, Shrewsbury, MA, Erickson SK. Comparison of binding and removal of remnants of triglyceride-rich lipoproteins of intestinal and hepatic origin by rat liver *in vitro*. Am J Physiol. 1982;243:G389–95.
109. Arbeeny CM, Rifici VA, Handley DA, Eder HA. Determinants of the uptake of very low density lipoprotein remnants by the perfused rat liver. Metabolism. 1987;36:1106–13.
110. Takahashi S, Kawarabayasi Y, Nakai T, Sakai J, Yamamoto T. Rabbit very low density lipoprotein receptor: a low density lipoprotein receptor-like protein with distinct ligand specificity. Proc Natl Acad Sci USA. 1992;89:9252–6.
111. Ellsworth JL, Erickson SK, Cooper AD. Very low and low density lipoprotein synthesis and secretion by the human hepatoma cell line Hep-G2: effects of free fatty acid. J Lipid Res. 1986;27:858–74.
112. Janus ED, Nicholl A, Wootton R *et al.* Quantitative studies of very low density lipoprotein: conversion to low density lipoprotein in normal controls and primary hyperlipidaemic states and the role of direct secretion of low density lipoprotein in heterozygous familial hypercholesterolaemia. Eur J Clin Invest. 1980;10:149.
113. Brown MS, Goldstein JL. A receptor-mediated pathway for cholesterol homeostasis. Science. 1986;232:34–47.
114. Kovanen PT, Basu SK, Goldstein JL *et al.* Low density lipoprotein receptors in bovine adrenal cortex. II. Low density lipoprotein binding to membranes prepared from fresh tissue. Endocrinology. 1979;104:610.

115. Fong LG, Bonney E, Kosek JC, Cooper AD. Immunohistochemical localization of low density lipoprotein receptors in adrenal gland, liver and intestine. J Clin. Invest. 1989;84:847–56.
116. Sudhof TC, Goldstein JL, Brown MS, Russell DW. The LDL receptor gene: a mosaic of exons shared with different proteins. Science. 1985;228:815–22.
117. Goldstein JL, Brown MS, Anderson RGW, Russell DW, Schneider WJ. Receptor-mediated endocytosis: concepts emerging from the LDL receptor system. Annu Rev Cell Biol. 1985;1:1–39.
118. Soutar AK, Harders-Spengel K, Wade DP *et al.* Detection and quantitation of low density lipoprotein (LDL) receptors in human liver by ligand blotting, immunoblotting, and radioimmunoassay. J Biol Chem. 1986;261:17127–33.
119. Sigurdsson G, Noel S-P, Havel RJ. Catabolism of the apoprotein of low density lipoproteins by the isolated perfused rat liver. J Lipid Res. 1978;19:628.
120. Pittman RC, Attie AD, Carew TE, Steinberg D. Tissue sites of degradation of low density lipoprotein: application of a method for determining the fate of plasma proteins. Proc Natl Acad. Sci USA. 1979;76:5343–9.
121. Bilheimer DW, Goldstein JL, Grundy SM, Starzl TE, Brown MS. Liver transplantation to provide low-density-lipoprotein receptors and lower plasma cholesterol ina child with homozygous familial hypercholesterolemia. N Engl J Med. 1984;311:1658–64.
122. Dietschy JM, Turley SD, Spady DK. Role of liver in the maintenance of cholesterol and low density lipoprotein homeostasis in different animal species, including humans. J Lipid Res. 1993;34:1637.
123. Kita T, Brown MS, Bilheimer DW, Goldstein JL. Delayed clearance of very low density and intermediate density lipoproteins with enhanced conversion to low density lipoproteins in WHHL rabbits. Proc Natl Acad Sci USA. 1982;79:5693–7.
124. Ellsworth JL, Chandrasekaran C, Cooper AD. Evidence of sterol-independent regulation of LDL receptors by a serum factor in Hep-G2 cells. Biochem J. 1991;279:175–87.
125. Grove RI, Mazzucco CF, Radka SF, Shoyab M, Kiener PA. Oncostatin M up-regulates low density lipoprotein receptors in HepG2 cells by a novel mechanism. J Biol Chem. 1991;266:18194–9.
126. Ellsworth JL, Brown C, Cooper AD. Stimulation of LDL receptor activity in HepG2 cells by a serum factor(s). J Cell Physiol. 1988;135:213–23.
127. Rudling M, Norstedt G, Olivecrona H, Reihnér E, Gustafsson J-Å, Angelin B. Importance of growth hormone for the induction of hepatic low density lipoprotein receptors. Proc Natl Acad Sci USA. 1992;89:6983–7.
128. Stopeck AT, Nicholson AC, Mancini FP, Hajjar DP. Cytokine regulation of low density lipoprotein receptor gene transcription in HepG2 cells. J Biol Chem. 1993;268:17489–94.
129. Wilson JM, Grossman M, Wu CH, Chowdhury NR, Wu GY, Chowdhury JR. Hepatocyte-directed gene transfer *in vivo* leads to transient improvement of hypercholesterolemia in low density lipoprotein receptor-deficient rabbits. J Biol Chem. 1992;267:963–7.
130. Krauss RM. Low-density lipoprotein subclasses and risk of coronary artery disease. Curr Opin Lipidol. 1991;2:248–52.
131. Glomset JA. The plasma lecithin: cholesterol acyltransferase reaction. J Lipid Res. 1968;9:155.
132. Barter P. High-density lipoproteins and reverse cholesterol transport. Curr Opin Lipidol. 1993;4:210–17.
133. Tall AR, and Small DM. Plasma high-density lipoproteins. N Engl J Med. 1978;299:1232–6.
134. Hamilton RL, Williams MC, Fielding CT *et al.* Discoidal bilayer structure of nascent high density lipoproteins from perfused rat liver. J Clin Invest. 1976;58:667.
135. Glomset JA, Mitchell CD, King WC *et al. In vitro* effects of lecithin : cholesterol acyltransferase on apolipoprotein distribution in familial lecithin : cholesterol acyltransferase deficiency. Proc NY Acad Sci. 1980;348:224.
136. Jonas A. Lecithin–cholesterol acyltransferase in the metabolism of high-density lipoproteins. Bioch Biophys Acta. 1991;1084:205–20.
137. Assmann G, von Eckardstein A, Funke H. Lecithin : cholesterol acyltransferase deficiency and fish-eye disease. Curr Opin Lipidol. 1991;2:110–17.
138. Fielding PE, Miida T, Fielding CJ. Metabolism of low-density lipoprotein free cholesterol by human plasma lecithin-cholesterol acyltransferase. Biochemistry. 1991;30:8551–7.
139. Miida T, Kawano M, Fielding CJ, Fielding PE. Regulation of the concentration of preβ high-density lipoprotein in normal plasma by cell membranes and lecithin–cholesterol acyltransferase activity. Biochemistry. 1992;31:11112–17.

140. Glomset JA, Norum KR, King WC. Plasma lipoproteins in familial lecithin : cholesterol acryltransferase deficiency. J Clin Invest. 1970;49:1827.
141. Gjone E, Skarbovik AJ, Blomhoff JP. Familial lecithin : cholesterol acyltransferase deficiency: report of a third Norwegian family with two afflicted members. Scand J Clin Lab Invest. 1974;33(suppl. 137):101.
142. Tall AR. Plasma lipid transfer proteins. J Lipid Res. 1986;27:361–7.
143. Agellon LB, Zhang P, Jiang XC, Mendelsohn L, Tall AR. The CCAAT/enhancer-binding protein *trans*-activates the human cholesteryl ester transfer protein gene promoter. J Biol Chem. 1992;267:22336–9.
144. Jiang XC, Agellon LB, Walsh A, Breslow JL, Tall A. Dietary cholesterol increases transcription of the human cholesteryl ester transfer protein gene in transgenic mice. Dependence on natural flanking sequences. J Clin Invest. 1992;90:1290–5.
145. Green PHR, Tall AR, Glickman RM. Rat intestine secretes discoid high density lipoprotein. J Clin Invest. 1978;61:528.
146. Schaefer EJ, Eisenberg S, and Levy RI. Lipoprotein apoprotein metabolism. J Lipid Res. 1978;19:667.
147. Fielding, CJ, and Fielding, PE. Molecular Physiology of Reverse Cholesterol Transport. J. Lipid Res. 1995;36:211–28.
148. Sigurdsson G, Noel S-P, Havel RJ. Quantification of the hepatic contribution to the catabolism of high density lipoproteins in the rat. J Lipid Res. 1979;20:316–24.
149. Andersen JM, Dietschy JM. Regulation of sterol synthesis in adrenal gland of the rat by both high and low density human plasma lipoproteins. Biochem Biophys Res Commun. 1976;72:880–5.
150. Glass C, Pittman RC, Civen M *et al.* Uptake of high-density lipoprotein-associated apoprotein A-I and cholesterol esters by 16 tissues of the rat *in vivo* and by adrenal cells and hepatocytes *in vitro*. J Biol Chem. 1985;260:744.
151. Schwartz CC, Halloran LG, Vlahcevic ZR *et al.* Preferential utilization of free cholesterol from high-density lipoproteins for biliary cholesterol secretion in man. Science. 1978;200:62–4.
152. McKnight GL, Reasoner J, Gilbert T *et al.* Cloning and expression of a cellular high density lipoprotein-binding protein that is up-regulated by cholesterol loading of cells. J Biol Chem. 1992;267:12131–41.

10
Induction of bile acid malabsorption for treatment of hypercholesterolaemia

K. A. EINARSSON

INTRODUCTION

The liver plays a central role in human cholesterol metabolism. A simplified schematic overview is shown in Fig. 1. The liver is thus a key element in regulating the amount of lipoprotein cholesterol in plasma and cholesterol excretion from the body, being the major site of cholesterol synthesis and the principal route for excretion of cholesterol from the body either direct as free cholesterol in the bile or after metabolism to bile acids[1]. About 50% of the endogenous cholesterol synthesis of the human body occurs in the liver, the process being regulated by the rate-limiting enzyme, 3-hydroxy-3-methylglutaryl coenzyme A (HMG-CoA) reductase. Most of the plasma LDL-cholesterol is cleared by the liver, mainly via active uptake by LDL receptors. Cholesterol is secreted into plasma as VLDL-cholesterol. A certain amount is also stored as cholesterol esters in the liver, the esterification reaction being catalysed by the enzyme acylcoenzyme A : cholesterol acyltransferase (ACAT).

The two bile acids primarily formed in human liver are cholic acid – a trihydroxy-bile acid – and chenodeoxycholic acid – a dihydroxy-bile acid – the ratio between the synthesis rates[2] being about 1.5–2. In the intestine the two bile acids are partly 7α-dehydroxylated by bacterial enzymes to give deoxycholic acid and lithocholic acid, respectively. Small amounts of chenodeoxycholic acid are converted into the 7β-epimer ursodeoxycholic acid by microbial enzymes in the intestine. From the intestine the di and trihydroxylated bile acids are very efficiently reabsorbed, mainly by an active process in the distal ileum but also by passive absorption along the whole intestine. The less polar dihydroxy-bile acids are especially taken up from the proximal part of the small intestine. Passive uptake of dihydroxy-bile acids apparently also occurs from the proximal colon. Lithocholic acid is very poorly reabsorbed from the intestine. The bile acids are transported to the liver via the portal vein. In the liver bile acids are very efficiently extracted – cholic acid to a higher extent than dihydroxy-bile acids –

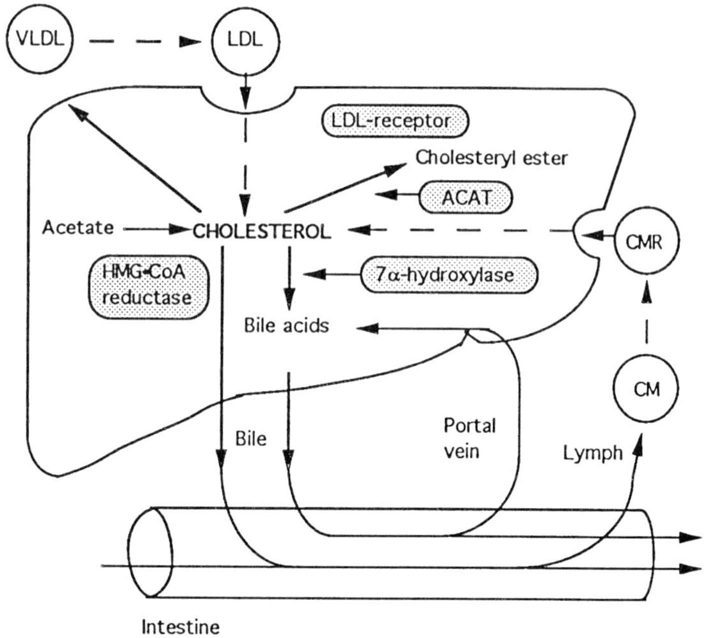

Fig. 1 Simplified scheme of hepatic cholesterol metabolism (see text). ACAT, acylcoenzyme A: cholesterol acyltransferase; 7α-hydroxylase, cholesterol 7α-hydroxylase; CM, chylomicrons; CMR, chylomicron remnants; HMG-CoA reductase, 3-hydroxy-3-methylglutaryl-CoA reductase; LDL, low density lipoproteins; VLDL, very low density lipoproteins

and re-excreted into the bile. The percentage composition of bile acids in human bile is: cholic acid 30–40%, chenodeoxycholic acid 30–40%, deoxycholic acid 20–25%, ursodeoxycholic acid 1–2%, and lithocholic acid 1–2% Because of the more efficient hepatic uptake of cholic acid, the dihydroxy-bile acids will dominate in the peripheral circulation.

The pool of bile acids circulates eight to 10 times a day in the enterohepatic circulation. Only small amounts of bile acids are lost and excreted with faeces per day. The losses are compensated for by new synthesis in the liver. The enterohepatic circulation of bile acids is thus very efficient, and under steady-state conditions the pools of bile acids are kept constant. The most important rate-limiting enzyme in bile acid synthesis is considered to be the hepatic cholesterol 7α-hydroxylase, which catalyses the first step in the conversion of cholesterol to bile acids[3]. The cholesterol 7α-hydroxylase is considered to be regulated by the portal inflow of bile acids to the liver by a sensitive feedback regulation. Not only the total concentration of bile acids in the portal vein but also the composition of individual bile acids is of importance for the regulation of enzyme activity. Thus, chenodeoxycholic acid is a much more potent regulator compared with ursodeoxycholic acid[4].

A partial or complete interruption by biliary drainage may cause a several-fold stimulation of bile acid synthesis. The enterohepatic circulation of bile acids is of great importance, not only for the feedback regulation of their own synthesis, but also for the overall metabolism of cholesterol in the liver. Interruption of the enterohepatic circulation of bile acids will therefore influence the hepatic metabolism of cholesterol in several ways.

This chapter summarizes how treatment with drugs, interfering with bile acid absorption in the intestine, will affect hepatic cholesterol metabolism and plasma lipoprotein levels in humans, with special reference to hypercholesterolaemic conditions.

BILE-ACID-BINDING RESINS

Bile-acid-binding resins have been used in the treatment of hypercholesterolaemia for several years. The two bile acid sequestrants available on the market in Sweden are cholestyramine and colestipol. They bind bile acids in the intestine, prevent their reabsorption and increase faecal bile acid excretion[5]. Both cholestyramine and colestipol have a greater affinity for dihydroxy bile acids than for trihydroxy bile acids *in vitro*[6,7]. Thus, the degree of interruption of the enterohepatic circulation will be higher for chenodeoxycholic acid and deoxycholic acid than for cholic acid. This effect will be further increased by the fact that chenodeoxycholic acid and deoxycholic acid are normally taken up more efficiently than cholic acid in the upper small intestine and thus circulate faster through the enterohepatic circulation[8,9]. This is demonstrated in Fig. 2, which shows that the postprandial serum concentrations of chenodeoxycholic acid and deoxycholic acid were reduced considerably in a healthy subject treated with cholestyramine, whereas the concentration of cholic acid was essentially unchanged. Cholestyramine treatment in a daily dose of 8 g t.i.d. did not change the fasting concentration of total bile acids in five healthy subjects, whereas the postprandial serum concentration of total bile acids was reduced by about 40% (Fig. 3). These results are in agreement with a previous report by Rossi *et al.*[11].

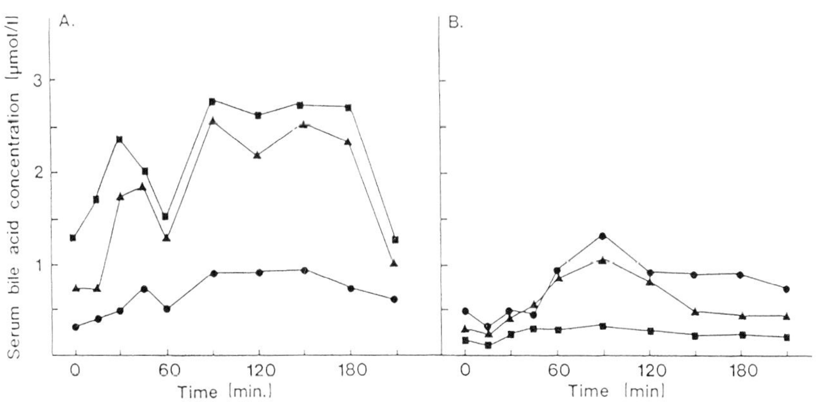

Fig. 2 Postprandial concentrations of cholic acid (●), chenodeoxycholic acid (▲), and deoxycholic acid (■) in a healthy subject during the control period (**A**) and during cholestyramine treatment (**B**). Reproduced with permission from ref. 10

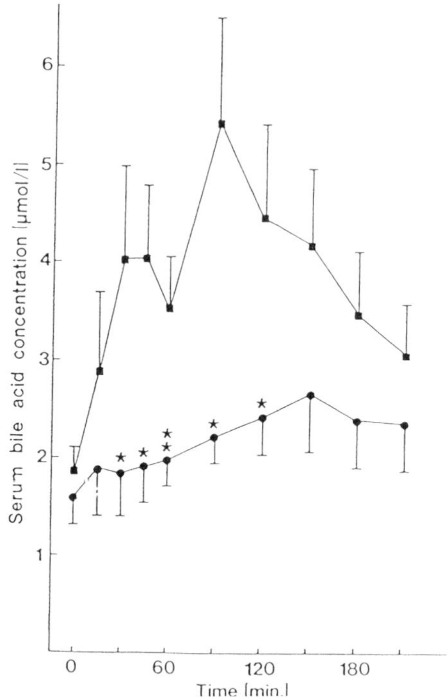

Fig. 3 Means of total postprandial serum bile-acid concentrations (sum of cholic acid, chenodeoxycholic acid, and deoxycholic acid) in eight healthy subjects during control period (■) and during cholestyramine treatment (•). Bars indicate SEM. *$p<0.05$, ** $p<0.01$. Reproduced with permission from ref. 10

These authors found that administration of the bile acid sequestrant colestipol in a daily dose of 5 g t.i.d. reduced the postprandial concentrations of serum bile acids by about 50% in five hypercholesterolaemic subjects. A reduction of the bile acid inflow to the liver by 40–50% is probably sufficient to promote maximal of near-maximal stimulation of bile acid synthesis at least during the day.

Effects on hepatic cholesterol metabolism

The increased faecal loss of bile acids during treatment with bile acid sequestrants is balanced by stimulation of bile acid synthesis[12,13]. This is due to a several-fold increase in the cholesterol 7α-hydroxylase activity as shown in Fig. 4[14]. Bertolotti *et al.*[15] have studied the influence of various doses of cholestyramine on the cholesterol 7α-hydroxylation by an *in-vivo* method. The hydroxylation rate was determined by measuring the increase in body water tritium after intravenous bolus of cholesterol tritiated at the 7α-position. The method assumes that labelled cholesterol mixes homogeneously with the hepatic

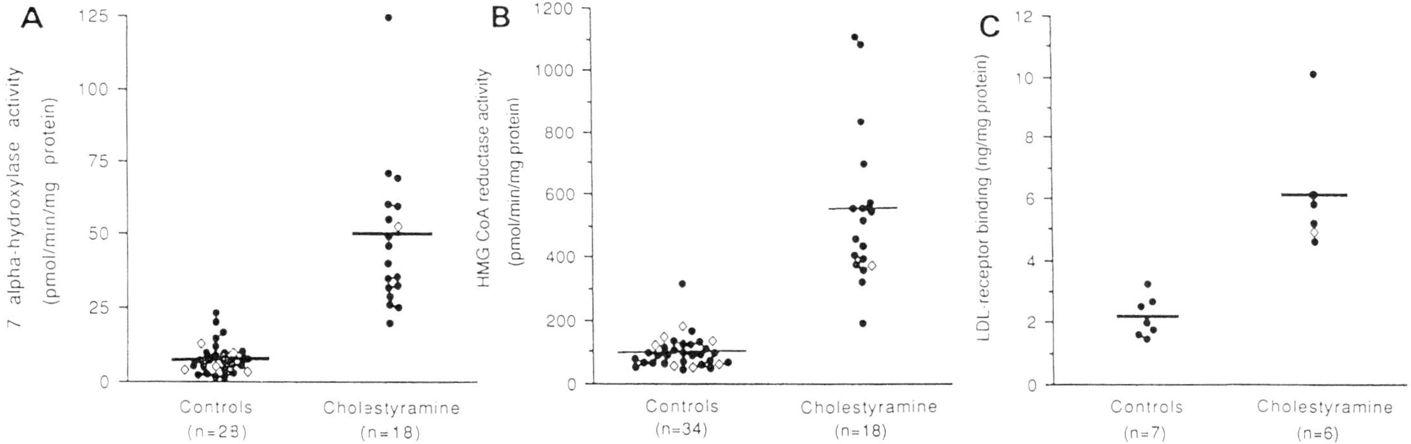

Fig. 4 **A**: Hepatic microsomal cholesterol 7α-hydroxylase activity; **B**: hepatic microsomal HMG-CoA reductase activity, and **C**: hepatic LDL-receptor binding activity in untreated and cholestyramine-treated patients with cholesterol gallstones. Open symbols, males. Horizontal bars indicate means within each group. Reproduced with permission from ref. 14

microsomal pool accessible to cholesterol 7α-hydroxylase. The authors found that cholestyramine induced a dose-related increase of the cholesterol 7α-hydroxylation rate. Recently, antibodies specific for the human cholesterol 7α-hydroxylase have been prepared, making it possible to quantitatively determine the protein mass of the enzyme[16]. In liver microsomes from cholestyramine-treated patients the level of cholesterol 7α-hydroxylase protein was about two-fold higher than those of liver microsomes from untreated patients, indicating a transcriptional control of the enzyme.

The increased bile acid formation causes an enhanced demand for cholesterol in the liver. The liver may respond to this situation in two ways: by an increased cholesterol synthesis and by an enhanced uptake of lipoprotein cholesterol via LDL-receptors. We have been able to examine in human liver the HMG-CoA reductase activity and LDL-receptor binding in relation to the cholesterol 7α-hydroxylase activity[14]. Our results established that cholestyramine treatment considerably stimulates HMG-CoA reductase activity in human liver (Fig. 4). Cholestyramine treatment also stimulates the LDL receptor binding activity (Fig. 4). As is evident from Fig. 4, the degree of stimulation is greater for the HMG-CoA reductase than for the LDL-receptor. From previous animal experiments it has been suggested that the rate of cholesterol synthesis and receptor-dependent LDL uptake in the liver are regulated independently. However, as shown in Fig. 5, our data suggest that the human liver responds to an enhanced demand of cholesterol by a concomitant increase of cholesterol synthesis and LDL receptor expression.

Effects on plasma lipoproteins

The expression of more LDL-receptors in the liver during treatment with cholestyramine and colestipol has been shown to be reflected in a higher frac-

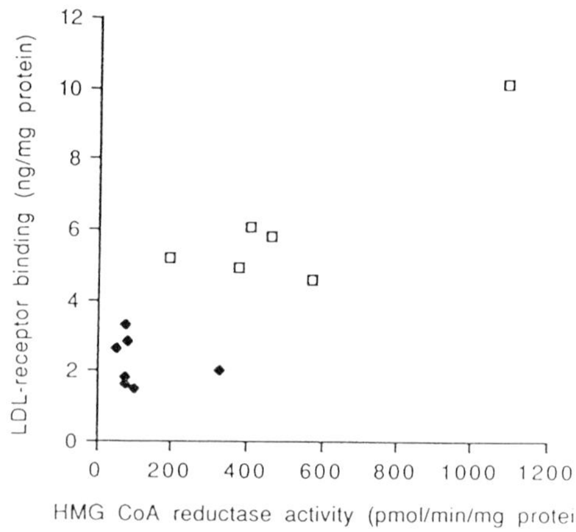

Fig. 5 Relationship between the heparin-sensitive binding activity of LDL and HMG-CoA reductase activity in human liver tissue in seven untreated (◆) and six cholestyramine-treated (□) gallstone patients ($r_s = 0.71$, $p<0.01$). Reproduced with permission from ref. 14

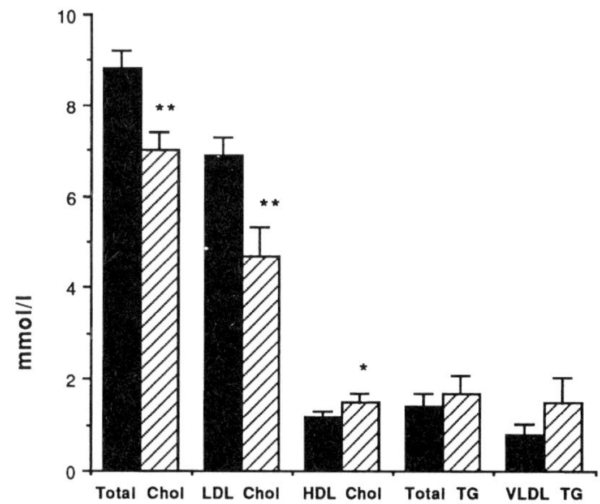

Fig. 6 Plasma lipoprotein profile in serum of patients with familial hypercholesterolaemia during basal conditions (■) and after 6 weeks of cholestyramine treatment at a dose of 8 g b.i.d. (▨). Means ± SEM. * $p<0.05$; ** $p<0.02$. Data from ref. 23

tional catabolic rate (FCR) of LDL in both hypercholesterolaemic patients[17,18] and normolipidaemic subjects[19]. As a consequence the plasma level of LDL-cholesterol may be reduced by up to 20–30% in patients with familial or non-familial hypercholesterolaemia[20–23], as exemplified in Fig. 6. The relatively moderate lowering of plasma LDL-cholesterol often observed during treatment with bile-acid-binding resins may be due to the fact that, in human liver, the capacity of the response is larger for the synthesis of cholesterol than for the expression of the LDL-receptors (Fig. 5).

Treatment with cholestyramine and colestipol is also associated with an increased secretion of VLDL particles into the plasma[23–25]. Simultaneously, the FCR of VLDL is increased, while usually only a moderate rise in the plasma concentration of triglycerides is observed[23,26,27] as demonstrated in Fig. 6. In most patients a compensatory increase in VLDL triglyceride removal occurs while the rise in plasma triglycerides often may be transient.

As mentioned above, treatment with cholestyramine and colestipol is usually associated with only a moderate decrease of the plasma level of LDL-cholesterol. This relative inefficiency of bile-acid-binding resins may have several explanations. First, the binding of bile acids by sequestrant resins is inefficient[28]. Successful treatment with bile acid sequestrants will therefore always need relatively large doses. Efforts to increase binding affinity and capacity, and to improve patient acceptance and compliance by new cholestyramine preparations have hitherto not been successful[29]. Secondly, recent experiments in rodents, by Lillienau *et al.*[30], indicate that maximal active ileal transport is regulated by feedback inhibition, being down-regulated by increased substrate load and up-regulated by decreased substrate load. The addition of cholestyramine to the diet caused an increase in maximal ileal transport of bile acids, the up-regulation requiring 3–4 days. Patients with hypercholesterolaemia who are treated with bile-acid-binding resins might well up-regulate ileal transport of bile acids, with the consequence that ileal absorption is greater for a given intraluminal bile acid concentration, thereby competing with the bile-acid-binding effect of the resins. Thirdly, as mentioned above, human liver responds to cholestyramine treatment with a greater stimulation of the hepatic synthesis of cholesterol compared with the receptor dependent uptake of plasma LDL-cholesterol.

URSODEOXYCHOLIC ACID

Administration of the naturally occurring bile acid ursodeoxycholic acid has also been shown to interfere with the absorption of common bile acids in the small intestine of humans. Thus, Stiehl *et al.*[31] reported that ursodeoxycholic acid given as a single dose of 500 mg decreases the absorption of cholic acid and chenodeoxycholic acid in patients with ileostomy. Previously Nilsell *et al.*[32] showed that feeding patients with ursodeoxycholic acid in a daily dose of 15 mg/kg body weight for 5–6 weeks increases the FCR of both cholic acid and chenodeoxycholic acid. In agreement with the results of Nilsell *et al.*, ursodeoxycholic acid has recently been shown to interfere with the uptake of the taurocholate analogue, SeHCAT (selenium homocholic acid taurine)[33,34]. SeHCAT behaves like the natural conjugated bile acid taurocholic acid in the enterohepatic circulation, with the exception that SeHCAT in only negligible amounts is deconjugated by intestinal bacteria. Eusufzai *et al.*[34] could demonstrate a dose-related interaction with the absorption of SeHCAT, indicating competitive inhibition of this bile acid (Fig. 7). According to two reports the synthesis rates of cholic acid and chenodeoxycholic acid are slightly stimulated following ursodeoxycholic acid administration[31,32].

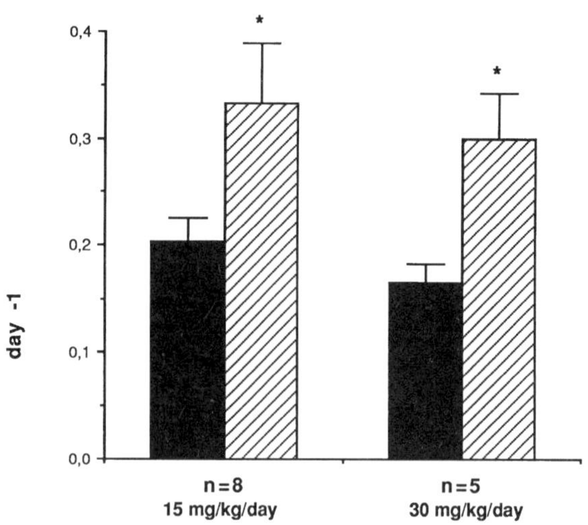

Fig. 7 Effects of treatment with ursodeoxycholic acid at two doses (▨) on fractional catabolic rate of SeHCAT in normal subjects. Means ± SEM * $p<0.05$. Data from ref. 34

Effects on hepatic cholesterol metabolism

Treatment of gallstone patients with ursodeoxycholic acid in a daily dose of 15 mg/kg body weight for 4 weeks prior to cholecystectomy does not significantly affect the cholesterol 7α-hydroxylase activity[4], as is shown in Fig. 8. Similar results have been obtained by Oda *et al.*[35], who treated gallstone patients with ursodeoxycholic acid (600 mg/day) for 7–10 days. In agreement with those results, Bertolotti *et al.*[15] obtained no effect on the 7α-hydroxylation rate of cholesterol in humans – as measured by an *in vivo* method – after ursodeoxycholic acid treatment (9–11 mg/kg body weight per day) for 4–6 weeks.

In a previous study by Angelin *et al.*[36], the administration of ursodeoxycholic acid to gallstone patients in a daily dose of 15 mg/kg body weight for 4 weeks did not significantly affect hepatic HMG-CoA reductase activity. In a more recent study, however, treatment of gallstone patients in the same dose for 3 weeks increased hepatic HMG-CoA reductase activity by about 50% (Fig. 9)[37]. Carulli *et al.*[38] reported that short-term treatment (1 week) with ursodeoxycholic acid treatment may stimulate hepatic HMG-CoA reductase activity in gallstone patients. On the other hand, Maton *et al.*[39] reported that long-term treatment of gallstone patients with ursodeoxycholic acid in a relatively low dose (4.5–7.2 mg/kg body weight per day) resulted in decreased HMG-CoA reductase activity.

To conclude, ursodeoxycholic acid treatment does not usually suppress cholesterol 7α-hydroxylase activity or hepatic HMG-CoA reductase activity. If anything, ursodeoxycholic acid may in some patients stimulate at least HMG-CoA reductase activity.

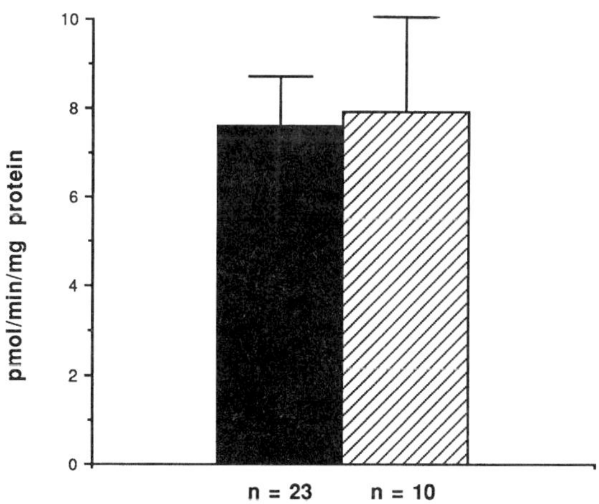

Fig. 8 Microsomal cholesterol 7α-hydroxylase activity in peroperative liver biopsies obtained from untreated gallstone patients (■) and from gallstone patients treated with ursodeoxycholic acid (▨) in a daily dose of 15 mg/kg body weight for 4 weeks prior to cholecystectomy. Means ± SEM. Data from ref. 4

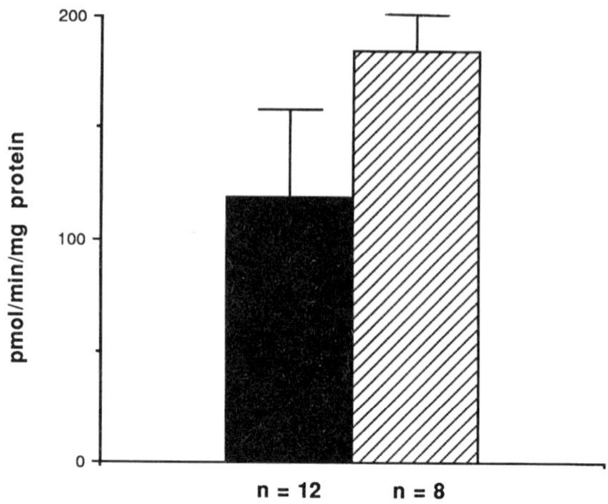

Fig. 9 Microsomal HMG CoA reductase activity in liver biopsies obtained from untreated gallstone patients (■) and gallstone patients treated with ursodeoxycholic acid (▨) in a daily dose of 15 mg/kg body weight for 3 weeks before cholecystectomy. Means ± SEM. Data from ref. 37

Effects on plasma lipoproteins

It has been reported that ursodeoxycholic treatment is associated with beneficial effects on plasma lipoproteins in humans[34,36]. Thus, Eusufzai *et al.*[34] found in healthy subjects that the plasma levels of total and LDL-cholesterol were reduced in a dose-related way[34] (Fig. 10). The plasma levels of HDL-cholesterol and triglycerides remained unchanged. In another study VLDL triglyceride kinetics and plasma lipoprotein levels were determined in nine subjects before

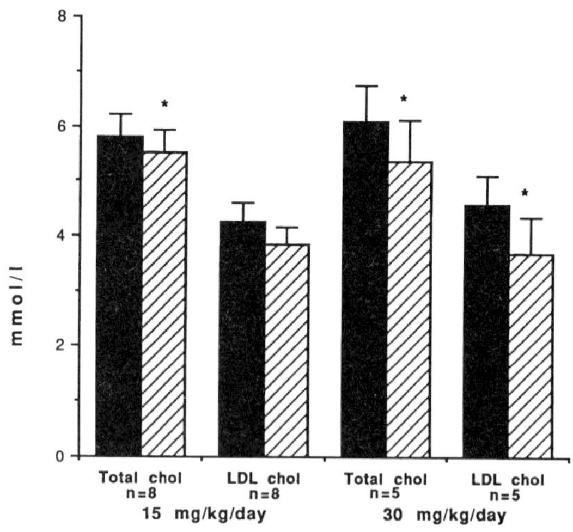

Fig. 10 Effects of treatment with UDCA at two doses (▨) on plasma cholesterol levels in normal subjects. Mean ± SEM. * $p<0.05$. Data from ref. 34

and after 4–6 weeks of treatment with ursodeoxycholic acid at a daily dose of 15 mg/kg body weight[40]. Plasma levels, FCR and formation of VLDL triglycerides were not significantly changed by the treatment.

Beneficial effects of ursodeoxycholic acid treatment on plasma lipoproteins have also been reported in patients with primary biliary cirrhosis (PBC)[41,42]. Although hyperlipoproteinaemia is probably not a risk factor for development of atherosclerosis in patients with PBC[43] it must be of value to know the long-term effects of ursodeoxycholic acid in such patients. In a 2-year placebo-controlled treatment study with ursodeoxycholic acid in 33 patients with PBC, Poupon *et al.*[42] found that ursodeoxycholic acid treatment lowered plasma levels of total cholesterol and LDL cholesterol by about 15% and 20% respectively (Fig. 11). Plasma triglycerides remained essentially unchanged. Similar results were recently reported by Miettinen *et al.*[44] from a randomized placebo-controlled 2-year study in 69 patients with PBC.

Further studies, however, are needed to evaluate the possible role of ursodeoxycholic acid as an adjunct in the treatment of hypercholesterolaemic conditions.

IIEAL BILE ACID TRANSPORT INHIBITORS

The active uptake of bile acids in the ileum is mediated by a sodium-dependent bile acid transport system located at the apical membrane of the ileal epithelial cells. Within the ileocyte, bile acids are transported to the basolateral membrane and secreted into the portal circulation via a sodium-independent organic anion exchange system. Dawson and collaborators have isolated and cloned a sodium-dependent bile acid transporter from hamster ileum[45]. Recently, Dawson also reported on the isolation and cloning of a similar human ileal bile acid transporter[46]. Based on the structure requirements for molecular recognition by the

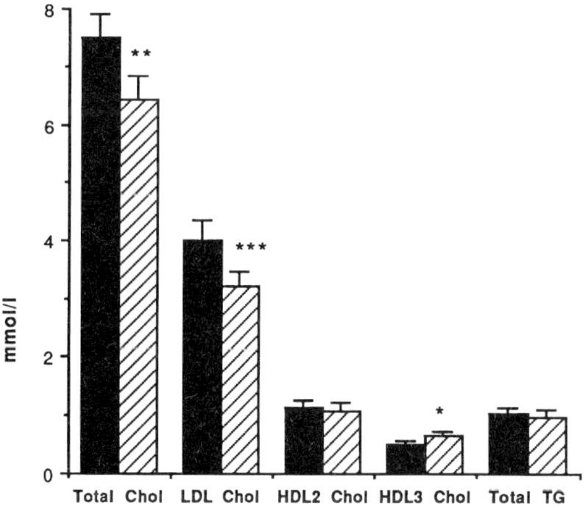

Fig. 11 Effects of treatment with ursodeoxycholic acid (▨) at a daily dose of 13–15 mg/kg body weight for 2 years in patients with primary biliary cirrhosis. Means ± SEM. * $p<0.03$; ** $p<0.02$; *** $p<0.01$. Data from ref. 42

ileal sodium-dependent bile acid transporter, Kramer *et al.* have designed and synthesized specific ileal transport inhibitors[46]. These compounds inhibit bile acid uptake without being absorbed. In the future such pharmacological agents may be developed for clinical use and hopefully may become a new and efficacious therapy for hypercholesterolaemia.

Acknowledgements

I am grateful to Mrs Monia Särd for typing the manuscript, and to the Swedish Medical Research Council (03X-4793) for financial support.

References

1. Turley SD, Dietschy JM. The metabolism and excretion of cholesterol by the liver. In: Arias I, Jacoby W, Popper H, Schachter D, Shafritz D, editors. The liver: biology and pathobiology, 2nd edn. New York: Raven Press; 1988:617–41.
2. Carey MC, Duane WC. Enterohepatic circulation. In: Arias IM, Boyer JL, Fausto N, Jacoby WB, Schachter DA, Shafritz DA, editors. The liver: biology and pathobiology, 3rd edn. New York: Raven Press; 1994:719–67.
3. Einarsson K, Angelin B, Ewerth S, Nilsell K, Björkhem I. Bile acid synthesis in man: assay of hepatic microsomal cholesterol 7α-hydroxylase activity by isotope dilution-mass spectrometry. J Lipid Res. 1986;27:82–8.
4. Reihnér E, Björkhem I, Angelin B, Ewerth S, Einarsson K. Bile acid synthesis in humans: regulation of hepatic microsomal cholesterol 7α-hydroxylase activity. Gastroenterology. 1989;97:1498–505.
5. Grundy SM, Ahrens EH Jr, Salen G. Interruption of the enterohepatic circulation of bile acids in man; comparative effects of cholestyramine and ileal exclusion on cholesterol metabolism. J Lab Clin Med. 1971;78:94–121.
6. Johns WH, Bates TR. Quantification of the binding tendencies of cholestyramine: I. Effect of structure and added electrolytes on the binding of unconjugated and conjugated bile-salt and anions. J Pharm Sci. 1969;58:179–83.
7. Thale M, Faergeman O. Binding of bile acids to anion-exchanging drugs in vitro. Scand J Gastronterol. 1978;13:353–6.
8. Angelin B, Einarsson K, Hellström K. Evidence for the absorption of bile acids in the proximal small intestine of normo- and hyperlipidemic subjects. Gut. 1976;17:420–5.
9. Einarsson KA, Grundy SM, Hardison WGM. Enterohepatic circulation rates of cholic acid and chenodeoxycholic acid in man. Gut. 1979;20:1078–82.
10. Angeline B, Björkhem I, Einarsson K. Ewerth S. Cholestyramine treatment reduces postprandial but not fasting serum bile acid levels in human. Gastroenterology. 1982;83:1097–101.
11. Rossi SS, Wayne ML, Smith RB, Wright CE, Andreadis NA, Hofmann AF. Effect of the bile-acid sequestrant colestipol on postprandial serum bile-acid concentration: evaluation by bioluminescent enzymatic analysis. Aliment Pharmacol Ther. 1989;3:41–6.
12. Einarsson K, Hellström K, Kallner M. The effect of cholestyramine on the elimination of cholesterol as bile acids in patients with hyperlipoproteinaemia type II and IV. Eur J Clin Invest. 1974;4:405–10.
13. Andersén E. The effect of cholestyramine on bile acid kinetics in healthy controls. Scand J Gastroenterol. 1979;14:657–62.
14. Reihnér E, Angelin B, Rudling M, Ewerth S, Björkhem I, Einarsson K. Regulation of hepatic cholesterol metabolism in man: stimulatory effect of cholestyramine on HMG CoA reductase activity and low density lipoprotein receptor expression in gallstone patients. J Lipid Res. 1990;31:2219–26.
15. Bertolotti M, Abate N, Loria P *et al.* Regulation of bile acid synthesis in humans: effect of treatment with bile acids, cholestyramine or simvastatin on cholesterol 7α-hydroxylation rates in vivo. Hepatology. 1991;14:830–7.
16. Maeda Y, Eggertsen G, Nyberg B *et al.* Immunochemical determination of human cholesterol 7α-hydroxylase. Eur J Biochem. 1995;228:144–8.

17. Shepherd J, Packard CJ, Bicker S, Lawrie TDV, Morgan HG. Cholestyramine promotes receptor-mediated low-density lipoprotein catabolism. N Engl J Med. 1980;302:1219–22.
18. Young SG, Witztum JL, Carew TE, Krauss RW, Lindgren FT. Colestipol-induced changes in LDL composition and metabolism. II. Studies in humans. J Lipid Res. 1989;30:225–38.
19. Ericsson S, Eriksson M, Vitols S, Einarsson K, Berglund L, Angelin B. Influence of age on the metabolism of plasma low density lipoproteins in healthy males. J Clin Invest. 1991;87:591–6.
20. Kane JP, Malloy MJ. Treatment of hypercholesterolemia. Med Clin N Am. 1982;66:537–50.
21. Angelin B, Einarsson K. Bile acid and lipoprotein metabolism. Atheroscler Rev. 1986;15:41–66.
22. Illingworth DR, Bacon S. Treatment of heterozygous familial hypercholesterolemia with lipid-lowering drugs. Arteriosclerosis. 1989;9:I-121–34.
23. Angelin B, Leijd B, Hultcrantz R, Einarsson K. Increased turnover of very low density lipoprotein triglyceride during treatment with cholestyramine in familial hypercholesterolaemia. J Intern Med. 1990;227:201–6.
24. Angelin B, Einarsson K, Hellström K. Leijd B. Effects of cholestyramine and chenodeoxycholic acid on the metabolism of endogenous triglyceride in hyperlipoproteinemia. J Lipid Res. 1978;19:1017–24.
25. Beil U, Crouse JR, Einarsson K, Grundy SM. Effects of interruption of the enterohepatic circulation of bile acids on the transport of very low density lipoprotein triglycerides. Metabolism. 1982;31:438–44.
26. Witztum JL, Schonfeld G, Weidman SW. The effects of colestipol on the metabolism of very-low-density lipoproteins in man. J Lab Clin Med. 1976;88:1008–18.
27. Packard CJ, Shepherd J. The hepatobiliary axis and lipoprotein metabolism; effects of bile acid sequestrants and ileal bypass surgery. J Lipid Res. 1982;23:1081–98.
28. Hofmann AF, Schteingart CD, Lillienau J. Biological and medical aspects of active ileal transport of bile acids. Ann Med. 1991;23:169–75.
29. Angelin B. Drugs acting in the gut. Curr Opin Lipidol. 1992;3:40–2.
30. Lillienau J, Crombie DL, Munoz J, Longmire-Cook SJ. Hagey LR, Hofmann AF. Negative feed-back regulation of the ileal bile acid transport systems in rodents. Gastroenterology. 1993;104:38–46.
31. Stiehl A, Raedsch R, Rudolph G. Acute effects of ursodeoxycholic acid and chenodeoxycholic acid on the small intestinal absorption of bile acids. Gastroenterology. 1990;98:420–8.
32. Nilsell K, Angelin B, Leijd B, Einarsson K. Comparative effects of ursodeoxycholic acid and chenodeoxycholic acid on bile acid kinetics and biliary lipid secretion in humans. Evidence for different modes of action on bile acid synthesis. Gastroenterology. 1983;85:1248–56.
33. Marteau P, Chazouillères O, Mayara A, Jian R, Ramboud JC, Poupon R. Effect of chronic administration of ursodeoxycholic acid on ileal absorption of endogenous bile acids in man. Hepatology. 1990;12:1206–8.
34. Eusufzai S, Ericsson S, Cederlund T, Einarsson K, Angelin B. Effects of ursodeoxycholic acid treatment on ileal absorption of bile acids in man as determined by the SeHCAT test. Gut. 1991;32:1044–8.
35. Oda H, Yamashita H, Kosadara K, Kuroki S, Nakayama F. Esterified and total 7α-hydroxy-cholesterol in human serum as an indicator for hepatic bile acid synthesis. J Lipid Res. 1990;31:2209–18.
36. Angelin B, Ewerth S, Einarsson K. Ursodeoxycholic acid treatment in cholesterol gallstone disease: effect on hepatic 3-hydroxy-3-methylglutaryl coenzyme A reductase activity, biliary lipid composition, and plasma lipid levels. J Lipid Res. 1983;24:461–8.
37. Sahlin S, Ahlberg J, Reihnér E, Ståhlberg D, Einarsson K. Cholesterol metabolism in human gallbladder mucosa: relationship to cholesterol gallstone disease and effects of chenodeoxycholic acid and ursodeoxycholic acid treatment. Hepatology. 1992;16:320–6.
38. Carulli N, Ponz de Leon M, Zironi F *et al.* Hepatic cholesterol and bile acid metabolism in subjects with gallstones: comparative effects of short-term feeding of chenodeoxycholic and ursodeoxycholic acid. J Lipid Res. 1980;21:35–43.
39. Maton PN, Ellis HJ, Higgins MJP, Dowling RH. Hepatic HMG CoA reductase in human cholelithiasis: effects of chenodeoxycholic and ursodeoxycholic acids. Eur J Clin Invest. 1980;10:325–32.
40. Angelin B, Nilsell K, Einarsson K. Ursodeoxycholic acid treatment in humans: effects on plasma and biliary lipid metbolism with special reference to very low density lipoprotein triglyceride and bile acid kinetics. Eur J Clin Invest. 1986;16:169–77.

41. Poupon RE, Bakkau B, Eschwège E, Poupon R and the UDCA-PBC Study Group. A multicenter trial of ursodiol for the treatment of primary biliary cirrhosis. N Engl J Med. 1991;324:1548–54.
42. Poupon RE, Ouguerram K, Chrétien Y *et al.* Cholesterol-lowering effect of ursodeoxycholic acid in patients with biliary cirrhosis. Hepatology. 1993;17:577–82.
43. Crippin JS, Lindor KD, Jörgenson R *et al.* Hypercholesterolemia and atherosclerosis in primary biliary cirrhosis: what is the risk? Hepatology. 1992;15:858–62.
44. Miettinen TA, Färkkilä M, Vuoristo M *et al.* Serum cholestanol, cholesterol precursors, and plant sterols during placebo-controlled treatment of primary biliary cirrhosis with ursodeoxycholic acid or colchicine. Hepatology. 1995;21:1261–8.
45. Wong MH, Oelkers P, Craddock AL, Dawson PA. Expression cloning and characterization of the hamster ileal sodium-dependent bile acid transporter. J Biol Chem. 1994;269:1340–7.
46. Stiehl A, Raedsch R, editors. XIII International Bile Acid Meeting. Bile Acids in Gastroenterology: Basic and Clinical Advances; 30 Sept–2 Oct 1994; San Diego. Congress Short Report, Falk Sympoium No. 80;1995:22.

11
Direct effects of bile acids on low-density lipoprotein cholesterol metabolism

H. FROMM, B. BOUSCAREL, S. CERYAK and M. MALAVOLTI

INTRODUCTION

Bile acid and cholesterol metabolism are closely connected. The most important connection relates to the fact that bile acids are synthesized from cholesterol. The rate of bile acid synthesis represents a major modulator of cholesterol catabolism. Increased intestinal bile acid loss – due to either ileal dysfunction (ileal disease/resection) or cholestyramine treatment – leads to a compensatory up-regulation of bile acid synthesis, with consequent stimulation of cholesterol synthesis and LDL receptor activity[1–3]. Although in some animal species, such as the rat, bile acid synthesis increases with cholesterol feeding, in humans the surplus cholesterol provides little stimulus to the rate of bile acid synthesis (albeit there are individual differences in responsiveness to a high-cholesterol diet). In other words, cholesterol synthesis increases with bile acid synthesis, but the reverse is generally not the case in humans.

While these relationships between bile acids and cholesterol are well appreciated, the existence of other important interactions between these two steroids have only relatively recently come into focus.

IN-VIVO EVIDENCE FOR DIRECT BILE ACID EFFECT

The original observations that suggested a direct action of certain bile acids on the LDL receptor were made in a hamster model[4]. Male golden Syrian hamsters were fed a 0.027% cholesterol rodent chow diet. Three groups of hamsters were studied. One received the diet alone for 4 weeks (control). The other two groups received, in addition, 0.1% chenodeoxycholic acid (CDCA) and ursodeoxycholic acid (UDCA), respectively. Light-microscopic examinations of the liver of randomly chosen animals from the different groups showed no significant histological abnormalities. Each study on a given day featured one animal from each group in a randomized sequence.

[^{14}C]Sucrose-labelled hamster LDL and methylated human LDL were studied. While hamster LDL is taken up in the tissues by both LDL receptor-dependent and LDL receptor-independent mechanisms, methylated human LDL is taken up through LDL receptor-independent pathways. Two types of LDL infusion experiments were conducted. In one study a bolus containing 20 μg of LDL proteins was injected, followed by a constant infusion for 1 h at a rate of 1 μg of protein in 70 μl/min. This infusion resulted in constant plasma levels of ^{14}C radioactivity. In order to study LDL uptake under conditions of optimal challenge to the LDL receptor, a second type of study was carried out. In these experiments the injection of a bolus of 5, 20, and 40 μg, respectively, of hamster LDL protein was followed by a 15-min constant infusion of [^{14}C]Sucrose-labelled hamster LDL at a rate of 0.25, 1.0, and 2.0 μg/min, respectively. Similar concentrations of [^{14}C]sucrose-labelled methylated human LDL were infused to assess the LDL receptor-independent uptake of LDL. [^{14}C]Sucrose-labelled albumin infusions were carried out to determine the albumin tissue space. The LDL tissue uptake was calculated by subtracting the [^{14}C]albumin tissue space from the [^{14}C]LDL tissue space.

In addition to the LDL uptake studies, both biliary and faecal bile acids were analysed by gas-liquid chromatography.

The results of the studies showed that, in the liver, which constituted by far the largest uptake of LDL in the body, the LDL receptor-dependent uptake was significantly higher in the UDCA-fed animals than in either the control or CDCA-fed hamsters.

It is of interest that, both in the CDCA- and UDCA-fed animals, CDCA became the major bile acid in bile, with mean values of 71% and 55%, respectively. The UDCA level in the UDCA-treated animals rose only to 17%, indicating marked biotransformation (epimerization) of UDCA to CDCA. As one would expect from the increase of CDCA in the enterohepatic circulation of the CDCA- and UDCA-treated animals, bile acid synthesis was markedly suppressed in these two animal groups, as evidenced by a marked reduction of total endogenous faecal bile acids (total faecal bile acids minus fed bile acids) in comparison to the control group.

Since UDCA induced a LDL receptor-dependent LDL uptake in the liver, in spite of a marked suppression of bile acid synthesis, the data suggest a direct effect of UDCA on the LDL receptor. UDCA feeding was also associated with a decrease in serum LDL. However, this decrease was not statistically significant. While serum HDL fell significantly in the CDCA-treated animals, it remained at the control level during UDCA treatment.

IN-VITRO EVIDENCE FOR DIRECT BILE ACID EFFECT

Freshly isolated hamster hepatocytes were used to test our hypothesis, derived from the *in-vivo* studies, that certain bile acids, such as UDCA, have the ability to exert a direct action on LDL uptake[5].

For *binding* experiments, hepatocytes were incubated at 4°C with increasing concentrations of [^{125}I]-labelled hamster LDL (1–70 μg/ml) in the presence and absence of the respective bile acid. Non-specific binding was determined by incubating the hepatocytes under the same conditions, but with an excess of unlabelled native human LDL (1.6 mg/ml). Experiments had shown that the results were similar regardless of whether native human LDL or hamster LDL was used to determine the non-specific binding. Specific binding was calculated by subtracting non-specific binding from total binding. Non-specific binding represented about 30% of total binding. In the presence of 1 mmol/l UDCA, the B_{max} of the specific LDL binding increased by 36% to 31.9 ± 1.5 ng/mg of cells without significant change in the K_d value. The effect of UDCA on specific LDL binding was transient, reversible, and concentration-dependent at a maximal level at 1 mmol/l.

Cell-associated LDL was measured at 37°C after incubation of hepatocytes with either [^{125}I]hamster LDL or [^{125}I]methylated human LDL, with or without the addition of the respective bile acid. Internalized LDL was distinguished from that specifically bound by further incubating the hepatocytes with Pronase for 1 h at 4°C. In the presence of 1 mmol/l UDCA the maximum binding and internalization of [^{125}I]hamster LDL increased significantly from a control level of 14 ± 3 ng/mg of cells to 23 ± 4 ng/mg of cells. Thus, UDCA increased cell-associated [^{125}I]hamster LDL by 60%. The effect of UDCA was concentration-dependent at a maximal level at 1 mmol/l. UDCA did not influence cell-associated [^{125}I]methylated human LDL.

LDL degradation was assessed by quantifying the radioactivity present in free iodotyrosine residues in the incubation medium, as described by Goldstein *et al.*[6]. The cellular degradation of LDL increased in a time-dependent manner and paralleled that of LDL uptake. With 1 mmol/l-UDCA it increased about 2 and 3.5 times, respectively, at 60 min and 120 min.

Several UDCA analogues were studied to assess the *structural requirements* for bile acids to affect [^{125}I](hamster LDL) binding and internalization. While the taurine and glycine conjugates of UDCA had effects very similar to those of free UDCA, nor-UDCA (lack of C-24), cholic acid and ursocholic acid did not increase LDL binding. These experiments indicate that, in addition to the presence of a 7β-hydroxy group, other very specific structural requirements have to be met for UDCA to affect LDL binding and uptake.

STUDIES OF THE MECHANISMS OF UDCA-INDUCED HEPATOCELLULAR LDL BINDING

Studies were also carried out in the hamster to gain information on the mechanism through which UDCA affects the LDL receptor[7]. These studies showed that chronic feeding of UDCA in this animal did not result in changes of the composition of the lipoprotein particle. There was also no change in either the release of lipids from the liver plasma membrane into the medium or in the hepatocellular lipid composition after 10 and 120 min incubation of the liver cells with UDCA. In isolated liver membrane fractions, UDCA increased both B_{max} and K_d for LDL by about 35%. These findings suggest that UDCA stimulates the LDL receptor at the plasma membrane level independent of an effect on LDL-receptor cycling. The action of UDCA could be explained by recruitment of cryptic receptors from a cellular membrane pool, possibly due to the unique localization of this bile acid in the plasma membrane lipid layer.

In summary, all *in-vivo* and *in-vitro* studies in the hamster model consistently show that UDCA stimulates the LDL-receptor. They also indicate this effect on the LDL-receptor to take place at the hepatocellular plasma membrane level without evidence for changes in the lipid composition of either the lipoprotein particle or liver membrane. Although relatively moderate, the effect of UDCA on the LDL-receptor may be important not only in relation to the induction of beneficial changes in LDL metabolism, but also in the context of membrane stabilization, which has been described by other authors to underlie the hepatoprotective action of UDCA[8].

References

1. Brown MS, Goldstein JL. Lipoprotein receptors in the liver: control signals for plasma cholesterol traffic. J Clin Invest. 1983;72:743–7.
2. Shepherd J, Packard CJ, Bicker S, Lawrie TDV, Morgan HG. Cholestyramine promotes receptor-mediated low density lipoprotein catabolism. N Engl J Med. 1980;302:1219–22.
3. Fromm H. Gallstone dissolution and the cholesterol–bile acid–lipoprotein axis. Propitious effects of ursodeoxycholic acid. Gastroenterology. 1984;87:229–33.
4. Malavolti M, Fromm H, Ceryak S, Roberts I. Modulation of low density lipoprotein receptor activity by bile acids: differential effects of chenodeoxycholic and ursodeoxycholic acids in the hamster. J Lipid Res. 1987;28:1281–95.
5. Bouscarel B, Fromm H, Ceryak S, Cassidy MM. Ursodeoxycholic acid increases low-density lipoprotein binding, uptake and degradation in isolated hamster hepatocytes. Biochem J. 1991;280:589–98.
6. Goldstein JL, Basu SK, Brown MS. Receptor-mediated endocytosis of low-density lipoproteins in cultured cells. Methods Enzymol. 1983;98:241–60.
7. Bouscarel B, Ceryak S, Robins S, Fromm H. Studies of the mechanism of the ursodeoxycholic acid-induced increase in hepatic low-density lipoprotein binding. Lipids. 1995 (In press)
8. Guldutuna S, Zimmer G, Imhof M, Bhatti S, You T, Leuschner U. Molecular aspects of membrane stabilization by ursodeoxycholic acid. Gastroenterology. 1993;104:1736–44.

Section IV
Pathogenesis of Cholesterol Gallstones

12 Formation and growth of cholesterol gallstones: the new synthesis

M. C. CAREY

INTRODUCTION

While the aetiologies of cholesterol gallstones are becoming clearer[1], the pathogenetic mechanisms for their formation are still uncertain[2–4]. A paradigm was introduced in 1989[5] that became something of a cliché rather than having a short half-life[6]. In the 'new paradigms'[5], a trinity of defects was proposed to explain cholesterol gallstone formation, namely cholesterol supersaturation, gallbladder hypomotility and rapid nucleation, all in the presence of a mucin gel[4]. Nonetheless, this older paradigm is non-durable in understanding cholesterol gallstone formation today and necessitates a conceptual and thematic revision to unify the pathophysiological model[7]. This has been prompted by several recent pathogenetic insights (reviewed in References 8 and 9) as well as by the identification of a triplet of *Lith* genes responsible for this complex trait in inbred mice[10]. It appears now that sustained cholesterol supersaturation of bile, an unambiguous hepatic defect[4,11,12], is responsible for most, but certainly not all, ancillary defects in the hepatobiliary tree[7]. These downstream defects include gallbladder hypomotility and accelerated nucleation and other perturbations in addition to the pathogenic trio[4,5] such as altered circulatory dynamics of the enterohepatic circulation of bile salts[12] and its corollary, profound changes in physicochemical properties of biliary lipids[4,9] that appear to augment the lithogenic state[7]. Moreover, the gallstone-susceptible mouse[10] is teaching us that one or more products of the *Lith* genes may influence gallbladder function as well as bile salt metabolism directly[9].

What follows is an attempt to place these evolutionary concepts in perspective and to marshall evidence that molecular cholesterol injury to the gallbladder mucosa and muscle has drastic homeostatic consequences on the functioning of the hepatobiliary system[7–9] as well as the enterohepatic circulation of bile salts[13,14]. In light of recent data[15], it is tempting to suggest that these influences may not only amplify the lithogenic state but could perpetuate it.

KEY ELEMENTS

In one way or another, it has been known for over 100 years that, in all gallstone disease (reviewed in Reference 16), bile is supersaturated because of metabolic defects in hepatic lipid processing. It was known also for a long time that there was stasis in the biliary tree, nucleation at 'interfaces' and accumulation of excess mucin. In modern pathophysiological parlance, this has been codified[4,5,7–9] for cholesterol stones (Figure 1) as sustained cholesterol supersaturation from hepatic hypersecretion, gallbladder hypomotility and rapid nucleation and phase transitions, all in the setting of accumulated mucin gel[7]. Each of these defects may vary in severity[17] but it is now believed that sustained cholesterol supersaturation is likely to set the vicious cycle in motion[7]. Although likely, it is not known whether a severe degree of cholesterol supersaturation will lead to heightened severity of the other defects. Nevertheless, molecular and pathophysiological explanations for all defects (Figure 1) are becoming clearer[7–9].

CHOLESTEROL SUPERSATURATION

This is caused by hepatic hypersecretion of cholesterol and not hyposecretion of bile salts[12,18]. The pie diagram (Figure 2) shows the solute composition of human gallbladder and hepatic bile in health. However, as shown by the quantitative biliary lipid compositions of gallbladder biles (Table 1) from two large studies[7,19], moles percent biliary cholesterol is 28% increased in biles of gall-

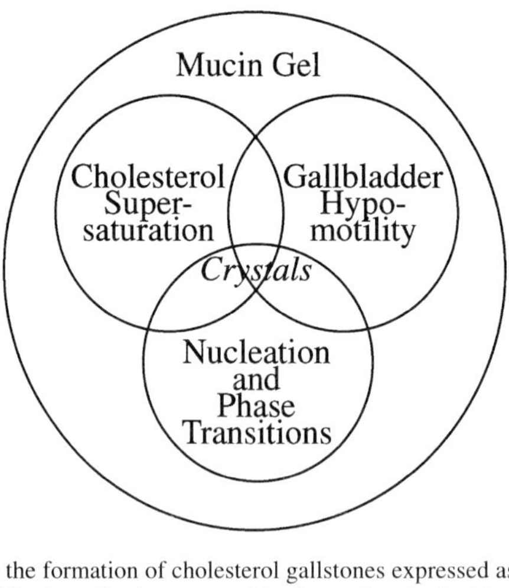

Fig. 1 Key elements in the formation of cholesterol gallstones expressed as a Venn diagram within a matrix of mucin gel. The hypothesis proposed in the review is that hepatic cholesterol hypersecretion into bile is the primary defect and is the outcome in part of a complex genetic trait[10]. The downstream effects of molecular cholesterol injury include gallbladder hypomotility and early nucleation and phase transitions. A major non-obvious result of gallbladder hypomotility is alteration in the kinetics of the enterohepatic circulation of bile salts (discussed in text)

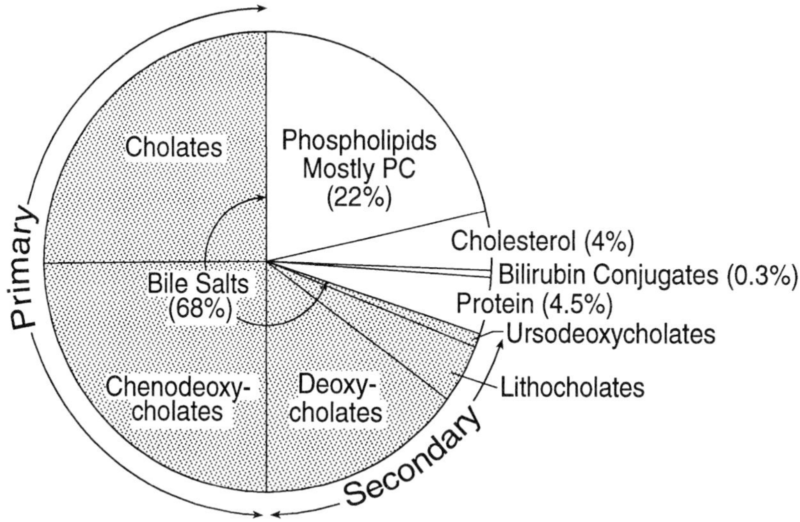

Fig. 2 Pie diagram showing proportions of the principal solutes in hepatic as well as gallbladder bile of humans. In the lithogenic state, the proportions of cholesterol are increased at the expense of total bile salt and phospholipid. In addition, hydrophobic secondary bile salts increase at the expense of their primary precursors. Proteins also expand in percentage and the pattern changes. Phospholipid molecular species and bilirubin conjugates appear to remain relatively stable (modified from Reference 12 with permission)

Table 1 Biliary lipid composition of gallbladder biles[a]

	Controls[b] (n = *545*)	*Stones*[b] (n = *196*)	*Controls*[c] (n = *23*)	*Stones*[c] (n = *48*)
Biliary lipid classes (moles %)				
Bile salts	72.0	70.5	71.6	69.2
Phospholipids (mostly PC)[d]	21.1	20.6	20.6	20.8
Cholesterol	6.9	8.8	7.8	10.0
Cholesterol saturation index	1.0	1.3	1.1	1.4
Ratios of lipid classes				
Cholesterol/phospholipid	0.34	0.45	0.38	0.48
Phospholipid/bile salt	0.30	0.30	0.29	0.30
Cholesterol/bile salt	0.10	0.13	0.11	0.14

[a]Adapted with permission from *American Journal of Surgery*[7];
[b]from Reference 19;
[c]from G. Salvioli and M. C. Carey (1982), unpublished observations;
[d]PC represents phosphatidylcholine

stone subjects compared with controls. The reciprocal decreases in the other lipids, bile salts and phosphatidylcholine (lecithin), the principal phospholipid of bile, is generally uniform. In gallstone disease, there are significant quantitative changes in other biliary components (Figure 2), particularly a reported increase in total protein content[20,21], definite increases in proportions of secondary bile salts[11,13], possibly qualitative changes in the pattern of biliary proteins[4] and variations in lecithin molecular species[4,22].

LIPID PARTICLES IN BILE

Bile is a complex fluid since none of the lipids are in true solution save for a small millimolar concentration of bile salts[23]. This monomeric concentration is distinct from 'the critical micellar concentration'[24] because it is the monomeric fraction of the inter-mixed micellar/vesicular bile salt concentration, i.e. that fraction of bile salts not associated with lecithin or cholesterol[25]. The majority of biliary lipids are heteroaggregated into three types of particles that are shown schematically in Figure 3[12,23]. The smallest of these, named simple micelles, are approximately 1–2 nm in radius[26]. They are composed principally of bile salt molecules with very small numbers of cholesterol and possibly a few lecithin molecules, all in an assembly of unknown structure. The medium-sized particles are mixed micelles of radius approximately 2–4 nm[26]. They are composed principally of lecithin molecules with smaller amounts of bile salt and modest numbers of cholesterol molecules[24]. Although shown here as block diagrams to suggest 'mixed disc' micelles[27], their fine structure is not known. Nevertheless, when mixed micelles enlarge, they elongate to rods[28,29] or 'worm-like'[30] particles in which the lecithin molecules are oriented radially like 'spokes-on-a-wheel' with bile salt molecules acting as both wedges between lecithin's head-groups and also serving as 'end-caps'[30]. Physiologically, unsaturated bile (Figure 3) is composed of a mixture of simple and mixed micelles[31,32]. Because

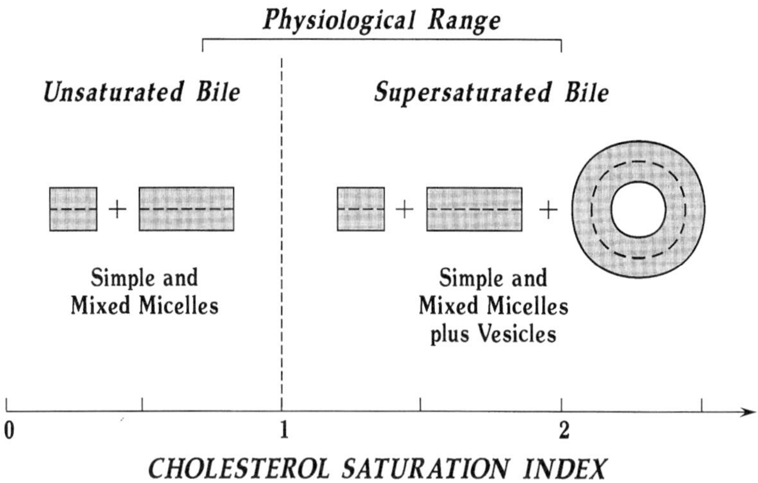

Fig. 3 Schematic block diagram to indicate distribution of lipid particles (simple micelles, mixed micelles and unilamellar vesicles) in human bile in relation to the physiological range of the cholesterol saturation index (CSI). Although supersaturated bile (CSI>1) is bile with persistent vesicles, vesicles can also be observed in all unsaturated biles (CSI<1) but they are transient (from Reference 11 with permission)

micelles are thermodynamically stable, they can never nucleate cholesterol molecules under any pathophysiological circumstance, provided temperature, pressure and composition are held constant[24]. The cholesterol saturation index (CSI) of such biles[33] is less than unity (Figure 3).

The third particle[34] responsible for the carriage of cholesterol in bile is a unilamellar vesicle (Figure 3). Before this was understood, the non-micellar state of cholesterol in model bile was called aptly a 'microprecipitate' particle[35]. The reported radii of vesicles in bile varies from 25 to 80 nm[36,37] but they are of uniform size in a particular bile. Clearly, vesicles are not only much bigger than micelles but have a distinct and well-accepted supramolecular structure[38]. Vesicles (Figure 3) are like miniscule golf balls composed of a spherical lipid shell enclosing a water core in which all the electrolytes of bile are dissolved[23]. As will be discussed below, bile is formed from vesicles which 'bud-off' the canalicular membrane at the level of the hepatocyte[39] and apparently they carry proteins from the canalicular membrane[40]. Although vesicles may be present transiently[41] in bile with a CSI ≤1, their persistence is the hallmark of supersaturated bile[42], i.e. bile with a CSI >1 (Figure 3). Vesicles that persist in hepatic and gallbladder biles are greatly enriched with cholesterol as was first shown for model systems[35]. For this reason, persistent vesicles are unstable in bile and are responsible for initiating the nucleation of cholesterol crystals[43] although it is likely that coexisting micelles play an auxillary role[44] because they are also supersaturated[42]. Supersaturation of vesicles means a cholesterol to phospholipid ratio >1 and supersaturation of micelles implies a cholesterol to phospholipid ratio >0.25–3[42].

CANALICULAR VESICLES AND BILE FORMATION

Figure 4 displays the morphology of biliary lipid secretion using ultrafast tissue-vitrification technology and electron spectroscopic imaging[39]. It is clear (Figure 4) that bile formation begins as vesicles on the luminal surfaces of the canalicular membranes, as was suspected previously[41]. The molecular mechanisms for vesicle formation on the luminal side of the membranes are not known, but a canalicular lecithin transmembrane translocator, the putative mdr2 P-glycoprotein of the mouse[45,46], apparently 'flips' biliary-specific lecithin molecules from inner to outer hemileaflets of the membrane. The activity of this so-called 'flippase' is likely to create localized high-pressure patches on the exoplasmic leaflet of the membrane, resulting in membrane asymmetry. These patches of lecithin molecules can easily buckle and vesiculate, particularly under the influence of a monomeric or micellar bile salt concentration which is present within the canalicular lumen[47,48]. It is believed that, following transport across the canalicular membrane as monomers by specific transporting proteins[12], bile salt molecules partition back in a 4 : 1 ratio into the lipids of the exoplasmic hemileaflet of the canalicular membrane[49] but are incapable of spontaneously 'flip-flopping'[50] to the cytoplasmic side. Therefore, just as detergents do in the 'laundering' process[51], bile salt molecules are capable of exerting a true detergent action on membrane phospholipids via a 'roll-up process' followed by the elution of biliary specific lecithins as unilamellar vesicles into the canalicular lumen[39,48].

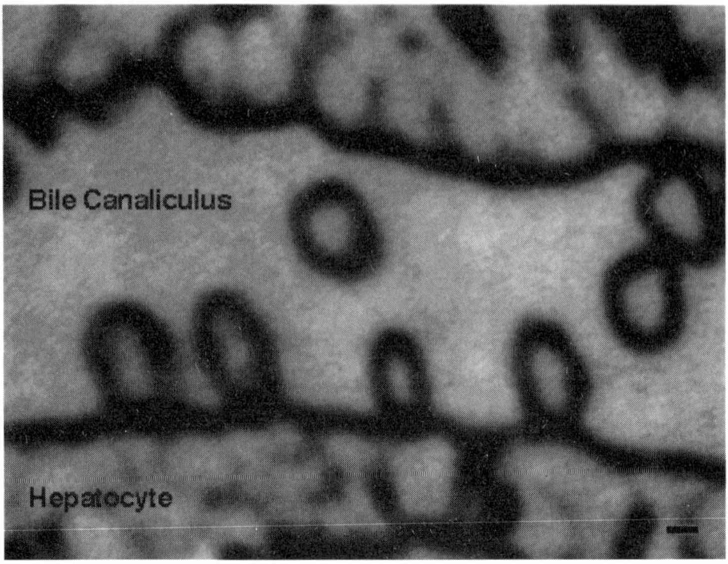

Fig. 4 Photomicrograph showing an electron spectroscopic image of a cryofixed canaliculus in a rat liver in the process of secreting biliary lipid vesicles. These are seen as ovals affixed to, and most likely formed from, the exoplasmic leaflet of the canalicular membrane. The bar represents 25 nm (From Reference 39 with permission)

FORMATION OF THE MATURE PHYSICAL STATE OF BILE

My colleagues and I have detailed elsewhere[52] the important role of the triangular phase diagram for bile salt–lecithin–water systems, established by Small and colleagues 30 years ago[53], in understanding the origin of the mature physical–chemical state of bile. Mixing of bile salt monomers and unilamellar vesicles in the canalicular space does not drastically affect vesicle morphology except for rendering the population of vesicles uniform in size[49]. However, with increases in lipid concentration, such as in the canals and collecting ductules that drain the canaliculi[12], vesicles are transformed first into rod-shaped particles followed by their size reduction to the radii (~1–4 nm) of micelles in mature hepatic and gallbladder biles[52]. If the overall composition of bile[33] has a CSI>1, then there is an insufficient bile salt concentration present to dissolve all vesicles produced at the canalicular level[48,54]. As displayed in Figure 5, this results in persistance of vesicles with increases in their cholesterol content by removal into mixed micelles of lecithin molecules in excess of cholesterol molecules[42,49]. This occurs simply because micelles have a 4-fold greater capacity for solubilization of phospholipid than cholesterol molecules. This is evidenced by the shape of the micellar zone in the corresponding triangular phase diagram for bile salt–lecithin–cholesterol systems at fixed percent H_2O[55]. As shown in Figure 5, more hydrophobic bile salts, by virtue of their lower critical micellar concentrations, are more efficient than hydrophilic bile salts in achieving these results[49]. A corollary to this is that vesicles with a

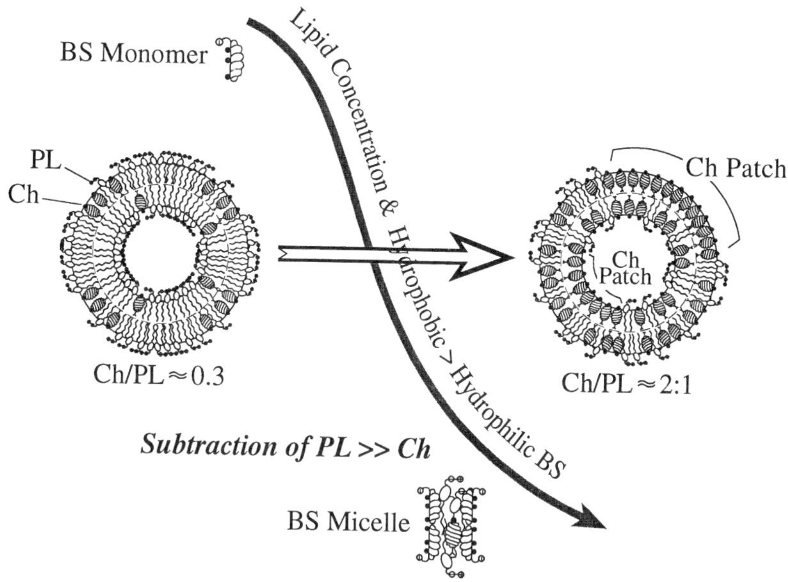

Fig. 5 Schematic depiction of the enrichment of cholesterol (Ch)-unsaturated biliary vesicles by bile salts (BS) by virtue of biliary phospholipid (PL) (lecithin) molecules being subtracted from vesicles and solubilized in micelles more efficiently than cholesterol molecules. This occurs in the proximal biliary tree when the total lipid concentration [TL] increases and bile salt micelles form. The process is more efficient for hydrophobic compared with hydrophilic bile salts. This schema is a logical result of the phase relationships of bile salt–lecithin–cholesterol–water systems described in Reference 55. The cholesterol supersaturated vesicles have a Ch/PL ratio (2 : 1) twice as large as the equimolar ratio observed at equilibrium[56]

cholesterol : phospholipid ratio of 0.34–0.38, typical of canalicular vesicles in health (Table 1), can metamorphose into vesicles with a 2 : 1 lipid ratio, i.e 100% supersaturation with cholesterol, in lithogenic gallbladder biles[56]. In cholesterol gallstone disease, cholesterol hypersecretion[18] which, at the canalicular level, is presumably via nascent vesicles[39] and possibly micelles[57], increases the overall cholesterol to phospholipid ratio of canalicular vesicles to values of 0.45–48 (Table 1). Hence, in the lithogenic state, vesicles in both hepatic and gallbladder biles should become supersaturated earlier, carry more cholesterol than in health, and be more populous than in normal bile. These simple facts are logical deductions from a knowledge of the degree of biliary cholesterol hypersecretion[18] and the phase equilibria of bile[55] but have not received the attention they deserve in understanding the instability of bile in cholesterol gallstone disease.

HEPATIC CHOLESTEROL METABOLISM

Although biliary cholesterol hypersecretion is clearly a hepatic defect (Figure 6), its cause is not understood[12]. In enzyme assays of microsomes prepared from liver biopsies obtained at surgery (peripheral mononuclear cells have been employed as a surrogate[58]), it is usually found that the activity of 3-hydroxy-3-methylglutaryl-CoA (HMGCoA) reductase, the rate-limiting enzyme in cholesterol synthesis, is increased significantly[58–62]. However, in three studies[63–65], no change was found, whereas, in two studies[66,67], there were significant reductions in HMGCoA reductase activity. The activity of microsomal cholesterol 7α-hydroxylase, the rate-limiting enzyme in bile salt synthesis was reported to be lower than controls in earlier studies[58–61], particularly on a high-cholesterol diet[58], but was normal[65] or significantly higher[67] in recent studies. The activity of acyl-CoA : cholesterol acyltransferase (ACAT) that catalyses cholesteryl ester synthesis for VLDL production (Figure 6) has been less well studied. ACAT assays of liver microsomes from cholesterol gallstone subjects have shown either no change[65] or a significant diminution[68] in activity compared with controls. However, three very important sources of cholesterol for the liver cell and potentially for bile have not yet been assayed (Figure 6); they are the receptors that draw cholesterol from blood into liver[69] and that control, therefore, the endocytosis of LDL, chylomicra remnants and absorption of the various components of HDL.

CHOLESTEROL GALLSTONE-SUSCEPTIBLE INBRED MOUSE

Together with colleagues at The Jackson Laboratory in Maine, we discovered by genetic analysis that susceptibility to cholesterol gallstone formation in the inbred laboratory mouse is the result of the combined action of three *Lith* genes[10] located on mouse chromosomes 2, 10 and 19. Presuming homology with the human genome, the *Lith* genes in gallstone patients should be on

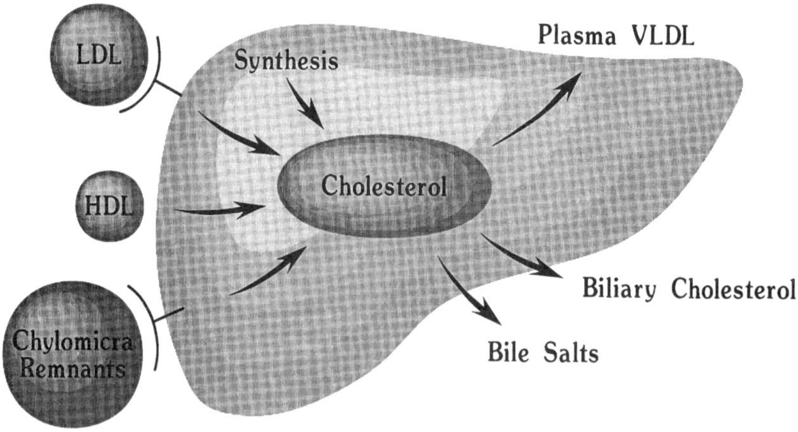

Fig. 6 Hepatic cholesterol metabolism: sources of hepatic cholesterol molecules are by means of plasma lipoproteins (LDL = low density lipoproteins, HDL = high density lipoproteins) and de-novo synthesis. Pathways for cholesterol disposition and secretion are via plasma VLDL (very low density lipoproteins) and the biliary steroids (discussed in text)

chromosomes 2, 6 and 10[8]. Currently, the functions of these genes are unknown but they do not appear to be structural genes for any lipid regulatory enzyme[10]. When fed a lithogenic diet containing 15% dairy fat, 1% cholesterol and 0.1% cholic acid for 4 weeks, mouse strains with the normal alleles do not supersaturate their biles but do accumulate small amounts of mucus gel and occasionally liquid crystals in their gallbladders[70]. However, the resistant mice do not acquire cholesterol crystals or gallstones even when fed the lithogenic diet for 18 weeks[10].

HEPATIC LIPID REGULATORY ENZYMES IN INBRED MICE

Table 2 lists the principal lipid regulatory enzyme activities in the livers of four strains of female inbred mice, two strains susceptible and two strains resistant to cholesterol gallstones after feeding the chow and lithogenic diets for six weeks[10]. Two aspects of the HMGCoA reductase activities are of note: in gallstone-susceptible strains, the HMGCoA reductase activites on the cholesterol-deficient (chow) diet do not upregulate to the levels seen in the resistant strains, and, on the lithogenic diet, they do not downregulate as they do in the gallstone-resistant strains. Whereas none of the *Lith* genes is the structural gene for HMGCoA reductase, these results imply that regulation of this important enzyme (Figure 6) is defective in the presence of *Lith* genes. This finding is reminiscent of the lack of strong physiological regulation of the human hepatic HMGCoA reductase in response to a dietary cholesterol challenge in gallstone patients as inferred from enzyme activities in peripheral mononuclear cells[58]. Table 2 also shows the expected increase in ACAT activities from the increased flux of dietary cholesterol reaching the liver in chylomicra remnants and the small decrease in cholesterol 7α-hydroxylase activities as expected for cholic acid in the diet[12]. As noted earlier, in the case of humans, studies on the activities of the important hepatic receptors for plasma lipoproteins in the inbred mouse strains (Figure 6) have yet to be carried out.

Table 2 Hepatic lipid regulatory enzyme activites in inbred mice[a]

Cholesterol gallstones	*Mouse strain*	*HMGR*[b](n=9) (*pmol min*$^{-1}$ (*mg protein*)$^{-1}$)			*ACAT*[b](n=5) (*nmol min*$^{-1}$ (*mg protein*)$^{-1}$)			C7H[b](n=9) (*pmol min*$^{-1}$ (*mg protein*)$^{-1}$)		
		Chow	*Lith*[c]	*p*[d]	*Chow*	*Lith*	p	*Chow*	*Lith*	p
Susceptible	C57L	28±7	22±3	NS	0.31±0.02	1.24±0.06	<0.001	11±1	6±1	0.03
Susceptible	SWR	24±6	30±3	NS	0.27±0.04	1.02±0.03	<0.001	11±1	9±2	NS
Resistant	SJL	51±5	14±3	<0.001	0.30±0.05	1.19±0.05	<0.001	14±1	8±2	0.02
Resistant	AKR	46±13	10±2	<0.001	0.22±0.02	1.00±0.04	<0.001	13±1	9±1	0.02

[a]From Reference 10; [b]HMGR = 3-hydroxy-3 methylglutaryl-CoA reductase, ACAT = acyl-CoA: cholesterol acyltransferase and C7H = cholesterol 7α -hydroxylase; [c]Lith = lithogenic diet, study carried out at 6 weeks of feeding diets to female inbred mice; [d]p = statistical probability by unpaired t-tests between Chow and Lith columns: NS = not significant

HEPATOBILIARY CONSEQUENCES OF SUSTAINED CHOLESTEROL SUPERSATURATION

The gallbladder is embryonally related to upper small intestinal mucosa and therefore has absorptive, storage and secretory functions[12]. Animal experiments have shown that biliary cholesterol is absorbed quite efficiently by the gallbladder mucosa, the rate being dependent on the absolute and relative cholesterol content of bile[71]. What is now becoming clear (Figure 7) is that, even in the healthy human, cholesterol molecules can be absorbed and apparently resecreted by gallbladder mucosa[72,73]. This is probably passive, occurring down concentration gradients, but could be via receptor-mediated facilitated diffusion as suggested for the upper small intestine[74,75]. Because of the normal diurnal variation (Figure 8) in biliary lipid composition[76], cholesterol absorption occurs during fasting, i.e. when bile is supersaturated, and back diffusion into bile occurs with feeding, i.e. when bile is unsaturated with cholesterol. Although diurnal oscillatory patterns persist in the lithogenic state (Figure 8), moles percent cholesterol is set higher in both fasting and fed states and sustained supersaturation occurs[76]. This appears to be accompanied by continued accumulation of cholesterol molecules in the gallbladder mucosa[73]. After absorption, cholesterol is esterified by mucosal ACAT which is activated by its substrate[77]. Thereafter, a key difference from small intestinal mucosa emerges in that the gallbladder mucosa cannot assemble cholesteryl esters into lipoproteins and export them to plasma so that they are stored in gallbladder tissues[78]. Possible fall-outs from this are that mucin is hypersecreted during early lithogenesis[79], cellular proliferation occurs in the submucosa[80,81] and invasion with inflammatory cells take place[82]. Small amounts of bile salts are absorbed by the gallbladder mucosa[78] and could poss-

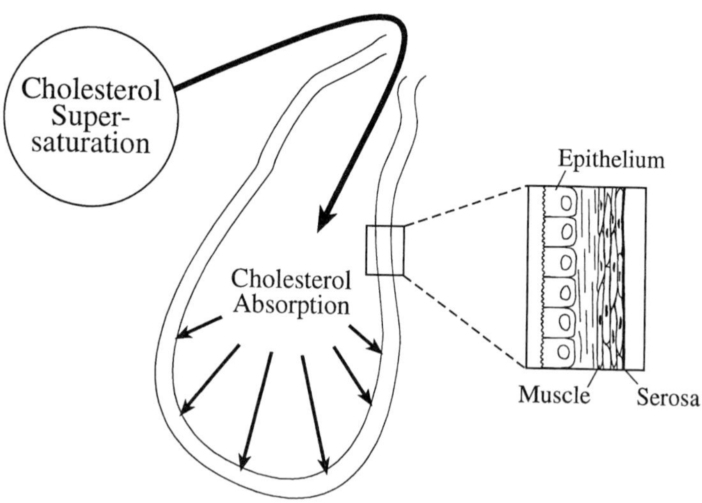

Fig. 7 Depiction of cholesterol absorption by the gallbladder mucosa from cholesterol supersaturated bile and the putative interactions of cholesterol molecules with absorptive (epithelial) cells, mucosa and muscle (muscularis propria) of the gallbladder tissue (discussed in text)

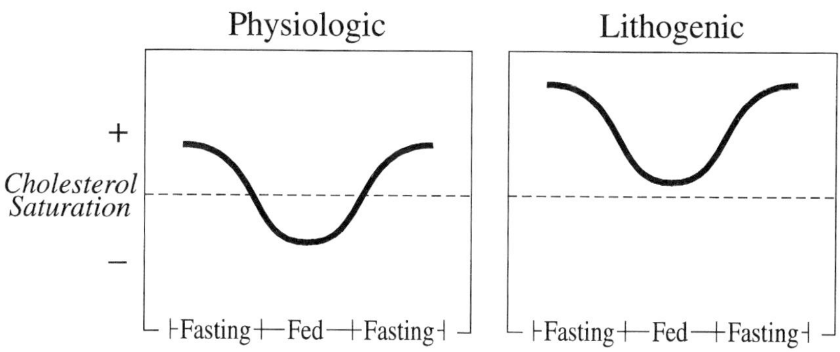

Fig. 8 Diurnal variation in biliary cholesterol saturation in physiological and lithogenic states. Plus (+) represents supersaturation, minus (–) represents unsaturation. With sustained cholesterol hypersecretion, the degree of cholesterol supersaturation is set at appreciably higher levels during fasting and does not unsaturate during feeding as in the physiological state. With respect to the gallbladder mucosa, it is likely that cholesterol molecules flow in both directions under physiological conditions but are 'trapped' in the mucosa under lithogenic conditions (data replotted from Reference 76)

ibly play a facilitating role in these events[83]. Enrichment of sarcolemmal membranes with unesterified cholesterol molecules apparently induces muscle failure[84]. Although intracellular contractile mechanisms of the muscle cells are intact[85,86], it has been shown, in cultures of lithogenic human gallbladder muscle cells as well as those from cholesterol-fed prairie dogs, that excess sarcolemmal cholesterol[87] impairs signal transduction when CCK binds to its plasma membrane receptor.

THE GALLBLADDER IN CHOLESTEROL GALLSTONE DISEASE

As inferred from animal studies[88], the lithogenic gallbladder becomes 'large, lax and lazy'[89] well before crystallization of cholesterol takes place or stones form (Figure 9). Although earlier isotopic studies suggested that disequilibrium existed between circulatory and stored bile salt pools[90], we know now that the cholesterol lithogenic gallbladder neither fills nor empties properly[14], and doesn't concentrate bile like a normal gallbladder[55,73]. As has been known to astute pathologists for years, loss of concentrating power is apparently an early event in gallstone disease[70] and persists for life[91]. Failure of the gallbladder to empty and fill properly, now well established in animals models[92,93], was proven only recently in humans by an ingenious combination of cholescintigraphy and ultrasonography[14]. By measuring gallbladder bile turnover, these authors[14] determined that, in cholesterol gallstone disease, the cholecystoduodenal division of hepatic bile changes from ≈50/50 in health[94] to ≈20/80 in favour of the small intestine in the lithogenic state (Figure 9). As will be discussed next, this pathophysiological alteration has profound consequences for the kinetics of the enterohepatic circulation of bile salts as first appreciated in lithogenic animals[95]. The duodenal diversion of hepatic bile augments the lithogenic state in many ways, principally because of anaerobic

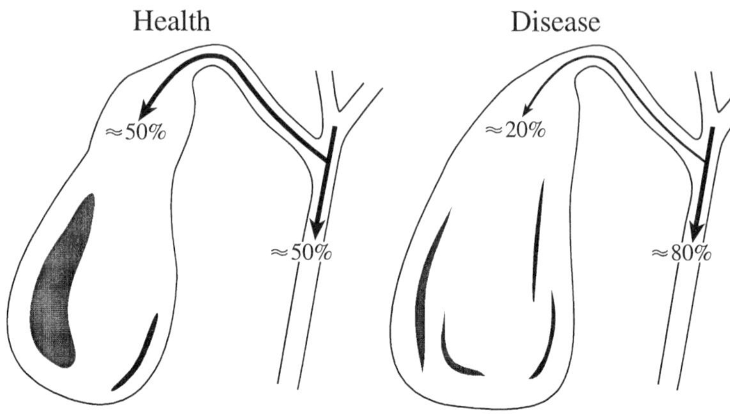

Fig. 9 In health, only 50% of the hepatic bile flow enters the gallbladder for concentration and storage. The 'large, lax and lazy' gallbladder of gallstone disease neither fills nor empties properly, usually directing up to 80% of hepatic bile into the duodenum. This has a profound influence of the enterohepatic circulatory dynamics of bile salts. With each enterohepatic cycle in the lithogenic state, more hepatic bile is delivered into the proximal small intestine and hence a greater exposure to the bile salt metabolizing microflora in the distal small and large intestines (based on concepts in Reference 14)

bacterial action in the distal small and large intestines on the chemistry of the bile salt's steroid nucleus[12].

ALTERED ENTEROHEPATIC CIRCULATION OF BILE SALTS

As far as we know, in cholesterol gallstone disease, the populations of anaerobic bacteria are distributed normally and colonize their usual anatomic sites in the distal ileum, caecum and colon[96]. Nevertheless, this may not be the case in all gallstone patients. In both human subjects[97] and lithogenic animals[98], it appears now that small bowel motility may also be impaired in cholesterol gallstone disease. In fact, direct exposure of ileal muscle to cholesterol-rich liposomes, as in the gallbladder, impairs their contractile response to CCK agonists[99]. The pathomechanics of impaired small bowel function may be distinct from the motor dysfunction of the gallbladder[14]. The intestinal defect may be secondary to increased spasmodic activity and impaired relaxation resulting in non-peristaltic activity[89,98]. This impaired relaxation is reminiscent of the diminished relaxant response of arterial smooth muscle to vasolidators observed in advanced hypercholesterolaemia in both rabbits[100] and humans[101] and may be a result of sustained 'hypercholesterobilia'[102]. If, as some indirect studies suggest[13,103,104], the anaerobic flora in gallstone patients colonizes the more proximal gut, then the intestinal component of lithogenesis could be viewed as an acquired 'endogenous infectious disease' amenable to antibiotic therapy[104]. If this line of reasoning is correct, the anaerobic flora then becomes an important silent partner in cholesterol gallstone disease[104,105] since a greater fraction of bile salts will be exposed to the intestinal microflora during every enterohepatic cycle (Figure 9). Furthermore, it is known that the bile salt metabolizing enzymes of some of these bacterial species are inducible[106]. In established cholesterol gallstone disease in humans, the levels of secondary bile salts particularly deoxycholates[103,105] in the bile salt pool, as well as lithocholates and lithocholate sulphates (Figure 2) are increased at the expense of their primary precursors, cholates and chenodeoxycholates[19,22,107]. When the sizes and kinetics of the bile salt pool are measured by isotopically-labelled bile salt dilution[108], it is not surprising that fractional turnover rates of the primary bile salts are increased[109], simply because the bile salt pool recycles more frequently[12]. Because of the high transhepatic flux of a more hydrophobic bile salt pool[110], there is some reduction in cholesterol 7α-hydroxylase activity[58–63] which is now reset to a new steady state level[111]. As a consequence, the bile salt pool becomes reduced significantly, often to 50% of control values[7,12,109,110].

Several other lines of evidence bolster the tenet that the altered kinetics of the enterohepatic circulation of bile salts is an acquired defect secondary to gallbladder dysfunction[7]. For example, even minor alterations in gallbladder structure or space-occupying lesions (e.g. prosthetic stones, pigment stones, mucin gel etc.) and, in the extreme case, cholecystectomy itself, give a true reduction in bile salt pool sizes as evaluated by the isotope dilution technique[90,112–114]. In fact, with established gallstones, trace levels of deoxycholate conjugates within stones are lowest at their centres and increase progressively toward the cortex and into the surrounding bile[115]; this argues in favour of the hypothesis that secondary bile salt levels become progressively abnormal with the development of gallbladder dysfunction and gallstone formation[7,11]. Biliary levels of deoxycholate conjugates are clearly a reflection of increased fractional turnover rates of primary bile salts and become elevated at puberty in humans[116], with prolonged intestinal transit times[103,105] as well as following cystic duct occlusion and cholecystectomy, especially if accompanied by sphincterotomy[117–120].

Although bile salt secretory rates are normal in gallstone disease because the small bile salt pool recycles more frequently[12,18], the change in recycling frequency and the higher content of hydrophobic secondary bile salts[105] appear to amplify the lithogenic state in several ways. In particular, increased deoxycholate conjugates in the bile salt pool:

1. Further increase cholesterol hypersecretion into bile[121,122],
2. Cause gallbladder mucosal injury[123], induce mucin hypersecretion[83] possibly by an ionophoric effect[124], e.g. Ca^{2+},
3. Are absorbed[78] and have a direct relaxant effect on the gallbladder's muscularis propria[125,126],
4. Are directly pronucleating in bile influencing phase equilibria and nucleation sequences thus shortening cholesterol crystallization times[44],
5. Increase canalicular and perhaps gallbladder protein secretion rates[127,128], and
6. Uncouple Na^+-linked gallbladder transport processes[129].

The induced changes in total biliary proteins and their patterns might be capable of tipping the anti-/pronucleation balance in bile toward crystallization, particularly when mild supersaturation is present[130].

OTHER EFFECTS OF CHOLESTEROL ON GALLBLADDER MUCOSA

From the aforegoing, it would appear that one of the most injurious agents to all tissues of the gallbladder are high concentrations either of cholesterol itself or cholesteryl ester from mucosal ACAT activity[73]. However, free cholesterol is probably the agent that leads to infiltration of the gallbladder mucosa with plasma cells[82] and hence IgA, IgG and IgM secretion from gallbladder mucosa into bile[131]. These immunoglobulins, particularly IgG which is markedly elevated in gallbladder bile of gallstone patients[131], have profound pro-nucleating potential[132], appear very early in lithogenesis[133] apparently from the gallbladder wall[134] and are also deposited in gallstones[135]. Despite recent data in a gallbladder cell line from the domestic dog which suggest that more hydrophobic bile salts are the pathophysiological stimulants to mucin hypersecretion[83], it is more likely that molecular cholesterol injury to mucosal cells, possibly promoted by bile salts, is responsible *in vivo*. Mucin accumulation is seen even in the gallstone-resistant mouse[70] in response to increases in biliary cholesterol levels that still fall within the micellar zone, i.e. unsaturated with cholesterol, and, further, the bile salt pool in the lithogenic mouse is hydrophilic. Perhaps molecular cholesterol or its ester in mucosal cells are also responsible for injury to the active transport mechanisms for gallbladder absorption of electrolytes and water that result in ineffectual lipid concentration of hepatic bile[24,44].

TIME-COURSE OF MUCIN HYPERSECRETION IN EXPERIMENTAL ANIMALS

As shown in Figure 10, mucin hypersecretion during the earliest stages of cholesterol gallstone formation was best documented using cultured explants of the gallbladder from the lithogenic prairie dog[79]. Mucin synthesis and secretion were monitored by means of [^{3}H]glucosamine radiotracer added to the culture medium. Two aspects of this experiment were notable (Figure 10):

1. Increased mucin synthesis and secretion to 40% of control was present at 3 days after initiating the lithogenic diet when bile was 75% saturated with cholesterol (Figure 10, left panel). This observation was confirmed in more recent work by finding mucin gel accumulation despite unsaturated bile in the gallstone-resistant inbred laboratory mouse[70].
2. When prairie dog bile became saturated with cholesterol at 5 days of feeding (Figure 10), mucin synthesis and secretion increased to 100 and 500% of control levels, respectively. Although cholesterol supersaturation of both gallbladder and hepatic bile was obvious at 8 and 14 days, and, as demonstrated by differences in CSIs between homogenized and centrifuged gallbladder bile (Figure 10), nucleation had occurred and mucin production showed a dramatic decline but did not reach basal rates, even at 14 days.

The most parsimonious interpretation of these findings is that absorbed cholesterol was the stimulus for increased mucus synthesis and secretion. Once

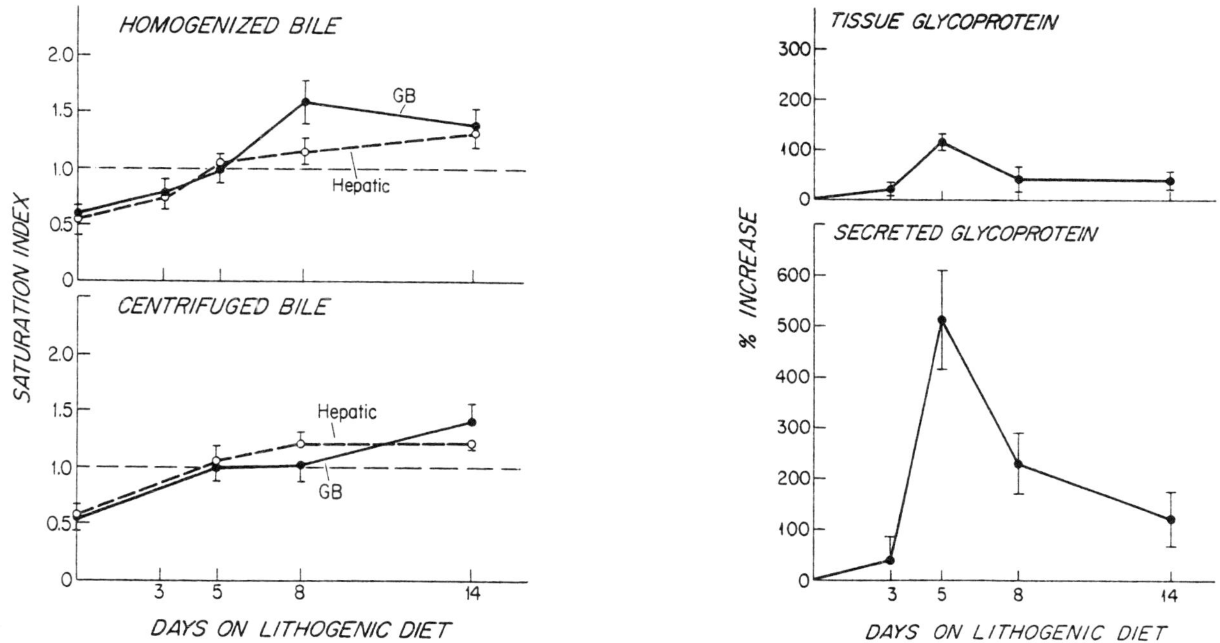

Fig. 10 The cholesterol saturation of bile of prairie dogs expressed as saturation index (CSI) and tissue and secreted mucin glycoproteins as functions of days on a lithogenic (1.2% cholesterol) diet. Mucin was monitored by the incorporation of [^{3}H]glucosamine employing gallbladder explants of the cholesterol-fed prairie dog. Note that mucin hypersecretion is maximal when bile just reaches saturation with cholesterol but declines with further increases in saturation index (discussed in text, from Reference 79 by copyright permission of The American Society for Clinical Investigation)

cholesterol nucleated and the degree of supersaturation of the mother bile decreased, and when mucin gel was sufficiently dense to act as a barrier to molecular diffusion, the cholesterol stimulus to gallbladder mucin hypersecretion abated, but was not completely eliminated[79].

NUCLEATION AND PHASE TRANSITIONS

Lithogenic bile produces cholesterol monohydrate crystals much faster than matched model biles or supersaturated bile from control subjects[136]. The original observation of Holan *et al.*[136] and many follow-on studies[4,7] do not clarify whether true nucleation is hastened, or whether crystallization and/or crystal growth is accelerated. In this 'nucleation' assay[136], native bile is forced to renucleate following removal of crystals and stones by centrifugation or filtration. Hence, if a 'critical nucleus' were present and was not removed because of its small size, then 'faster' nucleation compared with model or native control biles could present a 'lead-time' artifact. In fact, studies by de Bruijn *et al.*[137], suggest that a biliary 'lipoprotein' with a molecular weight of 80 kDa and isolated by concanavalin-A-affinity chromatography may be that 'critical nucleus'. This 'critical nucleus' probably originates in hepatic bile, and may be due to the greater cholesterol enrichment and concentration of biliary vesicles in lithogenic biles[4,7]. Of course, it is possible that faster crystal detection times could be due to changes in chemical composition of bile that had occurred since the initial crystallization process took place *in vivo*. These pronucleating factors include mucin gel[4,79], increased levels of deoxycholate conjugates[105], immunoglobulins from plasma cells in gallbladder mucosa[132,134] and pronucleating proteins from the liver[20,21,127] whose secretion may be promoted by a more hydrophobic and a more frequently recycling bile salt pool[7]. Moreover, in recent studies[138], we found that higher conjugated deoxycholate levels, high CSIs and higher total lipid concentrations could not explain fully the faster crystal detection times of gallstone bile, suggesting that other factors are involved.

CHOLESTEROL CRYSTALLIZATION PATHWAYS

It is known from *in-vivo*[139,140] as well as *in-vitro*[141] studies that a microscopic crystallization pathway begins in bile with the appearance of lamellar liquid crystals (multilamellar vesicles) which, in time, issue plate-like cholesterol monohydrate crystals from their structures. It is now known that, in both model and native biles, there is another crystallization pathway that involves filaments and arc-like crystals which appear to be composed of 'anhydrous' cholesterol molecules[142,143]. These crystals are followed by several intermediate forms, including right-handed helices and tubular crystals[144]. Figure 11 shows, on triangular co-ordinates, the positions of five separate crystallization pathways (labelled A–E) in bile as functions of physiological lecithin mole fractions for concentrated mixed bile salt–egg lecithin–cholesterol systems at pH 7.0, 0.15 mol/L NaCl and 37°C[44,138]. With dilution, cooling and increasing the hydrophilic–hydrophobic balance of the bile salt, the positions of the pathways

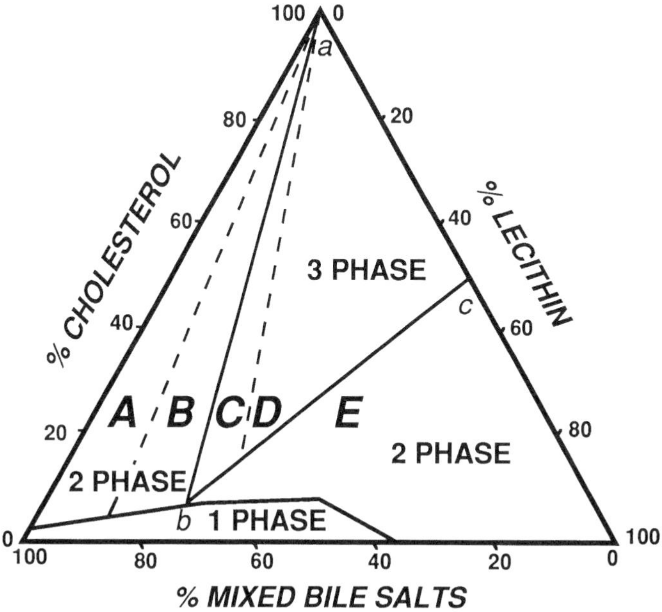

Fig. 11 Positions of five crystallization pathways (A–E) in bile plotted on triangular co-ordinates for mixed bile salts, lecithin and cholesterol in 0.15 mol/L NaCl (6.3 g/dl, 37°C, pH 7.0). The figure also indicates the number of phases that are present at equilibrium in these systems. The liquid and solid crystallization sequences corresponding to A–E are listed in Table 3

are shifted markedly to the left and the micellar zones become contracted[44]. Table 3 summarizes the crystallization sequences in each pathway as functions of increases in the lecithin mole fraction[44]. In general, at low lecithin contents, 'anhydrous' cholesterol crystals and the metastable intermediate crystals precede cholesterol monohydrate crystal formation. However, when the relative lipid compositions of bile increase toward higher lecithin contents, 'anhydrous' crystals postdate cholesterol monohydrate crystals (Table 3). When the composition of the mother liquor changes to zones C or D (Figure 11), then liquid crystals

Table 3 Cholesterol crystallization sequences in bile[a]

	Pathway				
	A	*B*	*C*	*D*	*E*
Lecithin mole fraction[b]	0–0.15	0.15–0.20	0.20–0.30	0.3–0.40	0.40–0.55
Sequence[c]	Ch"A"→ ChM	ChM→ Ch"A"	LC→ChM→ Ch"A"	LC→ChM	LC

[a]Model systems composed of mixed bile salts, egg lecithin and cholesterol ([TL] = 6.2 g/dl; 0.15 mol/L NaCl, pH = 7.0, 37°C); [b]molar lecithin:(lecithin plus bile salt) ratio; [c]Ch"A" = apparent anhydrous cholesterol; ChM = cholesterol monohydrate, LC = lamellar liquid crystals

invariably precede solid crystallization (Table 3). In zone E (Figure 11), liquid crystals precipitate rapidly but are stable and do not undergo a phase transition to solid crystals[44]. Lipid compositions of normal human gallbladder biles never plot in region E at 37°C[140]. However, the relative lipid composition of some highly dilute hepatic biles may do so because of the dilution-induced left shift in the positions of the crystallization pathways[44].

TWO PUTATIVE NUCLEATION MECHANISMS

Figure 12 presents two hypotheses for nucleation in bile which are based on a number of lines of evidence from our own work[44,144] (D. Q.-H. Wang, D. Ganz, D. M. Small, M. C. Carey, unpublished data) and the literature[137]. Aggregation and fusion of biliary vesicles to form multilamellar vesicles should result in cholesterol-to-cholesterol contact throughout the multilayered structure (Figure 12). Such an alignment of cholesterol molecules is not dissimilar from the bi-molecular packing of cholesterol monohydrate molecules in the solid state[145]. Because 'anhydrous' crystallization[146] appears to be induced in biles with low lecithin mole fractions (Table 3) and containing only unilamellar vesicles (Figure 11, zones A/B), then it is likely that internal nucleation ('implosion') of cholesterol molecules occurs within unilamellar vesicles to form an 'anhydrous' cholesterol core (Figure 12). If correct, this may engender a very large increase in intravesicular pressure, and filamentous

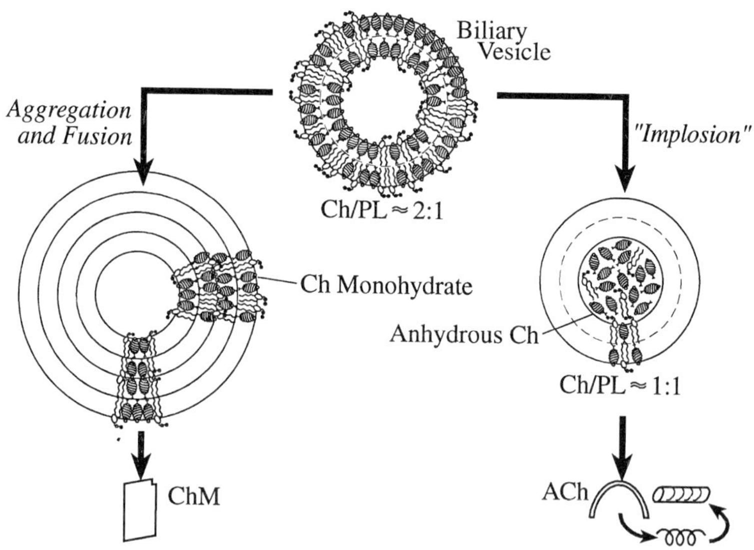

Fig. 12 Putative pathways for cholesterol nucleation in bile: hypothesized fusion and formation of multilamellar vesicles giving rise to cholesterol monohydrate (ChM) crystals. The author proposes that nucleation of 'anhydrous' cholesterol occurs internally as a liquid core in unilamellar vesicles and that this initiates 'anhydrous' cholesterol crystallization. Note that, with relief of supersaturation, the Ch/PL ratio (2 : 1) of vesicles reaches 1 : 1 at equilibrium

crystals could flow through the lipid bilayer into bulk bile like 'a stream of lava from under a volcano'. In bile, 'anhydrous' crystals appear to hydrate slowly[147] to form cholesterol monohydrate crystals and do so via a series of metastable intermediate structures[44,142,144], including helical and tubular crystals (Figure 12). These structures demonstrate the right-handed chirality of the cholesterol and lecithin molecules[144]. However, it should also be noted that thermodynamically-stable cholesterol monohydrate crystals may also arise de novo by a pathway (or pathways), especially in zone B (Figure 11, Table 3), that are independent of these events but little is known about them[44].

CHOLESTEROL GALLSTONE FORMATION – CONCEPTS OF PRIMARY, SECONDARY AND TERTIARY DEFECTS

This review has taken the position that the primary defect in cholesterol gallstone formation is hepatic cholesterol hypersecretion and sustained supersaturation of bile (Figure 13). This is probably the result of a genetic predisposition[10] triggered by an environmental perturbation[4]. A new concept is that sustained unphysiological supersaturation with cholesterol[12,17,18] can greatly impair the normal mechanical functioning of the organs downstream[88,89], including the

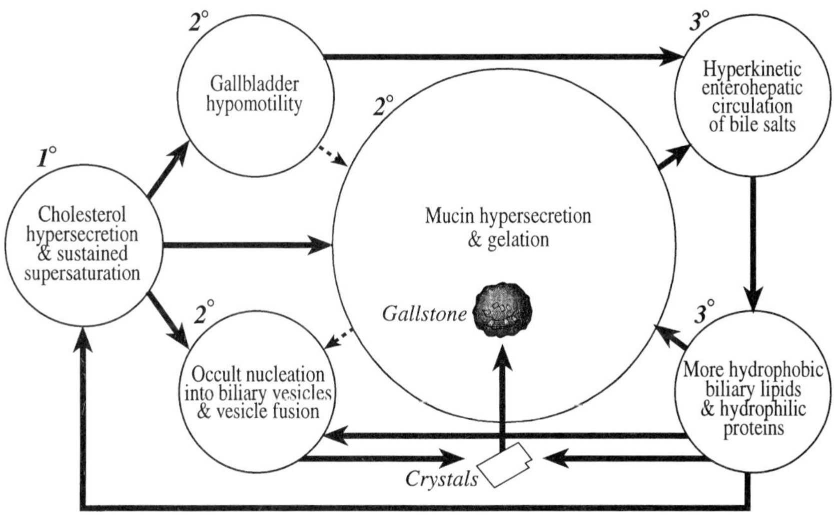

Fig. 13 A parsimonious hypothesis to summarize the pathogenesis of cholesterol gallstones. Cholesterol hypersecretion and sustained supersaturation is proposed at the primary defect (1°) from a genetic predisposition with environmental expression. Secondary defects (2°) are gallbladder hypomotility from muscle poisoning by cholesterol molecules (a genetic element is also possible) and occult nucleation into biliary vesicles and vesicle fusion probably in the hepatic ducts. Mucin hypersecretion and gelation are prominent 2° defects from cholesterol injury and precede crystallization. Tertiary defects (3°) result from a hyperkinetic enterohepatic circulation of bile salts from poor gallbladder filling and emptying which in turn initiates formation of more hydrophobic biliary lipids that promote secretion of more hydrophilic (pronucleating) bile proteins. The concept of a vicious circle is proposed

gallbladder and perhaps the upper small intestine[98], as well as inducing occult nucleation into biliary vesicles and vesicle fusion in hepatic bile (Figure 13). The gallbladder fails to pump or fill properly[14] and it is believed that this occurs secondary to molecular cholesterol 'poisoning' of the sarcolemmal membranes[87] although a genetic influence cannot be ruled out[10]. This leads to a tertiary defect (Figure 13) involving profound alterations in the enterohepatic circulation of bile salts[12] with the result that there are lipid and protein compositional changes in bile[22,40,82,105,109,127]. The changes in bile salt chemistry may be the result of a normal anaerobic flora in the distal ileum, caecum and colon[106] or a normal flora extending more proximally in the small intestine because of defective motility[13,15]. Simultaneously, the absorbed cholesterol molecules induce the mucosa of the gallbladder to undergo sterile inflammation[82,131] and produce secretory immunoglobulins[131–134]. Another secondary defect of cholesterol toxicity is that the mucosal cells hypersecrete mucin into bile which readily gels (Figure 13) even in the concentrated detergent environment[79–83]. These events all lead to other important tertiary effects – further promotion of protein secretion from the liver and gallbladder as well as augmenting the cholesterol hypersecretory state[4,7]. It is not beyond the bounds of reason that once the secondary and tertiary defects are in place they could be 'locked-in' by fibrotic repair of the gallbladder in response to mucosal injury. This response to chronic aseptic injury might prevent the full reversal of functional defects despite medically induced desaturation of bile and dissolution of stones. Patients who have early stones recurrence are known to have higher conjugated deoxycholate contents in bile[15] and a persistent glycoprotein pronucleating defect in hepatic bile[148]. All of these findings suggest that the hyperdynamic enterohepatic circulation of lithogenesis has not returned to normal, presumably because the secondary defects, principally gallbladder refilling and emptying as well as stability of hepatic bile (Figure 13), have not reverted to that of the pre-stone state[12].

AGGLOMERATION OF CRYSTALS AND GROWTH OF CHOLESTEROL GALLSTONES

This topic (Figure 14) has received little attention from investigators and a full analysis requires the approaches of modern chemical and biocrystallization techniques[149,150], microgravity[151] as well as cholesterol crystal growth in gel media[152] and sedimentary petrological approaches. Although not known for certain, it appears that the CSI can influence final crystal size[138] and mucin gels can influence crystal quality[153] but both subjects have not been systematically studied. It is also unknown why, in some gallbladders, cholesterol crystals can agglomerate and grow as a solitary gallstone, reaching sizes of 6–10 cm[16,154–156], and yet in others, tens of thousands of 1–15 mm separate gallstones are found[157]. Why other soluble as well as insolute components of bile should be deposited in and on cholesterol stones is also a mystery[16]. These include mucin and traces of several biliary proteins[16,158], bile pigment as calcium hydrogen bilirubinate[158,159], calcium carbonate and phosphate and many others[159]. One school[158] proposes that gallstone formation is initiated on a matrix of a small calcium-binding protein plus the canalicular enzyme aminopeptidase N, bound to mucin

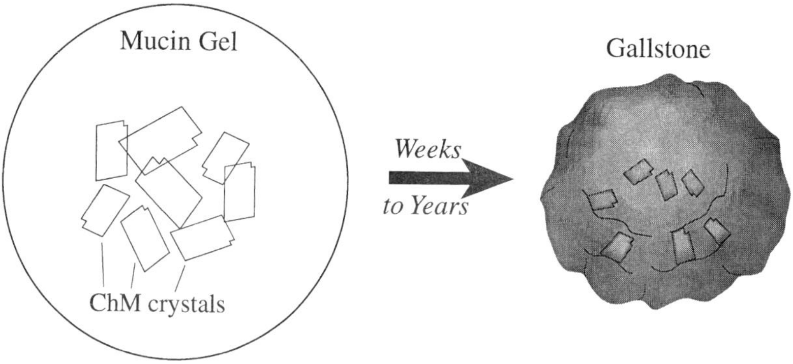

Fig. 14 The growth and agglomeration of crystals and growth of cholesterol gallstones is a neglected research subject. In the text, the key points in the relevant literature are summarized and critically evaluated

gel with calcium/pigment salts depositing on the bound metal-binding proteins and cholesterol crystallizing directly on the mucin.

In model bile studies[160], it was shown that, depending on the conditions, three patterns of crystal growth are possible with cholesterol monohydrate – screw dislocation at low saturation; two-dimensional growth at intermediate levels; and twining at high levels of cholesterol saturation. Osuga and colleagues[161,162] made a careful morphological study of cholesterol monohydrate crystal growth during nutritionally induced gallstone formation in squirrel monkeys and made comparisons with the human disease[163]. They found that, in gallbladder bile, crystals grow by layered growth (i.e. two-dimensional crystallization) as well as by random interactions and aggregation to form 'platy units' of 15–30 μm in size that constitute the building blocks of stones.

Contrary to popular belief, following cholesterol crystallization in the gallbladder, experimentally-induced gallstone formation or the natural process in humans is not rapid[153]. 'Biliary sludge', a dispersion of crystals in accumulated mucin gel is a key precursor, but can persist for years without transforming into gallstones[153]. Further, even in the inbred mouse carrying the three *Lith* genes, crystals precipitate quickly, yet gallstones, defined as small aggregates resistant to digital disintegration, can take weeks to form[70]. In a prospective cholecystographic study of lithogenic patients with initially stone-free gallbladders, Wolpers and Hofmann[164] noted that solitary gallstones developed after a precursor phase of over 2 years, during which time free-floating crystal laminae aggregated loosely and then compacted, presumably because of gallbladder contractions. Following cholecystectomy and stone analysis, it was found that about 10% of solitary stones had a pigment 'stone' in the centre. In contrast, multiple cholesterol gallstones formed without a precursor phase, with an abrupt onset of stepped aggregation from first-generation stones of 1 mm in size to coalesced facetted stones, often via multilobar or mulberry concretions[164]. The authors[164] were of the opinion that sealing of the gallstone surface by periods of supersaturation and deposition of calcium salts prevented further growth and afforded 'metamorphosis' of the stones' centres. It was hypothesized[164] that this occurred from temporary occlusion of the cystic duct and defective acidification of bile via the buffering effect of mucin[165]. The important work of Portman and his colleagues from the 70s[161–163] on the morphology of multiple gallstone formation in the squirrel monkey as well as in humans suggests that simple stones were formed by the aggregation of cholesterol microstones composed of 'platy units' to form 'sand-like' stones of ~400 μm size. As these enlarged, their interiors rearranged so that the constitutive crystals formed a simple radial pattern. Most macroscopic stones were either mulberry or multilobar which, interestingly, was verified by the prospective cholecystographic studies in humans[164]. One of the key differences between the two primate studies was that, in humans, the central nucleus of stones was frequently randomly arranged[162], often containing calcium (hydrogen) bilirubinate, mucin and calcium phosphate as well as cholesterol crystals[163].

Clearly necessary for stone formation are 'sticky' substances in bile to cement crystals together. The glycoprotein monomers of mucin gel are the most obvious candidates to play such an annealing role[153]. Nonetheless, 'anhydrous' cholesterol crystals, because of their extraordinary stickiness[142] and because they precipitate in native biles[44], could also play a major role. Whereas we have suggested[142] that 'anhydrous' cholesterol crystals constitute major components of cholesterol gallstones in the scorbutic (hypovitaminotic C) guinea-pigs fed a high-cholesterol diet[166], 'anhydrous' cholesterol crystals have not been detected rigorously in fresh human gallstones[167] except in one important study[168]. In the X-ray diffraction study[167], the so-called 'anhydrous' cholesterol variety appeared to be a decomposition artifact due to the efflorescence of the monohydrate crystal form during storage. The 'anhydrous' crystal structure has a reversible phase transition at 31.6±0.1°C not seen in crystals of cholesterol monohydrate[168] and its presence in fresh human gallstones has been proven by X-ray diffraction as well as calorimetry[168]. For stone formation in the human gallbladder, this hypothesis is attractive in that extremely sticky anhydrous crystals may precipitate periodically and, as they are remarkably stable in bile[44,70,137,141], they could induce sudden agglomeration of mixtures of cholesterol microliths.

It was estimated in 1986[169], on the basis of ^{14}C radiocarbon dating of gallstones from environmental release of $^{14}CO_2$ during nuclear weapons testing (late 1950s to early 1960s) that all gallbladder stones grow at similar rates, approximately 2.6±1.4 mm per year. A similar growth rate (95% confidence interval: 1.7–2.3 mm per year) was obtained by another group who based their sizes on surgically collected gallstones from whites, blacks and native American Indians in 10-year age bands[156]. In all racial groups, the proportion of subjects with single stones was similar (≈20%) and they averaged 0.5 cm larger than multiple stones. Mean gallstone size increased over time but stopped after the 4th decade when single stones became more frequent. Assuming linear growth rates from nucleation to the time of measurement, an extrapolation reveals that the earliest age at onset of stone formation in American Indian females was 8.3 years compared with 10.8 years in non-Indian females. If correct, this would place nucleation and crystallization at extremely early time points in cholesterol-gallstone-forming patients, heralded perhaps by the appearance of supersaturated bile in the earliest pubertal years[170]. Clearly, gallstone growth is a fascinating and revealing subject and the gallbladder a sublime milieu mineralogically for cholesterol precipitation and growth to occur. Obviously, an increase in the number of studies focused on this topic would allow this important 'Cinderella' of gallstone formation to emerge from its neglected status and reveal, like the rings in an old tree, the 'ebb and flow' of crystal growth and dissolution as well as interlocking configurations of crystals and admixture with 'dopants' that occur during human cholesterol gallstone formation.

Acknowledgements

The author is grateful to his associates in Boston and delegates at Falk Symposium No. 84 in Berlin for their continuing education and constructive criticisms. Original work in the author's laboratory is supported by National Institute of Health (USPHS) grants DK36588 and DK-34854. Administrative secretary Ms. Elaine O'Rourke prepared the manuscript and bibliography and Drs. David E. Cohen, Joanne M. Donovan, James M. Crawford and David Q.-H. Wang provided germinal ideas for many of the illustrations.

References

1. Sama C, Morselli-Labate AM, Tanoli F, Barbara L. Epidemiology and natural history of gallstone disease. Semin Liver Dis. 1990;10:149–58.
2. Paumgartner G, Sauerbruch T. Gallstones – pathogenesis. Lancet. 1991;338:1117–24.
3. Busch N, Matern S. Current concepts in cholesterol gallstone pathogenesis. Eur J Clin Invest. 1991;21:453–60.
4. LaMont JT, Carey MC. Cholesterol gallstone formation. 2. Pathobiology and pathomechanics. Prog Liver Dis. 1992;10:165–91.
5. Carey MC. Formation of cholesterol gallstones: The new paradigms. In: Paumgartner G, Stiehl A, Gerok W, eds. Trends in bile acid research. Dordrecht: Kluwer;1989:259–81.
6. Erlinger S. How is a cholesterol gallstone formed? Gastroenterol Clin Biol. 1994;18:984–7.
7. Carey MC. Pathogenesis of gallstones. Am J Surg. 1993;165:410–19.
8. Afdhal NH, Carey MC. New perspectives on gallstone pathogenesis and prevention. J Ir Coll Phys Surg. 1995;24:267–78.
9. Apstein MD, Carey MC. Pathogenesis of cholesterol gallstones: a parsimonious hypothesis. Eur J Clin Invest. [In press].
10. Khanuja B, Cheah Y-C, Hunt M *et al. Lith 1*, a major gene affecting cholesterol gallstone formation among inbred strains of mice. Proc Natl Acad Sci USA. 1995;92:7729–33.
11. Carey MC, LaMont JT. Cholesterol gallstone formation. 1. Physical-chemistry of bile and biliary lipid secretion. Prog Liver Dis. 1992;10:139–63.
12. Carey MC, Duane WC. Enterohepatic circulation. In: Arias IM, Boyer JL, Fausto N, Jakoby WB, Schachter D, Shafritz DA, eds. The liver, biology and pathobiology, 3rd Ed. New York: Raven Press; 1994:719–67.
13. Berr F, Pratschke E, Fischer S, Paumgartner G. Disorders of bile acid metabolism in cholesterol gallstone disease. J Clin Invest. 1992;90:859–68.
14. Jazrawi RP, Pazzi P, Petroni ML *et al.* Postprandial gallbladder motor function: Refilling and turnover of bile in health and cholelithiasis. Gastroenterology. 1995;109:582–91.
15. Berr F, Mayer M, Sackmann MF, Sauerbruch T, Holl J, Paumgartner G. Pathogenic factors in early recurrence of cholesterol gallstones. Gastroenterology. 1994;106:215–24.
16. Harding Rains AJ. Gallstones, causes and treatment. Springfield, IL: Charles C Thomas; 1964.
17. Hofmann AF. Primary and secondary prevention of gallstone disease: Implications for patient management and research priorities. Am J Surg. 1993;165:541–8.
18. Northfield TC, Hofmann AF. Biliary lipid output during three meals and an overnight fast. I. Relationship to bile acid pool size and cholesterol saturation of bile in gallstone and control subjects. Gut. 1975;16:1–11.
19. Hofmann AF, Grundy SM, Lachin *et al.* Pretreatment biliary lipid composition in white patients with radiolucent gallstones in the National Cooperative Gallstone Study. Gastroenterology. 1982;82:738–52.

20. Gallinger S, Harvey PRC, Petrunka CN, Ilson RG, Strasberg SM. Biliary proteins and the nucleation defect in cholesterol cholelithiasis. Gastroenterology. 1987;92:867–76.
21. Jüngst D, Lang T, von Ritter C, Paumgarter G. Role of high total protein in gallbladder bile in the formation of cholesterol gallstones. Gastroenterology. 1991;100:1724–9.
22. Hay DW, Cahalane MJ, Timofeyeva N, Carey MC. Molecular species of lecithins in human gallbladder biles. J Lipid Res. 1993;34:759–68.
23. Carey MC, Robins SJ. Bile production and secretion. In: Stein JH, ed. Internal medicine, 4th Ed. St. Louis: Mosby-Year Book Inc.; 1993:532–9.
24. Carey MC, Small DM. The characteristics of mixed micellar solutions with particular reference to bile. Am J Med. 1970;49:590–608.
25. Donovan JM, Timofeyeva N, Carey MC. Influence of total lipid concentration, bile salt:lecithin ratio, and cholesterol content on inter-mixed micellar/vesicular (non-lecithin-associated) bile salt concentration in model bile. J Lipid Res. 1991;32:1501–12.
26. Carey MC. Measurement of the physical–chemical properties of bile salt solutions. In: Barbara L, Dowling RH, Hofmann AF, Roda E, eds. Bile acids in gastroenterology. Lancaster: MTP Press; 1983:19–56.
27. Mazer NA, Benedek GB, Carey MC. Quasielastic light scattering studies of aqueous biliary lipid systems: Mixed micelle formation in bile salt–lecithin solutions. Biochemistry. 1980;19:601–15.
28. Hjelm RP, Thiyagarajan P, Sivia DS, Lindner P, Alkan H, Schwahn D. Small-angle neutron scattering from aqueous mixed colloids of lecithin and bile salt. Prog Coll Polymer Sci. 1990;81:225–31.
29. Long MA, Kaler EW, Lee SP. Structural characterization of the micelle–vesicle transition in lecithin–bile salt solutions. Biophys J. 1994;67:1733–42.
30. Cohen DE, Chamberlin RA, Thurston GM, Carey MC. Laser light scattering evidence for 'worm-like' mixed micelles in both cholanoyl (bile salt) in acyl (octylglucoside) detergent–long chain phosphatidylcholine aqueous systems: New insights on mixed micellar structure in bile. Biochemistry. [In press].
31. Cohen DE, Carey MC. Rapid (1 hour) high-performance gel filtration chromatography resolves coexisting simple micelles, mixed micelles and vesicles in bile. J Lipid Res. 1990;31:2103–12.
32. Mazer NA, Schurtenberger P, Carey MC, Preisig R, Weigand K, Känzig W. Quasielastic light scattering studies of native hepatic bile from the dog: Comparison with aggregative behavior of model biliary lipid systems. Biochemistry. 1984;23:1994–2005.
33. Carey MC. Critical tables for calculating the cholesterol saturation of native bile. J Lipid Res. 1978;19:945–55.
34. Sömjen GT, Gilat T. A non-micellar mode of cholesterol transport in human bile. FEBS Lett. 1983;156:265–8.
35. Mazer NA, Carey MC. Quasi-elastic light-scattering studies of aqueous biliary lipid systems: Cholesterol solubilization and precipitation in model bile solutions. Biochemistry. 1983;22:426–42.
36. Sömjen GJ, Marikovsky Y, Selkes P, Gilat T. Cholesterol-phospholipid vesicles in human bile: an ultrastructural study. Biochim Biophys Acta. 1986;879:14–21.
37. Cohen DE, Leighton LS, Carey MC. Bile salt hydrophobicity controls vesicle secretion rates and transformations in native bile. Am J Physiol. 1992;263:G386–95.
38. Huang C-h. Studies on phosphatidylcholine vesicles. Formation and physical characteristics. Biochemistry. 1969;8:344–51.
39. Crawford JM, Möckel GM, Crawford AR *et al.* Imaging biliary lipid secretion in the rat: Ultrastructural evidence for vesiculation of the hepatocyte canalicular membrane. J Lipid Res. 1995;36:2147–63.
40. Rigotti A, Nuñez L, Amigo L *et al.* Biliary lipid secretion – immunolocalization and identification of a protein associated with lamellar cholesterol carriers in supersaturated rat and human bile. J Lipid Res. 1993;34:1883–94.
41. Cohen DE, Angelico M, Carey MC. Quasielastic light scattering evidence for vesicular secretion of biliary lipids. Am J Physiol. 1989;257:G1–8.
42. Donovan JM, Carey MC. Separation and quantitation of cholesterol 'carriers' in bile. Hepatology. 1990;12:94S–105S.
43. Peled Y, Halpern Z, Eitan B, Goldman G, Konikoff F, Gilat T. Biliary micellar cholesterol nucleates via the vesicular pathway. Biochim Biophys Acta. 1989;1003:246–9.

44. Wang DQ-H, Carey MC. Complete mapping of the crystallization pathways during cholesterol nucleation from model biles. Influence of pathophysiologically-relevant physical–chemical variables and identification of a stable supersaturated liquid crystalline state in cold, dilute and hydrophilic bile salt containing systems. J Lipid Res. [In press].
45. Smit JJM, Schinkel AH, Oude Elferink RPJ *et al.* Homozygous disruption of the murine mdr2 P-glycoprotein gene leads to a complete absence of phospholipid from bile and to liver disease. Cell. 1993;75:451–62.
46. Higgins CF. To flip or not to flip? Curr Biol. 1994;4:259–60.
47. Coleman R, Igbal S, Godfrey PP, Billington D. Membranes and bile formation: Composition of several mammalian biles and their membrane-damaging properties. Biochem J. 1979;178:201–8.
48. Möckel GM, Gorti S, Tandon RK, Tanaka T, Carey MC. Microscope laser light scattering spectroscopy of vesicles within canaliculi of rat hepatocyte couplets. Am J Physiol. 1995;269:G73–84.
49. Cohen DE, Angelico M, Carey MC. Structural alterations in lecithin–cholesterol vesicles following interactions with monomeric and micellar bile salts. Physical chemical basis for subselection of biliary lecithin species and aggregative states of biliary lipids during bile formation. J Lipid Res. 1990;31:55–70.
50. Kamp F, Hamilton JA. Movement of fatty acids, fatty acid analogues, and bile acids across phospholipid bilayers. Biochemistry. 1993;32:11074–85.
51. Jones TG. Dirt removal. In: Durham K, ed. Surface activity and detergency. London: MacMillan & Co; 1961:72–118.
52. Cohen DE, Kaler EW, Carey MC. Cholesterol carriers in human bile: Are lamellae involved? Hepatology. 1993;18:1522–32.
53. Small DM, Bourgès MC, Dervichian DG. The biophysics of lipidic associations: I. The ternary systems lecithin–bile salt–water. Biochim Biophys Acta. 1966;125:563–80.
54. Pattinson N, Chapman B. Distribution of biliary cholesterol between mixed micelles and nonmicelles in relation to fasting and feeding in humans. Gastroenterology. 1986;91:697–702.
55. Carey MC, Small DM. Physical chemistry of cholesterol solubility in bile: Relationship to gallstone formation and dissolution in man. J Clin Invest. 1978;61:998–1026.
56. Lécuyer H, Dervichian DG. Structure of aqueous mixtures of lecithin and cholesterol. J Mol Biol. 1969;45:39–57.
57. Oude Elferink RPJ, Ottenhoff R, Van Wijland M, Smit JJM, Schinkel AH, Groen AK. Regulation of biliary lipid secretion by mdr2 P-glycoprotein in the mouse. J Clin Invest. 1995;95:31–8.
58. Kern F Jr. Effects of dietary cholesterol on cholesterol and bile acid homeostasis in patients with cholesterol gallstones. J Clin Invest. 1994;93:1186–94.
59. Salen G, Nicolau G, Shafer S, Mosbach EH. Hepatic cholesterol metabolism in patients with gallstones. Gastroenterology. 1975;69:676–84.
60. Coyne MJ, Bonorris GG, Goldstein LJ, Schoenfield LJ. Effect of chenodeoxycholic acid and phenobarbital on the rate-limiting enzymes of hepatic cholesterol and bile acid synthesis in patients with gallstones. J Lab Clin Med. 1976;87:281–91.
61. Maton PN, Ellis HJ, Higgins JP, Dowling RH. Hepatic HMG-CoA reductase in human cholelithiasis: Effects of chenodeoxycholic and ursodeoxycholic acids. Eur J Clin Invest. 1980;10:325–32.
62. Key PH, Bonorris GG, Marks JW, Chung A, Schoenfield LJ. Biliary lipid synthesis and secretion in gallstone patients before and during treatment with chenodeoxycholic acid. J Lab Clin Med. 1980;95:816–26.
63. Carulli N, Ponz de Leon M, Zironi F *et al.* Hepatic cholesterol and bile acid metabolism in subjects with gallstones: Comparative effects of short-term feeding of chenodeoxycholic and ursodeoxycholic acids. J Lipid Res. 1980;21:35–43.
64. Ahlberg J, Angelin B, Einarsson K. Hepatic 3-hydroxy-3-methylglutaryl coenzyme A reductase activity and biliary lipid composition in man: Relation to cholesterol gallstone disease and effect of cholic and chenodeoxycholic acid treatment. J Lipid Res. 1981;22:410–22.
65. Reihnér E, Angelin B, Björkhem I, Einarsson K. Hepatic cholesterol metabolism in cholesterol gallstone disease. J Lipid Res. 1991;32:469–75.
66. Angelin B, Backman L, Einarsson K, Eriksson L, Ewerth S. Hepatic cholesterol metabolism in obesity: activity of microsomal 3-hydroxy-3 methylglutaryl coenzyme A reductase. J Lipid Res. 1982;23:770–3.

67. Shoda J, He BF, Tanaka N *et al.* Increase of deoxycholate in supersaturated bile of patients with cholesterol gallstone disease and its correlation with de novo syntheses of cholesterol and bile acids in liver, gallbladder emptying, and small intestinal transit. Hepatology. 1995;21:1291–302.
68. Smith JL, Hardie IR, Pillay SP, de Jersey J. Hepatic acyl-coenzyme A: Cholesterol acyltransferase activity is decreased in patients with cholesterol gallstones. J Lipid Res. 1990;31:1993–2000.
69. Glickman RM, Sabesin SM. Lipoprotein metabolism. In: Arias IM, Boyer JL, Fausto N editors. The liver: biology and pathobiology. New York: Raven Press; 1994:391–414.
70. Wang DQ-H, Paigen B, Carey MC. Phenotypic characterization of *Lith* genes determining susceptibility to cholesterol gallstone formation in inbred mice. Hepatology. 1995;22:289A.
71. Neiderhiser DH, Harmon CK, Roth HP. Absorption of cholesterol by the gallbladder. J Lipid Res. 1976;17:117–24.
72. Jacyna MR, Ross PE, Baker MA, Hopwood A, Bouchier IAD. Characteristics of cholesterol absorption by human gallbladder; relevance to cholesterolosis. J Clin Pathol. 1987;40:524–8.
73. Sahlin S, Ståhlberg D, Einarsson K. Cholesterol metabolism in liver and gallbladder mucosa of patients with cholesterolosis. Hepatology. 1955;21:1269–75.
74. Thurnhofer H, Hauser H. The uptake of cholesterol by small intestine brush border membrane is protein-mediated. Biochemistry. 1990;29:2142–8.
75. Thurnhofer H, Schnabel J, Betz M, Lipka G, Pidgeon C, Hauser H. Cholesterol-transfer protein located in the intestinal brush border membrane. Partial purification and characterization. Biochim Biophys Acta. 1991;1064:275–86.
76. Metzger AL, Adler R, Heymsfield S, Grundy SM. Diurnal variation in biliary lipid composition. Possible role in cholesterol gallstone formation. N Engl J Med. 1973;288:333–6.
77. Goodman DS. Cholesterol ester metabolism. Physiol Rev. 1965;45:747–839.
78. Tilvis RS, Aro J, Stranberg TE, Lempinen M, Miettinen TA. Lipid composition of bile and gallbladder mucosa in patients with acalculous cholesterolosis. Gastroenterology. 1982;82:607–15.
79. Lee SP, LaMont JT, Carey MC. Role of gallbladder mucin hypersecretion in the evolution of cholesterol gallstones: Studies in the prairie dog. J Clin Invest. 1981;67:1712–23.
80. Lee SP, Scott AJ. The evolution of morphologic changes in the gallbladder before stone formation in mice fed a cholesterol-cholic acid diet. Am J Pathol. 1982;108:1–8.
81. Wahlin T. Effects of lithogenic diets on mouse gallbladder epithelium. A histochemical, cytochemical and morphometric study. Virchows Arch (B) Cell Pathol. 1976;22:273–86.
82. Lee SP, Nicholls JF. Nature and composition of biliary sludge. Gastroenterology. 1986;90:677–86.
83. Klinkspoor JH, Kuver R, Savard CE *et al.* Model bile and bile salts accelerate mucin secretion by cultured dog gallbladder epithelial cells. Gastroenterology. 1995;109:264–74.
84. Behar J, Lee KY, Thompson WR, Biancani P. Gallbladder contraction in patients with pigment and cholesterol stones. Gastroenterology. 1989;97:1479–84.
85. Behar J, Rhim BY, Thompson W, Biancani P. Inositol triphosphate restores impaired human gallbladder motility associated with cholesterol stones. Gastroenterology. 1993:104:563–8.
86. Yu P, Chen Q, Harnett K, Amaral J, Biancani P, Behar J. Direct G-protein activation reverses impaired CCK-signaling in human gallbladders with cholesterol stones. Am J Physiol. 1995;32:G659–G665.
87. Yu PR, Chen Q, Biancani P, Behar J. Excess membrane cholesterol impairs gallbladder muscle contraction. Gastroenterology. 1995;108:A442(Abstract).
88. LaMorte WW, Shoetz DJ, Birkett DH, Williams LF. The role of the gallbladder in the pathogenesis of cholesterol gallstones. Gastroenterology. 1979;77:580–92.
89. Shaffer EA. Motility of the gallbladder and biliary tree. In: 2nd International Conference on Gallstones: Causes and Management – Abstract booklet. Tel-Aviv: 1995:L5–L6.
90. Everson GT, Nemeth A, Kourourian S *et al.* Gallbladder function is altered in sickle hemoglobinopathy. Gastroenterology. 1989;96:1307–16.
91. Boyd W. Pathology for the physician. London: Kimpton; 1958.
92. Doty JE, Pitt HA, Kuchenbecker SL, DenBesten L. Impaired gallbladder emptying before gallstone formation in the prairie dog. Gastroenterology. 1983;85:168–74.
93. Roslyn JJ, Den Bensten L, Thompson JE, Cohen K. Chronic cholelithiasis and decreased bile salt pool size: cause or effect? Am J Surg. 1980;139:119–24.

94. Shaffer EA, Small DM. Gallstone disease: Pathogenesis and management. Current problems in surgery. Chicago: Year Book; 1976.
95. Meyer PD, DenBesten L, Gurll NJ. Effect of cholesterol gallstone induction on gallbladder function and bile salt pool size in the prairie dog. Surgery. 1978;83:595–604.
96. Simon GL, Gorbach SL. Intestinal flora and gastrointestinal function. In: Johnson LR, ed. Physiology of the gastrointestinal tract. New York: Raven Press; 1987:1729–47.
97. Heaton KW, Emmett PM, Symes CL, Braddon FEM. An explanation for gallstones in normal-weight women: slow intestinal transit. Lancet. 1993;341:8–10.
98. Xu QW, Scott RB, Tan DTM, Shaffer EA. Slow intestinal transit: An added motility disorder in cholesterol gallstone formation. Gastroenterology. 1995;108:A442(Abstract).
99. Yu P, Chen Q, Biancani P, Behar J. Cholesterol-rich liposome impairs gallbladder and ileal circular muscle cell contraction. Gastroenterology. 1994;106:A592(Abstract).
100. Creager MA, Cooke JP, Mendelsohn ME *et al.* Impaired vasolidation of forearm resistance vessels in hypercholesterolemic humans. J Clin Invest. 1990;86:228–34.
101. Schmidt K, Klatt P, Mayer B. Hypercholesterolemia is associated with a reduced response to smooth muscle guanylyl cyclase to nitrovasodilators. Arterioscler Thromb. 1993;13:1159–63.
102. Hussani SH, Murphy GM, Kennedy C, Besser GM, Wess JAH, Dowling RH. The role of bile composition and physical chemistry in the pathogenesis of octreotide-associated gallbladder stones. Gastroenterology. 1994;107:1503–13.
103. Marcus SN, Heaton KW. Intestinal transit, deoxycholic acid and the cholesterol saturation of bile: three inter-related factors. Gut. 1986;27:550–8.
104. Low-Beer TS, Nutter S. Colonic bacterial activity, biliary cholesterol saturation and pathogenesis of gallstones. Lancet. 1978;2:1063–5.
105. Marcus SN, Heaton KW. Deoxycholic acid and the pathogenesis of gallstones. Gut. 1988;29:522–33.
106. Hylemon PB. Metabolism of bile acids in intestinal microflora. In: Danielsson H, Sjövall J, eds. Sterols and bile acids (New comprehensive biochemistry), Vol. 12. Amsterdam: Elsevier; 1985:331–43.
107. Fisher MM, Yousef IM. Sex differences in the bile acid composition of human bile: studies in patients with and without gallstones. Can Med Assoc J. 1973;109:190–3.
108. Hofmann AF, Hoffman NE. Measurement of bile acid kinetics by isotope dilution in man. Gastroenterology. 1974;67:314–23.
109. Vlahcevic ZR, Bell CC, Buhac I, Farrar JT, Swell L. Diminished bile acid pool size in patients with gallstones. Gastroenterology. 1970;59:165–73.
110. Vlahcevic ZR, Bell CC, Gregory DH. Relationship of bile acid pool size to the formation of lithogenic bile in female Indians of the Southwest. Gastroenterology. 1972;62:73–83.
111. Vlahcevic ZR, Heuman DM, Hylemon PB. Regulation of bile acid synthesis. Hepatology. 1991;13:590–600.
112. Ho K-J, Ho C, Hsu S, Chen J. Bile acid pool size in relation to functional status of gallbladder and biliary lipid composition in Chinese. Am J Clin Nutr. 1980;33:1026–32.
113. Thurston OG, McDougall RM, Walker K. The effect of prosthetic gallstones on total bile acid pool size in dogs. Surg Gynecol Obstet. 1978;146:911–13.
114. Almond HR, Vlahcevic ZR, Bell CC, Gregory DH, Swell L. Bile acid pools, kinetics, and biliary lipid composition before and after cholecystectomy. N Engl J Med. 1973;289:1213–16.
115. Schoenfield LJ, Sjövall J, Sjövall K. Bile acid composition of gallstones from man. J Lab Clin Med. 1966;68:186–94.
116. Von Bergman K, Becker M, Leiss O. Biliary cholesterol saturation in non-obese women and non-obese men before and after puberty. Eur J Clin Invest. 1986;16:531–5.
117. Hepner GW, Hofmann AF, Malegelada JR, Szczepanik PA, Klein PD. Increased bacterial degradation of bile acids in cholecystectomized patients. Gastroenterology. 1974;66:556–64.
118. Chijiiwa K, Ogawa Y, Hirota I, Nakayama F. Biliary lipid and bile acid composition before and after endoscopic sphincterotomy. Hepato-Gastroenterology. 1990;37:510–12.
119. Berr F, Stellaard F, Pratschke E, Paumgartner G. Effects of cholecystectomy on the kinetics of primary and secondary bile acids. J Clin Invest. 1989;83:1541–50.
120. Sauerbruch T, Stellaard F, Paumgartner G. Effect of endoscopic sphincterotomy on bile acid pool size and bile lipid composition in man. Digestion. 1983;27:87–92.
121. Carulli N, Loria P, Bertolotti M *et al.* Effects of acute change of bile acid pool composition on biliary lipid secretion. J Clin Invest. 1984;74:614–24.

122. Low-Beer TS, Pomare EW. Can colonic bacterial metabolites predispose to cholesterol gall stones. Br Med J. 1995;22:438–40.
123. Chadwick VS, Gaginella TS, Carlson GL, Debongnie JC, Phillips SF, Hofmann AF. Effect of molecular structure on bile acid-induced alterations in absorptive function, permeability and morphology in the perfused rabbit colon. J Lab Clin Med. 1979;94:661–74.
124. Donovan JM, Jackson AA. Hydrophobic bile salts form low resistance membrane channels specific for both calcium and magnesium. Hepatology. 1994;20:A257(Abstract).
125. Xu Q, Shaffer EA. The influence of bile salts on small intestinal motility in the guinea pig in vitro. Gastroenterology. 1992;103:29–35.
126. Shaffer EA. Abnormalities in gallbladder functions in cholesterol gallstone disease: Bile and blood, mucosa and muscle – the list lengthens. Gastroenterology. 1992;102:1808–12.
127. Bozzoli M, Loria P, Concari M *et al.* Bile acid (BA) hydrophobicity and biliary secretion of total proteins and immunoglobulins G (IgG). Hepatology. 1992;16:254A(Abstract).
128. Lipsett PA, Fox-Talbot MK, Falconer SD *et al.* Biliary nonmucin glycoproteins in patients with and without gallstones. J Surg Res. 1995;58:386–90.
129. Beesley RC, Faust RG. Bile salt inhibition of sodium ion-coupled D-glucose and L-alanine accumulation by brush border membrane vesicles from hamster jejunum. Biochem J. 1980;190:731–6.
130. Strasberg SM, Tolt JL, Gallinger S, Harvey PRC. High protein and total lipid concentration are associated with reduced metastability of bile in an early stage of cholesterol gallstone formation. Gastroenterology. 1990;98:739–46.
131. Nuñez L, Amigo L, Miquel JF *et al.* Role of biliary immunoglobulins on cholesterol gallstone disease: marked increase of IgG in gallbladder bile of gallstone patients. Gastroenterology. 1995;108:A1135(Abstract).
132. Harvey PRC, Upadhya GA, Strasberg SM. Immunoglobulins as nucleating proteins in the gallbladder bile of patients with cholesterol gallstones. J Biol Chem. 1991;266:13996–4003.
133. Lipsett P, Kaufman HS, Shermack MA, Fox-Talbot MK, Lillemoe KD, Pitt HA. Early appearances of biliary non-mucin glycoproteins in cholesterol-fed prairie dogs. Gastroenterology. 1992;102:A320(Abstract).
134. Johnston S, Nakeeb A, Barnes SA, Lillemoe KD, Pitt HA, Lipsett PA. Immunoglobulins in gallstone pathogenesis: A systemic or a local phenomenon? Gastroenterology. 1995;108:A1092(Abstract).
135. Lipsett PA, Hildrett J, Kaufman HS, Lillemoe KD, Pitt HA. Human gallstones contain pronucleating non-mucin glycoproteins that are immunoglobulins. Gastroenterology. 1992;102:A320(Abstract).
136. Holan KR, Holzbach RT, Hermann RE, Cooperman AM, Claffey WJ. Nucleation time: A key factor in the pathogenesis of cholesterol gallstone disease. Gastroenterology. 1979;77:611–17.
137. deBruijn J, Mok K, Domingo N, Lafont H, Tytgat GN, Groen AK. Further characterization of the cholesterol crystallization promoting lipoprotein in biliary Con-A binding proteins. Gastroenterology. 1992;102:A310(Abstract).
138. Wang DQ-H, Carey MC. Nucleation pathways during cholesterol crystallization from human gallbladder bile: Pathway identity with corresponding model biles but faster crystallization rates and phase transitions. J Lipid Res. [In press].
139. Holzbach RT, Corbusier C, Marsh M, Naito HK. The process of cholesterol cholelithiasis induced by diet in the prairie dog. A physicochemical characterization. J Lab Clin Med. 1976;87:987–98.
140. Halpern Z, Dudley MA, Kibe A, Lynn MP, Breuer AC, Holzbach RT. Rapid vesicle formation and aggregation in abnormal human bile: A time-lapse video-enhanced contrast microscopy study. Gastroenterology. 1986;90:875–85.
141. Halpern Z, Dudley MA, Lynn MP, Nader JM, Breuer AC, Holzbach RT. Vesicle aggregation in model systems of supersaturated bile: Relation to crystal nucleation and lipid composition of the vesicular phase. J Lipid Res. 1986;27:295–306.
142. Konikoff FM, Chung DS, Donovan JM, Small DM, Carey MC. Filamentous, helical and tubular microstructures during cholesterol crystallization from bile: Evidence that biliary cholesterol does not nucleate classic monohydrate plates. J Clin Invest. 1992;90:1155–60.
143. Konikoff FM, Carey MC. Cholesterol crystallization from a dilute bile salt-rich model bile. J Cryst Growth. 1994;144:79–86.

144. Chung DS, Benedek GB, Konikoff FM, Donovan JM. Elastic free energy of anisotropic helical ribbons as metastable intermediates in the crystallization of cholesterol. Proc Natl Acad Sci USA. 1993;90:11341–5.
145. Craven BM. Crystal structure of cholesterol monohydrate. Nature. 1976;260:727–9.
146. Shieh HS, Hoard LG, Nordman CE. Crystal structure of anhydrous cholesterol. Nature. 1977;267:287–9.
147. Loomis CR, Shipley GG, Small DM. The phase behavior of hydrated cholesterol. J Lipid Res. 1979;20:525–35.
148. Groen AK, Stout JPJ, Drapers JAG, Hoek FJ, Grijm R, Tytgat GNJ. Cholesterol nucleation-influencing activity in T-tube bile. Hepatology. 1988;8:347–52.
149. Weissbuch I, Addadi L, Lahav M, Leiserowitz L. Molecular recognition at crystal interfaces. Science. 1991;253:637–45.
150. Hulliger J. Chemistry and crystal growth. Angew Chem Int Ed Engl. 1994;33:143–62.
151. Koszelak S, Day J, Leja C, Cudney R, McPherson A. Protein and virus crystal growth on International Microgravity Laboratory-2. Biophys J. 1995;69:13–19.
152. Karniewicz J, Wiktorowska B. The crystal growth in gels. Kristall Technik. 1980;15:1227–35.
153. Carey MC, Cahalane MJ. Whither biliary sludge? Gastroenterology. 1988;95:508–23.
154. Walter FA. Anatomisches Museum. Berlin: Belilz und Braun;1796.
155. Wolpers C. Morphologie der gallensteine. Leber Magen Darm. 1974;4:43–57.
156. Lowenfels AB, Walker AM, Althaust DP, Townsend G, Domellöf L. Gallstone growth, size and risk of gallbladder cancer: an interracial study. Int J Epidemiol. 1989;18:50–4.
157. Martin KW, Jackson BT. Record number of gallstones. Br J Surg. 1987:74:704.
158. Lechene de la Porte P, Domingo N, Van Wijland MJA, Groen AK, Ostrow JD, Lafont H. Localization of biliary proteins Ca, Cu, P, S., in the pigment and cholesterol zone of mixed gallstones. In: 2nd International Conference in Gallstones: Causes and Management. Tel Aviv: Abstract Booklet; 1995:56.
159. Cahalane MJ, Neubrand MW, Carey MC. Physical–chemical pathogenesis of pigment gallstones. Semin Liver Dis. 1988;8:317–28.
160. Toor EW, Evans DF, Cussler EL. Cholesterol monohydrate growth in model bile solutions. Proc Natl Acad Sci USA. 1978;75:6230–4.
161. Osuga T, Portman OW, Mitamura K, Alexander M. A morphologic study of gallstone development in the squirrel monkey. Lab Invest. 1994;30:486–93.
162. Osuga T, Mitamura K, Miyagawa S, Sato N, Kintaka S, Portman OW. A scanning electron microscopic study of gallstone development in man. Lab Invest. 1974;31:696–704.
163. Portman OW, Osuga T, Tanaka N. Biliary lipids and cholesterol gallstone formation. Adv Lipid Res. 1975;13:135–94.
164. Wolpers C, Hofmann AF. Solitary versus multiple cholesterol gallbladder stones – Mechanisms of formation and growth. Clin Invest. 1993;71:423–34.
165. Shiffman ML, Sugerman HJ, Kellum JM, Moore EW. Changes in gallbladder bile composition following gallstone formation and weight reduction. Gastroenterology. 192;103:213–21.
166. Jenkins SA. Biliary lipids, bile acids and gallstone formation in hypovitaminotic C guinea-pigs. Br J Nutr. 1978;40:317–26.
167. Sutor DJ, Wooley SE. X-ray diffraction studies of the composition of gallstones from English and Australian patients. Gut. 1969;10:681–3.
168. Hsu L-Y, Nordman CE. Phase transition and crystal structure of the 37°C form of cholesterol. Science. 1983;220:604–6.
169. Mok HYI, Druffel ERM, Rampone WM. Chronology of cholelithiasis. Dating gallstones from atmospheric radiocarbon produced by nuclear bomb explosions. N Engl J Med. 1986;314:1075–7.
170. Bennion JL, Knowler WC, Mott DM, Spagnola AM, Bennett PH. Development of lithogenic bile during puberty in Pima Indians. N Engl J Med. 1979;300:873–6.

13
Modifications in biliary lipid secretion and bile acid kinetics in the pathogenesis of cholesterol gallstones

E. RODA, A. CIPOLLA, F. BAZZOLI, N. VILLANOVA, G. MAZZELLA and A. RODA

Cholesterol gallstones form as a result of three main factors: supersaturation, gallbladder hypomotility and accelerated nucleation[1]. Supersaturation of bile, usually from cholesterol hypersecretion is the oldest and most well-known of the three elements. However, despite several studies, the exact mechanisms that determine this disorder are still unknown.

This paper will focus on the relationship between biliary lipid secretion, bile acid kinetics (pool, synthesis and fractional turnover rate) and enterohepatic circulation of bile acids in the pathogenesis of cholesterol gallstones. Non-obese normolipidaemic cholesterol gallstone patients and obese patients (potential 'gallstone formers') will be used as models to better understand cholesterol gallstone pathogenesis.

Non-obese patients with gallstones have supersaturated bile due to an excessive cholesterol secretion rate[2]. Reduced bile acid pool, normal hepatic bile acid synthesis, increased recycling frequency and increased percent molar of deoxycholic acid (DCA) in bile are other features that are found in these patients (Table 1). Recycling frequency is inversely proportional to bile acid pool size and directly correlated to DCA secretion rate. There is also a very close relationship between cholesterol and DCA secretion rates[2] (Figure 1A).

Obese patients (potential gallstone formers) have some characteristics, with regard to their biliary lipids secretion, that are similar to those of gallstone patients[3]. Supersaturation of bile is due mainly to increased biliary cholesterol secretion. There is also an increased recycling frequency and normal synthesis rate but, unlike gallstone patients, bile acid pool size is not reduced even when body weight is accounted for. As with the gallstone group, these patients have a high DCA secretion rate which is correlated with recycling frequency and cholesterol secretion (Figure 1B).

Table 1 Parameters of biliary lipid metabolism

	Normal subjects	Gallstone-free obese subjects	Non-obese gallstone patients
CSI	1.05	1.27	1.55
Biliary lipid secretion			
Cholesterol (μmol/h)	175	233	195
Bile acid (mmol/h)	2.6	2.7	2.3
Phospholipid (mmol/h)	0.4	0.7	0.4
Bile acid synthesis (mg/day)	290	340	285
Bile acid pool size (mmol)	2.3	2.6	1.8
Recycling frequency (day^{-1})	9.3	11.6	14.0
Bile acid composition (%)			
CA	40	35	39
CDCA	44	38	40
DCA	16	26	21

DCA: deoxycholic acid

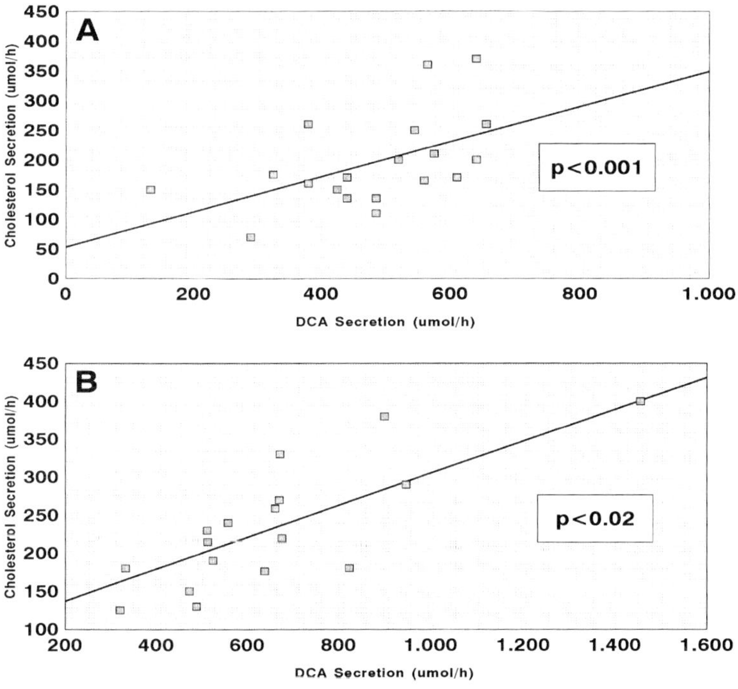

Fig. 1 Relationship between deoxycholic acid secretion and cholesterol secretion in non-obese normolipidaemic gallstone patients (A) and in obese subjects (B)

In the past, it has been shown that, in gallstone patients, there is an increased fractional turnover rate of cholic and chenodeoxycholic acids[4] with greater intestinal exposure of the bile acid pool to intestinal bacterial flora[5]. Recent studies in obese patients have reported the presence of prolonged

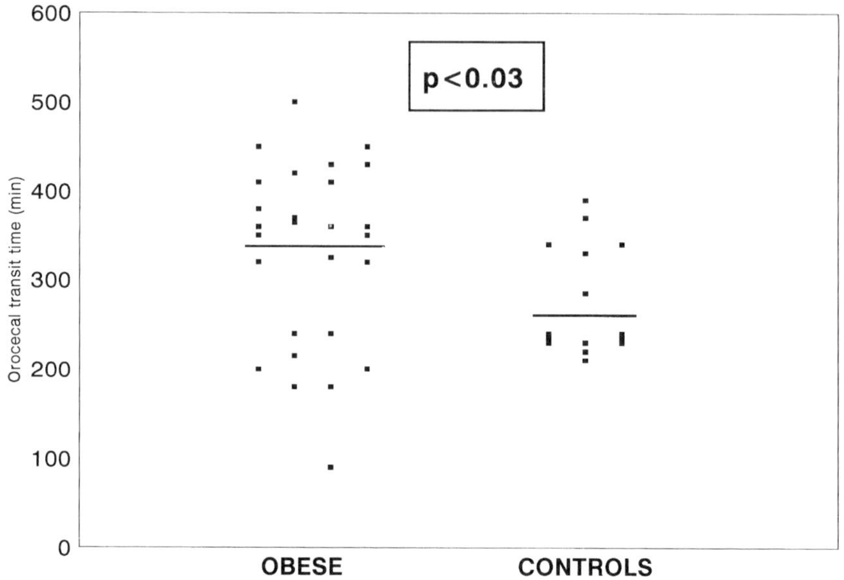

Fig. 2 Orocaecal intestinal transit time measured by starch H_2 breath test in normal and obese subjects

intestinal transit times in these subjects[6] (Figure 2). These data suggest a possible primary role of the intestine in generating cholesterol hypersecretion. In the hypotonic intestine, bile acids are held up and exposed to intestinal bacterial flora for longer than normal periods of time. These bacteria catabolize primary bile acids and this leads to an increase in fractional turnover rate and recycling frequency (in part due to unconjugated bile acid shunting via passive diffusion in the small intestine). Intestinal hypomotility may also cause slight bile acid malabsorption that induces reduction of total bile acid pool; thus, reduced pool size may be considered a secondary phenomenon. Gallbladder dismotility also contributes and integrates this defect. These events finally lead to an expansion of DCA pool size which induces hepatic cholesterol hypersecretion into bile.

This sequence of events does not necessarily exclude other factors from the pathogenesis of cholesterol hypersecretion. Genetically induced differences in cholesterol and bile acid synthesis may nevertheless play an important role and help to explain racial differences.

The fact that cholesterol gallstone disease is a very frequent condition in developed nations must lead us to take a better look into the relationships that exist between diet, intestinal function and biliary lipid secretion.

References

1. Admirand WH, Small DM. The physicochemical basis of cholesterol gallstone formation in man. J Clin Invest. 1968;47:1043–52.

2. Bazzoli F, Mazzella G, Parini P *et al.* Bile acid metabolism and enterohepatic dynamics in non-obese normolipidemic patients with cholesterol gallstones. Gastroenterology. 1991;100:A309.
3. Mazzella G, Bazzoli F, Festi D *et al.* Comparative evaluation of chenodeoxycholic and ursodeoxycholic acids in obese patients. Effects on biliary lipid metabolism during weight maintenance and weight reduction. Gastroenterology. 1991;101:490–6.
4. Nilsell K, Angelin B, Lilejeqvist L, Einarsson K. Biliary lipid output and bile acid kinetics in cholesterol gallstone disease. Evidence for an increased hepatic secretion of cholesterol in Swedish patients. Gastroenterology. 1985;89:287–93.
5. Roda E, Aldini R, Mazzella G *et al.* Enterohepatic circulation of bile acids after cholecystectomy. Gut. 1978;19:640–9.
6. Ventrucci M, Villanova N, Conci T, Cornia GL, Roda E. Investigation of intestinal transit time and absorption of starch in obesity. Gastroenterology. 1993;104:A65

14
Role of gallbladder dysmotility in gallstone formation

P. PORTINCASA, K.J. VAN ERPECUM, M.F.J.K. STOLK and G.P. VAN BERGE-HENEGOUWEN

INTRODUCTION

Cholesterol (XOL)-rich gallstones comprise about 75–80% of gallstones in Western countries. XOL gallstone disease may be regarded as an abnormal disposal of XOL in bile. For XOL gallstones to occur, *at least* three simultaneous defects must be present: XOL supersaturation of bile (with formation of XOL-rich unstable vesicles); rapid crystallization of XDL in bile (due to kinetic defects, such as a shortage of crystallization-inhibiting or an abundance of crystallization-promoting factors, glycoproteins in particular); and prolonged gallbladder stasis (due to impaired gallbladder motility) (Fig. 1). The final result is the early *nucleation* of XOL molecules[1] from XOL-rich vesicles and the subsequent *crystallization* of XOL[2], which eventually conglomerates into micro- and macroscopic gallstones.

This chapter will focus on the role of gallbladder motility in the pathogenesis of XOL cholelithiasis.

GALLBLADDER MOTILITY AND XOL GALLSTONES: CURRENT OPINIONS

Increased fasting gallbladder volume at sonography is frequently found in gallstone patients[3–8]. We confirmed this finding in two large epidemiological–clinical studies[9,10] and showed that about 15% of gallstone patients had a fasting gallbladder volume greater than 43 ml, which represented the 97.5th percentile or upper limit of gallstone-free controls[10]. An efficient gallbladder emptying (i.e. small gallbladder residue volume) after a test meal or exogenous stimulation with cholecystokinin (CCK) is found in the majority (60–80%) of patients with gallstones (also referred to as *strong contractors* or *contractors*)[6–8,11–14]. In this case the absolute amount of bile evacuated in the duodenum can be even greater than that of healthy subjects, especially if fasting gallbladder volume is increased[8,10]. By contrast,

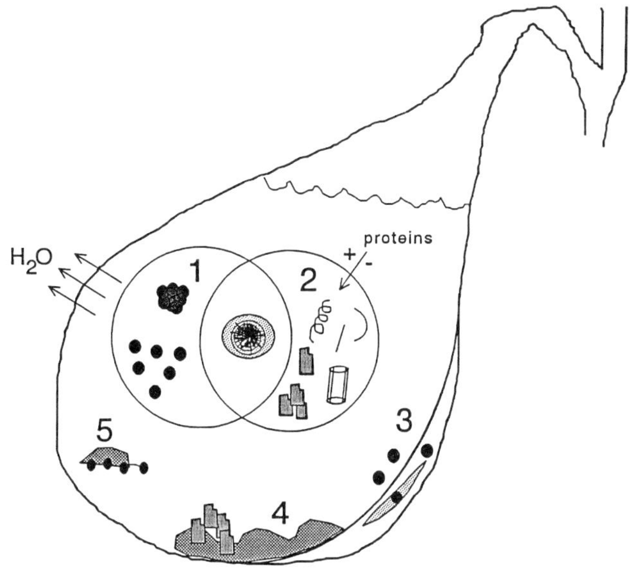

Fig. 1 Current concepts of the multiple defects in the pathogenesis of XOL gallstones. (1) Supersaturation of bile with XOL (•) and formation of XOL-rich unstable vesicles; (2) shortage of inhibiting or abundance of promoting biliary proteins leading to rapid crystallization of XOL (as classical plates and other shapes such as spirals, needles, arcs, tubules and aggregates of plates); (3) impaired smooth muscle contractility (myotoxicity of XOL?); (4) XOL crystal trapping by mucosal mucin; (5) increased percentage of the hydrophobic bile salt deoxycholate. The diagram of Venn shows two of the multiple defects. Another circle is the gallbladder itself (impaired motility), where all these events occur (adapted from ref. 128)

impaired gallbladder emptying (i.e. decreased ejection volume *and* increased residual gallbladder volume) is typically found in *weak contractors* (or *hypocontractors*)[6–8,10]. We[10] and others[15,16] have shown that differences in contractility between strong and weak contractors also exist *in vitro* when gallbladder smooth muscle strips are incubated with CCK, the physiological mediator of gallbladder contraction.

The gallbladder motility defect found in XOL cholelithiasis might occur early. In animal experiments with lithogenic diet the impairment of both gallbladder contractility[17] and emptying[18] is found *prior to* gallstone formation. Increased fasting and postprandial gallbladder residual volume will promote stasis of concentrated bile (see below). This, in turn, may cause enrichment in nucleating agents and subsequent XOL crystallization. Several factors such as interdigestive intestinal motility, CCK release, gallbladder innervation, inflammation, gallstones and bile composition should be examined when considering the pathogenesis of impaired gallbladder motility in cholelithiasis.

A physiological gallbladder emptying (30–40% of fasting volume) is observed during the late phase II of the migrating motor complex (MMC), a cyclic triphasic pattern of gastrointestinal contractile activity with a frequency of 1–3 h, occurring during the fasting or interdigestive state[19]. However, impairment of gastrointestinal motility frequently occurs in cholelithiasis, including slow transit time of the whole gut[20]. In a recent study we employed ambulatory overnight six-channel antroduodenal manometry and gallbladder sonography in XOL gallstone patients. Compared to healthy subjects we found that gallstone patients had longer MMC cycles and disruption of motilin release pattern. Interestingly, interdigestive gallbladder emptying was greatly reduced since there was no significant fluctuation of fasting gallbladder volume[21]. Thus, an abnormal interdigestive gallbladder emptying, in addition to the postprandial defect, might also be an important pathogenetic factor in XOL gallstone patients by providing time for the gallbladder mucosa to concentrate the residue in the gallbladder[22].

CCK has a key role in postprandial gallbladder contraction[12,23–25] and in the maintenance of fasting gallbladder volume[26,27]. A decreased release of endogenous CCK might therefore contribute to the pathogenesis of the gallbladder hypomotility in gallstone patients. However, postprandial CCK plasma levels in gallstone patients have been found either normal[5,7,28] or diminished in patients with a good gallbladder emptying, and increased (and similar to controls) in those with a poor gallbladder emptying[12]. Van Erpecum *et al.*[6] found increased postprandial CCK plasma levels only in weak contractor gallstone patients.

Either qualitative or quantitative changes in the gallbladder innervation may contribute to one or more events leading to cholelithiasis. Intact cholinergic pathways are essential for the full physiological effect of CCK on the gallbladder[29]. Vagotomy predisposes to gallbladder stasis and this, in turn, increases the risk of cholelithiasis[30,31]. Chronic inflammation of the gallbladder wall or biliary changes might affect intramural neurons[32]. Gallbladders excised from gallstone patients had decreased intramural neuronal density as compared to control tissues[33]. Gallbladder stasis might also facilitate the adverse effect of more hydrophobic bile salts (e.g. deoxycholate) on cholinergic nerve membranes in the gallbladder wall[34].

Large stones might physically impede gallbladder evacuation. The influence of stones *per se* in the unobstructed viscus, however, is very limited. In the experimental animal, impaired gallbladder motility antedates gallstone formation[35–38] and the implantation of prosthetic gallstones diminishes *in vitro* gallbladder contractility only by 20% without changing bile composition[39]. In humans, gallbladder hypomotility is also found with a small gallstone[10,11,40–45], and does not improve after shock-wave lithotripsy and successful stone clearance[46–48] (see also below).

Chronic cholecystitis is common during cholelithiasis[49], and phlogistic changes can antedate gallstone formation[16]. However, gallbladder inflammation is often mild[13,14]. We have shown, using a specific histological scoring system, that the degree of gallbladder inflammation was moderate and similar between strong and weak contractor gallstone patients[8,10].

Qualitative changes of bile might also influence gallbladder smooth-muscle function in XOL cholelithiasis. The gallbladder is able to absorb biliary XOL[50], which might act as a direct myotoxic agent causing gallbladder smooth-muscle stiffness and functional impairment[51]. The toxic effect of XOL in situations with supersaturated bile could potentially cause this so-called ‘XOL shock’ on the smooth muscle at a very early stage. Muscle strips from human specimens with XOL stones or cholesterolosis have reduced *in vitro* CCK-induced contractility compared with muscle strips from specimens with pigment stones[10,52]. Impaired gallbladder emptying is also found in gallstone-free patients with excess biliary XOL[53,54]. The gallbladder smooth muscle CCK-receptor has been analysed[13,55–58]. Upp *et al.* reported that CCK-receptor-binding affinity was lower in a subgroup of gallstone patients with a weak gallbladder contraction[13]. In another study, however, no difference in CCK-receptor capacity/affinity between controls and gallstone patients was found[57]. Excess biliary XOL might also affect the signal transduction *across* smooth muscle plasma membrane, leading to impaired production of intracellular second messengers (e.g. phosphoinositols)[59] with defective release of intracellular calcium and contractility[60–63]. Interestingly, it has been recently shown that direct manipulation of XOL content in muscle membranes of prairie dog gallbladder incubated with XOL-containing liposomes impaired CCK-induced muscle contraction[64]. More hydrophobic biliary bile salts are also able to directly impair the contractility of the gallbladder *in vitro*[65]. It is possible that, during gallbladder stasis, bile salts might have an adverse effect on gallbladder musculature, since bile salts can also be absorbed in small amounts by the gallbladder wall[66]. We have shown[67] that minute amounts of hydrophobic bile salts (10^{-6} mol/l deoxycholate) can inhibit acetylcholine-induced contractility of human gallbladder smooth muscle *in vitro*. Furthermore, a detrimental effect on human gallbladder emptying *in vivo* has been reported during bile acid therapy with CDCA[28,68] and, for UDCA, by some[4,5,68] but not all[28] studies.

EXPERIMENTAL WORKS

Bile concentration

XOL nucleation and crystallization from a supersaturated bile are important steps preceding the aggregation of solid XOL crystals into stones. The overall process might be facilitated when bile is being concentrated in the gallbladder. The effect of bile concentration on XOL crystallization is already evident in gallstone-free subjects with XOL crystals in their fresh gallbladder bile: the nucleation time of typical XOL plate-like crystals is shorter in concentrated bile than in dilute bile of gallstone-free patients with crystals in fresh bile[69]. We[70] and others[69,71,72] have shown that this difference in nucleation behaviour of XOL (according to bile concentration) also occurs in gallstone patients[70]. Recently we have extended these observations in gallbladder biles from 50 XOL gallstone patients[73]. Dilute bile (total lipid concentration 3.7 ± 0.2 g/dl, $n = 16$) had a higher cholesterol saturation index (CSI) (1.7 ± 0.14 vs 1.3 ± 0.6, $p = 0.020$), and a longer nucleation time for classical XOL plates (8.3 ± 2.0 vs 4.2 ± 0.6 days, $p = 0.02$) than concentrated bile (total lipid concentration >5 g/dl, 9.9 ± 0.6 g/dl, $n = 34$). Interestingly, the nucleation time of novel crystal forms such as arcs and needles (most likely non-hydrated XOL[74]) was also longer for dilute than concentrated bile (10.8 ± 2.2 vs 5.2 ± 1.0 days, $p = 0.01$). XOL transport and solubilization in bile is accomplished through the formation of XOL–phospholipid–bile salt mixed micelles[75] and XOL–phospholipid vesicles[76,77]. Thus, our data confirm that bile concentration – through formation of XOL-rich and unstable vesicles which tend to aggregate – facilitates the nucleation of monohydrate XOL crystals[69,71,72,78–80]. Furthermore, it seems that bile concentration hastens the growth of other XOL crystal forms – namely non-hydrated XOL – which precede or are associated with classical monohydrate XOL crystals.

In our study a negative correlation was found between total bile salt concentration and mol% phospholipids or mol% XOL, and a positive correlation between total bile salt concentration and mol% bile salts. The fact that CSI decreases at increasing bile concentration[70,71,81,82] depends on the method used for calculation of CSI (which takes into account only micellar XOL solubilization and ignores vesicular XOL solubilization[83]). This explains why CSI increases in more dilute biles, even if mol% XOL, phospholipid and bile salts are unchanged. Furthermore, mol% XOL and phospholipid decrease, and mol% bile salt increases, at increasing bile concentration. This results in a lower CSI at increasing bile concentration. Decreased mol% XOL and phospholipid are probably caused by XOL[50,84] and phospholipid absorption in the gallbladder[85,86], possibly as XOL–phospholipid vesicles. Further studies were planned by our group in order to further address this issue (see below).

Gallbladder motility and gallbladder bile composition

Little is known about the mechanisms by which gallbladder emptying can influence bile composition and XOL crystallization. We have recently characterized the relationship between gallbladder emptying, lipid composition and crystallization of biliary XOL in 30 gallstone patients undergoing elective cholecystectomy for symptomatic XOL gallstones[8]. The sonographic study of postprandial gallbladder emptying (mixed meal, 30 g of fat) identified 22 strong contractors (postprandial emptying ≥50%) and eight weak contractors (postprandial emptying <50%). Hypocontractors had a residual gallbladder volume (after a test meal) which was 2- and 5-fold increased, compared to strong contractors and to 20 healthy subjects, respectively.

The analysis of gallbladder bile (which had a total lipid concentration >5 g/dl in all patients) showed that bile salt concentration in weak contractors was 2-fold higher (235 ± 25 vs 130 ± 11 mmol/l, $p<0.001$) and phospholipid concentration was 1.5-fold higher than strong contractors. XOL concentration was comparable between weak and strong contractors. This biliary lipid profile resulted in a 1.7-fold increase of total lipid concentration but a 56% decrease of CSI (0.90 ± 0.08 vs 1.61 ± 0.17) in weak contractors. Neither the percentage of vesicular XOL, nor bile salt species, molecular species of phosphatidylcholine nor the degree of gallbladder wall inflammation were significantly different between weak and strong contracting gallstone patients. Weak contractors tended to have a longer nucleation time (i.e. XOL plate observation time in ultrafiltered bile, 5 ± 2 days vs 3 ± 0.6) than weak contractors, but the difference did not attain statistical significance. These findings suggest that different patterns of postprandial gallbladder emptying might differently influence bile composition, providing different pathogenetic mechanisms for XOL gallstone formation:

1. In strong contractors, hypersecretion and high saturation of XOL appear to be major pathogenetic mechanisms for precipitation–crystallization of biliary XOL. Although in these patients the gallbladder motility defect

might be moderate, the increase of fasting and residual gallbladder volume[8,10,48] may further enhance the chance for XOL crystal aggregation.
2. In weak contractors the important gallbladder motility defect (with major increase of residual volume) provides enough residence time for biliary changes to occur. Stasis of bile is followed by increased absorption of water, XOL and phospholipid (possibly as vesicles[86]) across the gallbladder wall[50,84,87]. These events lead to increased concentration of total lipids and bile salts, and to enhanced XOL precipitation *despite* a less supersaturated bile.

Gallbladder motility in extracorporeal shock-wave lithotripsy (ESWL)

Impaired gallbladder emptying may cause incomplete[88] or delayed[89,90] fragment clearance after ESWL. The gallbladder motility defect has also been suggested to be an important co-factor for the recurrence of gallstones after ESWL[47]. Within a larger trial[48] we studied gallbladder motility, gallstone clearance and recurrence in a group of 49 gallstone patients successfully treated with ESWL + adjuvant bile salt dissolution therapy (Ursofalk® and Chenofalk®, each 7–8 mg kg^{-1} day^{-1}, Tramedico, The Netherlands). Median follow-up period after ESWL was 42 months (range 9–62 months). All patients (67% with solitary stones, mean diameter of largest stone 15.0 ± 0.94 mm) achieved complete gallstone clearance (two consecutive negative ultrasound) after 6 months (median, range 0.2–27). Stone recurrence (sonography) was documented at ultrasound in 17 patients after 15 months (median, range 3–50). Gallbladder volume was measured by sonography in the fasting state and during 2 h after a standard test meal[91]. Twenty-three healthy subjects served as control. Of the 49 patients, 24 had a good postprandial gallbladder emptying (arbitrarily defined as a residual volume ≤6 ml) while 25 had a poor gallbladder emptying (residual volume >6 ml).

1. We found that a small residual gallbladder volume after a standard stimulus was associated with fast gallstone clearance after ESWL. Median time to observe 50% patients free of gallstones was shorter in patients with good than poor gallbladder emptying (3.4 vs 10 months, log-rank statistics; $p<0.004$). Residual gallbladder volume tended to correlate positively with clearance time ($r = +0.32$, $n = 49$, $p = 0.055$), especially in patients with initial multiple gallstone (Fig. 2). Our findings integrate previous studies on this topic[89,90,92]. Furthermore, we also observed that fragment clearance was faster in those patients with initial solitary gallstones and good fragmentation after ESWL (fragment size ≤5 mm). This is also in agreement with previous studies[92–95].
2. Gallbladder motility was impaired in gallstone patients, especially in those with gallstone recurrence (Table 1). Fasting gallbladder volume was comparable between controls and patients without recurrence, but was 20–30% greater in those patients with recurrence ($p<0.05$). Residual gallbladder volume was 3-fold and 1.9-fold in patients with recurrence and no recurrence, respectively, as compared to controls ($p<0.05$). The ejection gallbladder volume (Δvol max%) was decreased by 26% and 35% in patients without and with gallstone recurrence, respectively ($p<0.05$ vs controls).

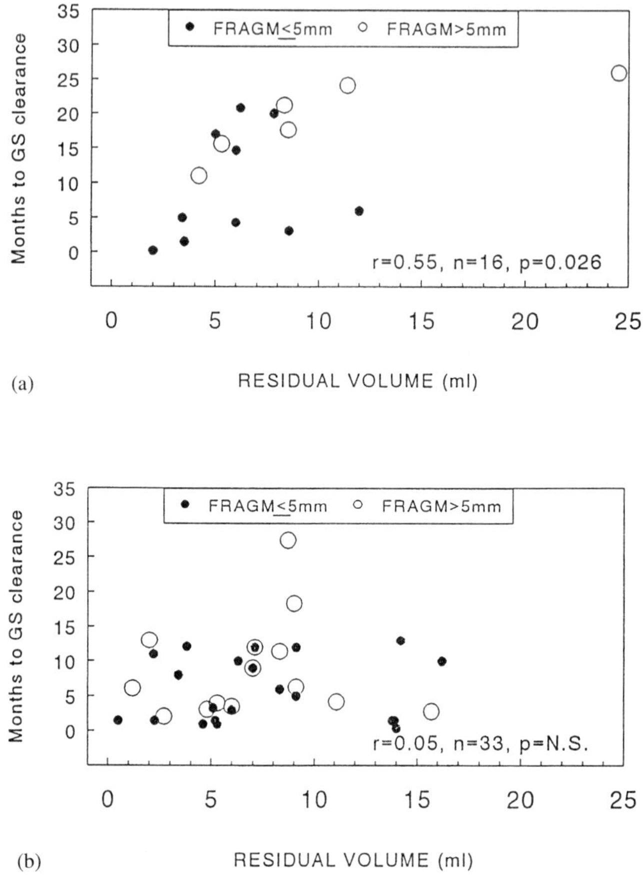

Fig. 2 Relationship between residual gallbladder volume and time to become gallstone-free in 49 patients with initial multiple (**a**) and solitary (**b**) stones. Fragment size at first ultrasound after ESWL (≤ or >5 mm) is indicated as an additional factor influencing speed of clearance

Table 1 Indices of gallbladder motility in gallstone patients without and with stone recurrence and healthy controls

	Controls (n = 23)	*No recurrence* (n = 32)	*Recurrence* (n = 17)
Fasting volume (ml)	25.4±1.7	24.6±1.4	31.3±2.8*†
Residual volume (ml)	3.2±0.7	6.2±0.7*	9.5±1.3*†
Residual volume (%)	12.7±2.2	26.6±2.4*	34.1±5.2*
Δvol max (%)	87.3±2.3	73.4±2.4*	65.9±5.2*

*p<0.05 vs controls; †p<0.05 vs no recurrence (nominal p value; ANOVA followed by Fisher's LSD); residual volume is the smallest postprandial gallbladder volume measured postprandially during 120 min; Δvol max indicates ejection volume. Indices are given as millilitres and as percentage of initial fasting gallbladder volume

There were more recurrences in the group of patients with poor gallbladder emptying (residual volume >6 ml) than in those with good gallbladder (residual volume ≤6 ml) (52% vs 21%, $p = 0.023$). Accordingly, gallstone recurrence rate at 57 months by actuarial analysis was much greater in patients with poor gallbladder emptying than good gallbladder emptying (45.2 ± 23.0% vs 78.0 ± 17.0%, log-rank statistics; $p = 0.020$). This study shows that impaired gallbladder motility (particularly an increased residual gallbladder volume) after ESWL is associated with a high gallstone recurrence rate. The median postprandial residual gallbladder volumes of patients with and without recurrence was close to that reported after CCK infusion by the group of Munich[47]. The increase of fasting gallbladder volume in patients with gallstone recurrence, however, has not been reported before and might point to a more complex motility defect.

CORRECTION OF THE GALLBLADDER MOTILITY DEFECT: WHICH ROLE?

Animal experiments suggest that gallstone formation can be prevented by improving gallbladder emptying[96–98]. Following the above-mentioned considerations it is tempting to speculate that the correction of gallbladder stasis in selected patients might improve the enterohepatic circulation of bile salts, the composition of bile[99] and the clearance of gallstone fragments, and impede the recurrence of stones.

Several drugs are of potential interest in this respect. In humans, daily intravenous CCK prevents gallbladder stasis and sludge/gallstone formation during long-term total parenteral nutrition[100,101]. Cerulein, the CCK analogue, accelerated post-ESWL fragment clearance, at least in patients with small solitary gallstones[102]. Cholestyramine, the non-adsorbable bile acid sequestrant resin, interrupts the physiological negative feedback between duodenal bile salts and endogenous CCK release[103,104]. It is of interest that this resin at low doses (4–8 g) induces a major decrease of gallbladder volume when ingested alone, or with an oral[105] or intraduodenal test meal[106]. We recently showed that the effect of cholestyramine on fasting gallbladder volume is sustained, and does not induce a change of antroduodenal motility from fasting to postprandial state[107]. In two previous studies we found that only 4 g oral cholestyramine given with 12 g fat greatly increased gallbladder emptying, and reduced the residual volume in both gallstone patients[108] and obese subjects[109] with gallbladder hypomotility. Intravenous amino acid solutions also promote gallbladder emptying in healthy subjects[110], possible through endogenous CCK release[111]. Thus, giving aminoacids by the intravenous route might help in recipients of parenteral nutrition with gallbladder stasis[111,112] and at risk for formation of sludge and gallstones[100,111,113]. CCK-induced release by only 10 g of dietary fats completely restored gallbladder emptying and prevented the formation of gallstones in obese people during very low-calorie dieting[114,115]. Erythromycin (a motilin analogue), induced a significant reduction of fasting and postprandial residual gallbladder volumes in both healthy subjects and gallstone patients after acute and chronic administration[116–118]. In an animal model of XOL gallstone disease, adding erythromycin restored impaired gallbladder contractility in the XOL diet group, possibly via a more rapid enterohepatic circulation of bile salts, increased bile salt secretion and XOL solubility in bile[119]. In the same animal model a similar effect has been reported for cisapride, a pro-cholinergic drug[99]. Cisapride also improved gallbladder hypokinesia in chronically dyspeptic patients[120,121]. Although this prokinetic might induce CCK release, most probably via an atropine-sensitive mechanism, chronic treatment resulted in diminished postprandial CCK release[122]. A detrimental effect of cisapride on gallbladder dynamics has been also described in healthy volunteers[123]. Non-steroidal anti-inflammatory drugs might also affect gallbladder motility[124]. Chronic indomethacin improved gallbladder emptying in gallstone patients[125]. However, in healthy volunteers acute ingestion of both indomethacin and misoprostol did not do so[126]. Levosulpiride (a dopaminergic DA_2-receptor antagonist), has been reported to accelerate gallbladder emptying in dyspeptic patients[127].

CONCLUSIONS

The gallbladder motility defect in XOL gallstone disease is an early condition which facilitates a series of pathological events in the gallbladder such as bile concentration and enrichment of nucleating proteins which enhance XOL crystal growth and aggregation. In gallstone patients, differences in postprandial gallbladder emptying pattern can be linked to differences in bile composition, providing different pathogenetic mechanisms for XOL gallstone formation. Effective gallbladder emptying is important for fast fragment clearance, and to decrease gallstone recurrence rate after ESWL. We speculate that XOL crystallization, gallstone clearance and recurrence might be modulated by improving gallbladder motility in selected patients. Prospective studies need to address this issue further.

References

1. Holzbach RT. Nucleation of cholesterol crystals in native bile. Hepatology. 1990;12:155S–61S.
2. Holan KR, Holzbach RT, Hermann RE, Cooperman AM, Claffey W. Nucleation time: a key factor in the pathogenesis of cholesterol gallstone disease. Gastroenterology. 1979;77:611–17.
3. Kishk SMA, Darweesh RMA, Dodds WJ *et al.* Sonographic evaluation of resting gallbladder volume and postprandial emptying in patients with gallstones. AJR. 1987; 148:875–9.
4. Festi D, Frabboni R, Bazzoli F *et al.* Gallbladder motility in cholesterol gallstone disease. Effect of ursodeoxycholic acid administration and gallstone dissolution. Gastroenterology. 1990;99:1779–85.
5. Forgacs IC, Murphy GM, Dowling RH. Influence of gallstones and UDCA on gallbladder emptying. Gastroenterology. 1984;87:299–307.
6. Van Erpecum KJ, vanBerge-Henegouwen GP, Stolk MFJ, Hopman WPM, Jansen JBMJ, Lamers CBHW. Fasting gallbladder volume, postprandial emptying and cholecystokinin release in gallstone patients and normal subjects. J Hepatol. 1992;14:194–202.
7. Pauletzki J, Cicala M, Holl J, Sauerbruch T, Schafmayer A, Paumgartner G. Correlation between gallbladder fasting volume and postprandial emptying in patients with gallstones and healthy controls. Gut. 1993;34:1443–7.
8. Stolk MFJ, Van Erpecum KJ, Renooij W, Portincasa P, van de Heijning BJM, vanBerge-Henegouwen GP. Gallbladder emptying *in vivo*, bile composition and nucleation of cholesterol crystals in patients with cholesterol gallstones. Gastroenterology. 1995;108:1882–8.

9. Palasciano G, Serio G, Portincasa P *et al.* Gallbladder volume in adults and relationship to age, sex, body mass index and gallstones: a sonographic population study. Am J Gastroenterol. 1992;87:493–7.
10. Portincasa P, Di Ciaula A, Baldassarre G *et al.* Gallbladder motor function in gallstones patients: sonographic and *in vitro* studies on the role of gallstones, smooth muscle function and gallbladder wall inflammation. J Hepatol. 1994;21:430–40.
11. Pomeranz IS, Shaffer EA. Abnormal gallbladder emptying in a subgroup of patients with gallstones. Gastroenterology. 1985;88:787–91.
12. Thompson JC, Fried GM, Ogden WD *et al.* Correlation between release of cholecystokinin and contraction of the gallbladder in patients with gallstones. Ann Surg. 1982;195:670–6.
13. Upp JR, Jr, Nealon WH, Singh P *et al.* Correlation of cholecystokinin receptors with gallbladder contractility in patients with gallstones. Ann Surg. 1987;205:641–8.
14. Masclee AA, Jansen JB, Driessen WM, Geuskens LM, Lamers CB. Plasma cholecystokinin and gallbladder responses to intraduodenal fat in gallstone patients. Dig Dis Sci. 1989;34:353–9.
15. Shulz M, Hanisch E, Guldutuna S. *In vitro*-kontraktilitatsverhalten humaner muskulatur von gallenblasen mit und ohne steinerkrankung – Relevanz des prostaglandin-systems fur die CCK-regulierte motorik. Z Gastroenterol. 1993;31:376–87.
16. Zhu XG, Greeley GH, Newman J, Wiener I, Fagan CJ, Thompson JC. Correlation of *in vitro* measurements of contractility of the gallbladder with *in vivo* ultrasonographic findings in patients with gallstones. Surg Gynecol Obstet. 1985;161:470–2.
17. Fridhandler TM, Davison JS, Shaffer EA. Defective gallbladder contractility in the ground squirrel and prairie dog during the early stages of cholesterol gallstone formation. Gastroenterology. 1983;85:830–6.
18. Pellegrini CA, Ryan T, Broderick W, Way LW. Gallbladder filling and emptying during cholesterol gallstone formation in the prairie dog. A cholescintigraphic study. Gastroenterology. 1986;90:143–9.
19. Stolk MFJ, van Erpecum KJ, Smout AJP, *et al.* Motor cycles with phase III in antrum are associated with high motilin levels and prolonged gallbladder emptying. Am J Physiol. 1993;264:G596–G600.
20. Heaton KW, Emmett PM, Symes CL, Braddon FEM. An explanation for gallstones in normal-weight woman: slow intestinal transit. Lancet. 1993;341:8–10.
21. Stolk MFJ, Van Erpecum KJ, Samson M *et al.* Interdigestive gallbladder emptying, antroduodenal motility and motilin release in cholesterol gallstone patients. In: Stolk MFJ, Pathogenesis of cholesterol gallstones. Utrecht, Thesis, Universiteit Utrecht; 1993:65–78.
22. Itoh Z, Takahashi I, Nakaya M, Suzuki T, Arai H, Wakabayashi K. Interdigestive gallbladder bile concentration in relation to periodic contraction of gallbladder in the dog. Gastroenterology. 1982;83:645–51.
23. Wiener I, Inoue K, Fagan CJ, Lilja P, Watson LC, Thompson JC. Release of CCK in man: correlation of blood levels with gallbladder contraction. Ann Surg. 1981;194:321–27.
24. Hildebrand P, Berlinger C, Gyr K *et al.* Effects of a cholecystokinin antagonist on intestinal phase of pancreatic and biliary responses in man. J Clin Invest. 1990;85:640–6.
25. Meyer BM, Werth BA, Beglinger C *et al.* Role of cholecystokinin in regulation of gastrointestinal motor functions. Lancet. 1989;2:12–15.
26. Niederau C, Heintges T, Rovati L, Strohmeyer G. Effects of loxiglumide on gallbladder emptying in healthy volunteers. Gastroenterology. 1989;97:1331–6.
27. Konturek JW, Konturek SJ, Kurek A, Bogdal J, Olesky J, Rovati L. CCK receptor antagonism by loxiglumide and gallbladder contractions in response to cholecystokinin, sham feeding and ordinary feeding in man. Nippon Heikatsukin Gakkai Zasshi. 1989;25:360–2.
28. Van Erpecum KJ, vanBerge-Henegouwen GP, Stolk MFJ, Hopman WP, Jansen JB, Lamers CB. Effects of ursodeoxycholic acid on gallbladder contraction and cholecystokinin release in gallstone patients and normal subjects. Gastroenterology. 1990;99:836–42.
29. Takahashi T, May DO. Cholinergic dependence of gallbladder response to cholecystokinin in the guinea pig *in vivo*. Am J Physiol. 1991;261:G565–9.
30. Baxter JN, Grime JS, Critchley M, Jenkins SA, Shields P. Relationship between gastric emptying of a solid meal and emptying of the gallbladder before and after vagotomy. Gut. 1987;28:855–63.
31. Fisher RS, Rock E, Malmud LS. Gallbladder emptying in response to sham feeding in humans. Gastroenterology. 1986;90:1854–7.

32. McKirdy ML, Johnson CD, McKirdy HC. Inflammation impairs neurally mediated responses to electrical field stimulation in isolated strips of human gallbladder muscle. Dig Dis Sci. 1994;39:2229–34.
33. Conte VP. Normal neuronal features of the human gallbladder and structural changes in cholelithiasis patients. Rev Hosp Clin Fac Med Sao Paulo. 1989;44:211–13.
34. Xu QW, Shaffer EA. The influence of bile salts on cholinergically mediated gallbladder contraction. Gastroenterology. 1993;102:948A.
35. Meyer PD, DenBesten L, Gurll NJ. Effects of cholesterol gallstone induction on gallbladder function and bile salt pool size in the prairie dog model. Surgery. 1978;83:599–604.
36. Roslyn JJ, DenBesten L, Thompson JE, Cohen K. Chronic cholelithiasis and decreased bile salt pool size: cause or effect?. Am J Surg. 1980;139:119–24.
37. Gurll NJ, Meyer PD, DenBesten L. Effect of cholesterol crystals on gallbladder function in cholelithiasis. Surg Forum. 1977;28:412–13.
38. Doty JE, Pitt HA, Kuchenbecker SL, DenBesten L. Impaired gallbladder emptying before gallstone formation in prairie dog. Gastroenterology. 1983;85:168–74.
39. Pomeranz IS, Davison JS, Shaffer EA. The effects of prosthetic gallstones on gallbladder function and bile composition. J Surg Res. 1986;41:47–52.
40. Konikoff FM, Cohen DE, Carey MC. Phospholipid molecular species influence crystal habits and transition sequences of metastable intermediates during cholesterol crystallization from bile salt-rich model bile. J Lipid Res. 1994;35:60–70.
41. Fisher RS, Stelzer F, Rock E, Malmud LS. Abnormal gallbladder emptying in patients with gallstones. Dig Dis Sci. 1982;27:1019–24.
42. Forgacs IC, Hilson AJM, Maisey MN, Murphy GM, Dowling RH. Ursodeoxycholic acid (UDCA) treatment reduces gallbladder contraction in response to exogenous CCK. A possible explanation for relief of biliary pain during therapy. Clin Sci. 1981;61:21P.
43. Forgacs IC, Maisey MN, Murphy GM, Dowling RH. New radioimmunoassay for cholecystokinin (CCK): relationship between post-prandial CCK levels and gall bladder contraction. Gut. 1982;23:906A.
44. Krishnamurthy GT, Bobba VR, McConnel D, Turner F, Mesgarzdeh M, Kingston E. Quantitative biliary dynamics: introduction of a non-invasive scintigraphic technique. J Nucl Med. 1983;24:217–23.
45. Shaffer EA, McOrmond P, Duggan H. Quantitative cholescintigraphy: assessment of gallbladder filling and emptying and duodenogastric reflux. Gastroenterology. 1980;79:899–906.
46. Spengler U, Sackmann M, Sauerbruch T, Holl J, Paumgartner G. Gallbladder motility before and after extracorporeal shock-wave lithotripsy. Gastroenterology. 1989;96:860–3.
47. Berr F, Mayer M, Sackmann M, Sauerbruch T, Holl J, Paumgartner G. Pathogenic factors in early recurrence of cholesterol gallstones. Gastroenterology. 1994;106:215–24.
48. Portincasa P, Van Erpecum KJ, van de Meeberg PC, vanBerge-Henegouwen GP. Gallbladder (GB) motility is important for gallstone (GS) clearance and recurrence after extracorporeal shock-wave lithotripsy (ESWL). Neth J Med. 1995 (In press).
49. Edlund Y, Zettergren L. Histopathology of the gallbladder in gallstone disease related to clinical data. Acta Chir Scand. 1959;116:450–60.
50. Jacyna MR, Ross PE, Bakar MA *et al.* Characteristics of cholesterol absorption by human gallbladder: relevance to cholesterolosis. J Clin Pharmacol. 1987;40:524–9.
51. LaMont JT, Carey MC. Cholesterol gallstone formation. 2. Pathobiology and pathomechanics. Prog Liver Dis. 1992;10:165–91.
52. Behar J, Lee KY, Thompson WR, Biancani P. Gallbladder contraction in patients with pigment and cholesterol stones. Gastroenterology. 1989;97:1479–84.
53. Brugge WR, Brand DL, Atkins H, Lane B, Abel WG. Gallbladder dyskinesia in chronic acalculous cholecystitis. Dig Dis Sci. 1986;31:461–7.
54. van der Werf SD, vanBerge-Henegouwen GP, Palsma DM, Ruben AT. Motor function of the gallbladder and cholesterol saturation of duodenal bile. Neth J Med. 1987;30:160–71.
55. Portincasa P, Howard A, Murphy GM, Dowling RH. Cholecystokinin receptor binding by human gallbladder myocyte membranes. Gut. 1986;27:1261A.
56. Portincasa P, Murphy GM, Dowling RH, Palasciano G, Albano O. A method proposed for the preparation of plasma membranes from myocytes of human gallbladders, In: Gorrod JW, Albano O, Papa S, editors. Molecular aspect of human disease. London: Ellis Horwood; 1988:241–9.

57. Schjoldager B, Molero X, Miller LJ. Functional and biochemical characterization of the human gallbladder muscularis cholecystokinin receptor. Gastroenterology. 1989;96:1119–25.
58. Steigerwalt RW, Goldfine ID, Williams JA. Characterization of cholecystokinin receptors on bovine gallbladder membranes. Am J Physiol. 1984;247:G709–14.
59. Yu P, Chen Q, Harnett K, Biancani P, Behar J. Impaired IP3 and DAG production in human gallbladder muscle with cholesterol stones. Gastroenterology. 1994;107:A1220–30.
60. Behar J, Rhim BY, Thompson W, Biancani P. Inositol trisphosphate restores impaired human gallbladder motility associated with cholesterol stones. Gastroenterology. 1993;104:563–8.
61. Taylor EL, Jr, Harrington TM. Cholecystitis and cholelithiasis. Prim Care. 1988;15:147–56.
62. Xu QW, Shaffer EA. The influence of bile salts on small intestinal motility in the guinea pig in vitro. Gastroenterology. 1992;103:29–35.
63. Yu P, De Petris G, Biancani P, Amaral J, Behar J. Cholecystokinin-coupled intracellular signaling in human gallbladder muscle. Gastroenterology. 1994;106:763–70.
64. Yu P, Chen Q, Biancani P, Behar J. Excess membrane cholesterol impairs gallbladder muscle contraction. Gastroenterology. 1995;108:A442.
65. Shaffer EA, Lax H, Bomzon A, Harrington K, Freedman S. Hydrophobic bile salts directly impair gallbladder contractility to cholecystokinin. Gastroenterology. 1990;98:A262.
66. Ostrow JD. Absorption by the gallbladder of bile acid salts, sulfobromophthalein and iodipamide. J Lab Clin Med. 1969;74:482–94.
67. Stolk MFJ, van de Heijning BJM, Van Erpecum KJ, Verheem A, Akkermans LMA, vanBerge-Henegouwen GP. A preliminary study on the effects of bile salts on *in vitro* gallbladder motility. In: Stolk MFJ. Pathogenesis of cholesterol gallstones. Ph. D. thesis, University of Utrecht, 1993:143–53.
68. Sylwestrowicz TA, Shaffer EA. Gallbladder function during gallstone dissolution. Effect of bile acid therapy in patients with gallstones. Gastroenterology. 1988;95:740–8.
69. Strasberg SM, Toth JL, Gallinger S, Harvey PR. High protein and total lipid concentration are associated with reduced metastability of bile in an early stage of cholesterol gallstone formation. Gastroenterology. 1990;98:739–46.
70. Van Erpecum KJ, vanBerge-Henegouwen GP, Stoelwinder B, Schmidt YMG, Willekens FLH. Bile concentration is a key factor for nucleation of cholesterol crystals and cholesterol saturation index in gallbladder bile of gallstone patients. Hepatology. 1990;11:1–6.
71. Halpern Z, Dudley MA, Lynn MP, Nader JM, Breuer AC, Holzbach RT. Vesicle aggregation in model systems of supersaturated bile: relation to crystal nucleation and lipid composition of the vesicular phase. J Lipid Res. 1986;27:295–306.
72. Van Erpecum KJ, Stolk MFJ, van den Broek AMWC, Renooij W, van de Heijning BJM, vanBerge-Henegouwen GP. Bile concentration promotes nucleation of cholesterol monohydrate crystals by increasing the cholesterol concentration in the vesicles. Eur J Clin Invest. 1993;23:283–8.
73. Portincasa P, Van Erpecum KJ, Jansen A, Renooij W, Gadellaa M, vanBerge-Henegouwen GP. Nucleation behaviour of various cholesterol (xol) crystals in bile from gallstone patients. Gastroenterology. 1995;108:A1150.
74. Konikoff FM, Chung DS, Donovan JM, Small DM, Carey MC. Filamentous, helical and tubular microstructures during cholesterol crystallization from bile. Evidence that biliary cholesterol does not nucleate classic monohydrate plates. J Clin Invest. 1992;90:1156–61.
75. Carey MC, Small DM. The physical chemistry of cholesterol solubility in bile. Relation to gallstone formation and dissolution in man. J Clin Invest. 1978;61:998–1026.
76. Harvey PRC, Sömjen G, Lichtenberg MS, Petrunka C, Gilat T, Strasberg SM. Nucleation of cholesterol from vesicles isolated from bile of patients with and without cholesterol gallstones. Biochim Biophys Acta. 1987;921:198–204.
77. Lee SP, Park HZ, Madani H, Kaler EW. Partial characterization of a nonmicellar system of cholesterol solubilization in bile. Am J Physiol. 1987;252:G384–8.
78. O'Leary DP. Biliary cholesterol transport and the nucleation defect on cholesterol gallstone formation. J Hepatol. 1995;22:239–46.
79. Harvey PR, Somjen GJ, Gilat T, Gallinger S, Strasberg SM. Vesicular cholesterol in bile. Relationship to protein concentration and nucleation time. Biochim Biophys Acta. 1988;958:10–18.
80. Conter RL, Roslyn JJ, Porter-Fink V, DenBesten L. Gallbladder absorption increases during early cholesterol gallstone formation. Am J Surg. 1986;151:184–92.

81. Jungst D, Lang T, von Ritter C, Pratschke E, Paumgartner G. Cholesterol nucleation time in gallbladder bile of patients with solitary or multiple cholesterol gallstones. Hepatology. 1992;15:804–8.
82. Van Erpecum KJ, vanBerge-Henegouwen GP, Stoelwinder B, Stolk MFJ, Eggink WF, Govaert WHA. Cholesterol and pigment gallstone disease: comparison of the reliability of three bile tests for differentiation between the two stone types. Scand J Gastroenterol. 1988;23:948–54.
83. Carey MC. Critical tables for calculating the cholesterol saturation of native bile. J Lipid Res. 1978;19:945–55.
84. Neiderhiser DH, Roth HP. Absorption of cholesterol by the gallbladder. J Lipid Res. 1976;17:117–24.
85. Neiderhiser DH, Morningstar WA, Roth H. Absorption of lecithin and lysolecithin by the gallbladder. J Lab Clin Med. 1973;82:891–7.
86. Purdum PP, Shamburek RD, Hylemon PB, Moore EW. Rapid phospholipid transfer across cultured human gallbladder epithelia. Gastroenterology. 1992;102:A871.
87. Ross PE, Butt AN, Gallacher C. Cholesterol absorption by the gallbladder. J Clin Pathol. 1990;43:572–5.
88. Sackmann M, Eder H, Spengler U *et al.* Gallbladder emptying is an important factor in fragment disappearance after shock wave lithotripsy. J Hepatol. 1993;17:62–6.
89. Pauletzki J, Sailer C, Klueppelberg U *et al.* Gallbladder emptying determines early gallstone clearance after shock-wave lithotripsy. Gastroenterology. 1994;107:1496–502.
90. Greiner L, Munks C, Heil W, Jakobeit C. Gallbladder stone fragments in feces after biliary extracorporeal shock wave lithotripsy. Gastroenterology. 1990;98:1620–4.
91. Everson GT, Braverman DZ, Johnson ML, Kern F, Jr. A critical evaluation of real-time ultrasonography for the study of gallbladder volume and contraction. Gastroenterology. 1980;79:40–6.
92. Buttmann A, Adamek HE, Weber J, Riemann JF. ESWL and oral dissolution therapy: what factors influence results? Dig Dis Sci. 1993;38:1702–11.
93. Gleeson D, Ruppin CD, Saunders A, Murphy GM, Dowling RH. Final outcome of ursodeoxycholic treatment in 126 patients with radiolucent gallstones. Q J Med. 1990;76:711–29.
94. Sackmann M, Pauletzki J, Sauerbruch T, Holl J, Schelling G, Paumgartner G. The Munich gallbladder lithotripsy study: results of the first 5 years with 711 patients. Ann Intern Med. 1991;114:290–6.
95. Tint SG, Dyrszke H, Sanghavi B *et al.* Lithotripsy plus ursodiol is superior to ursodiol alone for cholesterol gallstones. Gastroenterology. 1992;102:2042–9.
96. Poston GJ, Draviam EJ, Yao CZ, Townsend CM, Jr., Thompson JC. Effect of age and sensitivity to cholecystokinin on gallstone formation in the guinea pig. Gastroenterology. 1990;98:993–9.
97. Roslyn J, DenBesten L, Thompson JE, Jr. Effects of periodic emptying of gallbladder on gallbladder function and formation of cholesterol gallstone. Surg Forum. 1979;30:403–4.
98. Roslyn JJ, DenBesten L, Pitt HA, Kuchenbecker SL, Polarek JW. Effects of cholecystokinin on gallbladder stasis and cholesterol gallstone formation. J Surg Res. 1981;30:200–4.
99. Xu QW, Shaffer EA. Cisapride improves gallbladder contractility in bile lipid composition in an animal model. Gastroenterology. 1993;105:1184–91.
100. Stizmann JV, Pitt HA, Steinborn PA, Pasha ZR, Sanders RC. Cholecystokinin prevents parenteral nutrition induced biliary sludge in humans. Surg Gynecol Obstet. 1990;170:25–31.
101. Doty JE, Pitt HA, Porter Fink V, DenBesten L. Cholecystokinin prophylaxis of parenteral nutrition-induced gallbladder disease. Ann Surg. 1985;201:76–80.
102. Ziegenhagen DJ, Zehnter E, Kruis W, Pohl C. Induced gallbladder contraction accelerates fragment clearance after extracorporeal shockwave lithotripsy. J Gastroenterol Hepatol. 1993;8:406–9.
103. Gomez G, Upp JR, Lluis F *et al.* Regulation of the release of cholecystokinin by bile salts in dogs and humans. Gastroenterology. 1988;94:1036–46.
104. Koop I, Fellgiebel A, Koop H, Schafmayer A, Arnold R. Effect of cholestyramine on plasma cholecystokinin and pancreatic polypeptide levels and exocrine pancreatic secretion. Eur J Clin Invest. 1988;18:517–23.
105. Palasciano G, Portincasa P, Belfiore A, Baldassarre G, Albano O. Opposite effects of cholestyramine and loxiglumide on gallbladder dynamics in humans. Gastroenterology. 1992;102:633–9.

106. Strom BL, West SL. The epidemiology of cholesterol gallstone disease. In: Cohen S, Soloway RD, editors. Gallstones. New York: Churchill Livingstone; 1985:1–26.
107. Portincasa P, van de Meeberg PC, Van Erpecum KJ *et al.* Marked effects of acute but not chronic oral cholestyramine (CH) on gallbladder (GB) and antroduodenal motility. Gastroenterology. 1995;108:A432.
108. Portincasa P, Di Ciaula A, Palmieri V, Baldassarre G, Palasciano G. Enhancement of gallbladder emptying in gallstone patients after oral cholestyramine. Am J Gastroenterol. 1994;6:909–14.
109. Portincasa P, Di Ciaula A, Palmieri V, vanBerge-Henegouwen GP, Palasciano G. Effects of cholestyramine on gallbladder and gastric emptying in obese and lean subjects. Eur J Clin Invest. 1995 (In press).
110. Nealon WH, Upp JR, Jr, Alexander RW, Gomez G, Townsend CM, Jr., Thompson JC. Intravenous amino acids stimulate human gallbladder emptying and hormone release. Am J Physiol. 1990;259:G173–8.
111. Zoli G, Ballinger A, Healy J, O'Donnell LJ, Clark M, Farthing MJ. Promotion of gallbladder emptying by intravenous aminoacids. Lancet. 1993;341:1240–1.
112. Cano N, Cicero F, Ranier F *et al.* Ultrasonographic study of gallbladder motility during total parenteral nutrition. Gastroenterology. 1986;91:313–17.
113. Messing B, Bories C, Kunstlinger F, Bernier JJ. Does total parenteral nutrition induce gallbladder sludge formation and lithiasis? Gastroenterology. 1983;84:1012–19.
114. Festi D, Orsini M, LiBassi S *et al.* Risk of gallstone formation during rapid weight loss: protective role of gallbladder motility. Gastroenterology. 1992;102:A311.
115. Stone BG, Ansel HJ, Peterson FJ, Gebhard RL. Gallbladder emptying stimuli in obese and normal-weight subjects. Hepatology. 1992;15:795–8.
116. Jebbink MC, Masclee AA, van der Kleij FG *et al.* Effect of loxiglumide and atropine on erythromycin-induced reduction in gallbladder volume in human subjects. Hepatology. 1992;16:937–42.
117. Catnach SM, Fairclough PD, Trembath RC *et al.* Effect of oral erythromycin on gallbladder motility in normal subjects and subjects with gallstones. Gastroenterology. 1992;102:2071–6.
118. Catnach SM, Ballinger AB, Law PA, Nellans H, Fairclough PD. Dose-dependent stimulation of gallbladder contraction by intravenous erythromycin in man. Aliment Pharmacol Ther. 1993;7:55–9.
119. Xu QW, Scott RB, Tan DTM, Shaffer EA. Erythromycin as a prokinetic agent in an animal model of cholesterol gallstone disease. Gastroenterology. 1995;108:A441.
120. Marzio L, Neri M, De Angelis C *et al.* Effect of cisapride on gallbladder kinetics in normals and patients with decreased gallbladder response to a liquid meal. Curr Ther Res. 1987;42:895–900.
121. Marzio L, DiFelice F, Laico MG, Imbimbo B, Lapenna D, Cuccurullo F. Gallbladder hypokinesia and normal gastric emptying of liquids in patients with dyspeptic symptoms. A double-blind placebo-controlled clinical trial with cisapride. Dig Dis Sci. 1992;37:262–7.
122. Koop H, Moennikes H, Koop I, Donysious J, Schwarz C, Arnold R. Effects of the prokinetic drug cisapride on gastrointestinal hormone release. Scand J Gastroenterol. 1986;97:1331–6.
123. Ziegenhagen DJ, Glimm E, Kruis W, Zehnter E. Oral cisapride increases gallbladder volume in volunteers. J Gastrointest Mot. 1992,4:119–23.
124. Brotschi EA, LaMorte WW, Williams LFJ. Effect of dietary cholesterol and indomethacin on cholelithiasis and gallbladder motility in guinea pig. Dig Dis Sci. 1984;29:1050–6.
125. O'Donnell LJ, Wilson P, Guest P *et al.* Indomethacin and postprandial gallbladder emptying. Lancet. 1992;339:269–71.
126. Murray FE, Stinchcombe SJ, Hawkey CJ. Effect of indomethacin and misoprostol on fasted gallbladder volume and meal-induced gallbladder contractility in humans. Dig Dis Sci. 1992;37:1228–31.
127. Arienti V, Corazza R, Sorge M *et al.* Effect of levosulpiride on gastric and gallbladder emptying in functional dyspepsia. Hepatogastroenterology. 1993;23:A277.
128. Portincasa P. Gallbladder and bile in health and gallstone disease. The role of motility, gallstones and bile lipid composition. Ph. D. thesis, Utrecht University, 1995.

15 Imbalance of biliary pronucleating and antinucleating factors in cholesterol gallstone formation

N. BUSCH, F. LAMMERT and S. MATERN

INTRODUCTION

Cholesterol gallstone formation involves multiple steps including secretion of lithogenic bile and nucleation and growth of cholesterol crystals within the gallbladder followed by agglomeration of crystals into mature stones[1].

Besides cholesterol supersaturation, defining the solubility defect[2–5], and gallbladder dysmotility, determining the residence time defect[6,7], kinetic factors, inhibiting or promoting cholesterol crystallization, are assumed to play a key role in cholesterol gallstone pathogenesis (Figure 1).

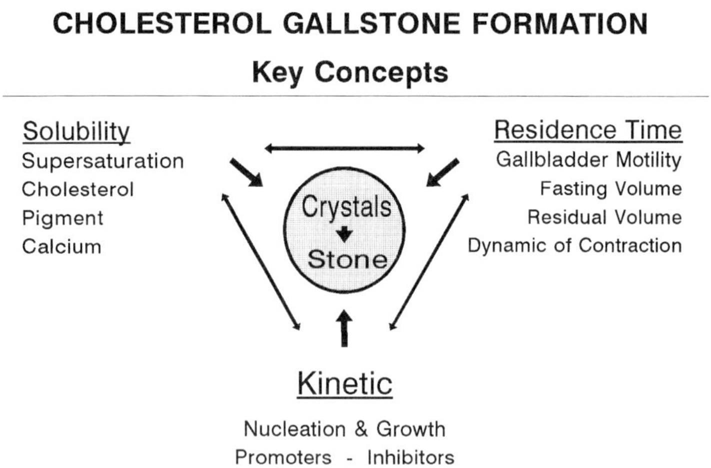

Fig. 1 Representation of the three pivotal defects in cholesterol gallstone pathogenesis according to the current understanding of the molecular mechanisms involved

In 1979, Holzbach's group reported that normal bile, although supersaturated, nucleates cholesterol crystals significantly less rapidly than either equally saturated bile of gallstone patients or model bile prepared in the laboratory[8,9]. Thus, it was believed by some that normal bile contains a factor that retards nucleation and that the nucleation defect was the lack of the antinucleating factor in bile of patients with cholesterol gallstones[10].

Some years later, evidence was provided that bile of gallstone patients contains a potent pronucleating factor[11]. Using a mixing design experiment, it was observed that normal bile samples, when mixed with crystal-free abnormal bile, nucleate cholesterol as rapidly as the abnormal parent bile. Mucous glycoproteins had been proposed as a pronucleating factor[12–15]. Subsequent studies proved additional smaller-molecular-weight pronucleators to exist in abnormal bile[16], some of which were isolated by affinity chromatography to Concanavalin A[17]. Lectin affinity chromatography was also successfully applied to isolate inhibitor proteins of cholesterol crystallization from normal and abnormal bile[18]. These studies also showed that pronucleating and antinucleating proteins coexist in human bile. It is assumed that a balance of the antagonistic kinetic protein factors in bile defines health and an imbalance defines disease[19].

KINETIC FACTORS OF CHOLESTEROL CRYSTALLIZATION

Since the introduction of the kinetic concept of cholesterol crystallization in bile, many factors have been reported to influence cholesterol nucleation and crystal growth. Nuclei of cholesterol in bile are submicroscopic aggregates of several hundred cholesterol molecules which form and redissolve continuously[5]. When these nuclei reach a certain critical size, molecular association rate overcomes dissociation rate followed by growth into microscopic crystals.

Two types of nucleation can be distinguished depending on the degree of supersaturation and the composition of the solute. In highly supersaturated solutions containing only the solute and the solvent, thermodynamic activity is sufficient to overcome the energy barriers for homogeneous nucleation to occur. Numerous nuclei form spontaneously followed by precipitation of multiple small crystals from the solution. This type of nucleation is more common in simple systems like model solutions. In complex biological systems like native bile, with a comparable low degree of supersaturation (typically 100–200%), heterogeneous nucleation occurs more commonly. In this process, nucleating agents or kinetic factors are required to overcome the energy barriers. These factors promote crystallization. Conversely, factors impeding the traversing of these energy barriers inhibit crystallization[19].

Influence on nucleation can be assessed using the nucleation time assay measuring the time of first appearance of cholesterol monohydrate crystals by polarizing light microscopy[8]. This time, better referred to as crystal detection time, represents a sequence of several events including fusion and/or aggregation of vesicles, nucleation and subsequent growth of solid cholesterol crystals to a microscopically detectable size (about 200 nm). The nucleation time represents one time point of a crystal growth curve[20]. Experimental determination of the nucleation process itself is precluded because of detection limits.

Among the non-protein factors, besides cholesterol supersaturation, biliary lipid composition, hydrophobicity of bile salts, and total lipid concentration as well as elevated concentrations of total calcium ions have been proven to modulate nucleation[21–23]. Their influences are directly predicated by physical chemistry of charged colloids and by restraints of phase equilibria[24,25].

Biliary proteins were shown to play a major role in cholesterol crystallization[26]. Inhibiting activity was directly attributable to the presence of a crude protein fraction isolated from normal gallbladder bile by cumbersome methods[10]. On the other hand, abnormal bile was shown to contain potent pronucleating activity[11]. Total protein concentration in gallbladder bile was found to be significantly higher in cholesterol gallstone patients[16], and very high biliary protein (>10 g/L) was nearly always associated with cholesterol crystals irrespective of the concentrations of total lipids, bile salts and phospholipids[27].

CHOLESTEROL CRYSTALLIZATION PROMOTING PROTEINS

During the last few years, several promoter proteins have been isolated from human bile. Gallbladder mucin was shown to be an important promoting factor in cholesterol crystallization and stone formation. Purified mucin accelerates cholesterol crystal detection times in model bile at concentrations in the mg/ml range[14,15]. In animal models of cholesterol gallstone disease, hypersecretion of mucus precedes the appearance of cholesterol crystals. The development of a mucin gel on the gallbladder wall and its accumulation in gallbladder sludge is assumed to be of primary importance in accelerating crystal and gallstone formation[28].

Introducing lectin affinity chromatography, progress has been made in isolation of non-mucous promoter proteins. Potent promoting activity was found in the biliary protein fraction bound to Concanavalin A[17]. The activity has been attributed to a 130-kDa glycoprotein recently identified to be aminopeptidase N[29]. Additional Concanavalin A reactive promoter proteins separated from human bile were identified to be immunoglobulins[30], phospholipase C[31], and α_1-acid glycoprotein[32]. Other potential pronucleating proteins are low-molecular-weight acidic calcium-binding proteins isolated from cholesterol and pigment gallstones[33–35].

CHOLESTEROL CRYSTALLIZATION INHIBITING PROTEINS

Apolipoproteins A-I and A-II are present in bile as intact peptides. Because of their known ability to solubilize and transport lipids, the influence of human serum apolipoproteins on cholesterol crystallization was tested in model bile. Apo A-I and A-II, at concentrations found in gallbladder bile, inhibited nucleation[36]. These studies demonstrated that protein factors may act as inhibitors. The modest effect of apolipoproteins on nucleation times tested in model biles and the lack of differences in concentrations of Apo A-I and A-II between normal and gallstone patients, however, was not sufficient to explain the much longer nucleation times of native normal gallbladder bile[8,37].

Using various lectin-affinity chromatography columns, mixtures of inhibiting and promoting proteins have been partially purified from normal human gallbladder bile[18]. All lectin-bound biliary protein mixtures exhibited either a promoting or an inhibiting effect on cholesterol crystal growth depending on the total protein concentration tested. The Concanavalin A-reactive fraction proved to be enriched in promoting activity while the *Helix pomatia*-reactive fraction was mostly enriched in inhibiting activity[18]. From the *Helix pomatia*-bound fraction, the first specific inhibitor, a ~120-kDa glycoprotein with subunits of 58/63 kDa, has been isolated from bile[38].

Isolation of inhibiting and promoting proteins from identical model bile suggests that a balance of antagonistic factors is important in cholesterol gallstone formation. In normal bile, this balance is in favour of inhibition of cholesterol crystallization. In abnormal bile, an imbalance of kinetic factors induced by either a deficiency of inhibitors or an excess of promoters may facilitate nucleation and cholesterol crystal growth[1,39,40]. Utilizing binding to cholesterol crystals, a subgroup of four protein bands having molecular weights of about 74, 63, 28 and 16 kDa was isolated from the lectin-bound biliary protein mixture. All proteins of this subgroup proved to be potent inhibitors of cholesterol crystallization[41]. These protein bands were suggested to be the secretory component and the heavy and light chains of biliary immunoglobulin A[42,43].

BILIARY PROTEINS: EFFECT ON CHOLESTEROL CRYSTALLIZATION AND STONE FORMATION

Evidence has been provided that promoter proteins interact with biliary vesicles: the vesicular carrier of biliary lipids was found to have a well-defined protein profile with a potent cholesterol crystallization promoting activity. Immunoglobulins, albumin and four different hydrophobic glycoproteins with a molecular weight of 130, 114, 86 and 62–67 kDa were associated with purified hepatic biliary vesicles[44].

In another study, the interaction of mucin and Concanavalin A-binding proteins isolated from human bile with cholesterol/phospholipid vesicles was investigated. Using resonance energy transfer, destabilization of the vesicles instead of protein-induced fusion was observed, as monitored by release of entrapped carboxyfluorescein. The extent of fluorescein leakage was well correlated with nucleation-promoting activity of the Concanavalin A-binding proteins, indicating that protein-induced destabilization of vesicles precedes cholesterol crystallization[45].

On the other hand, scanning electron microscopy studies demonstrated that cholesterol crystal morphology was changed when crystals were grown in model bile under the influence of biliary proteins bound to various lectin columns. With proteins, predominance of euhedral crystals with smooth surfaces was observed, forming orderly aligned aggregates and compact microliths. In contrast, without effector proteins, mainly polycyclic crystals with stepwise dislocations were found, forming irregular aggregates and clusters of about 200 μm with radially arranged polycyclic plates opening up into space[41]. These results fit well to earlier scanning EM studies of cholesterol gallstones, demonstrating a well-ordered alignment of platelike cholesterol crystals in slowly growing solitary gallstones and an unsettled arrangement of crystals in fast-growing multiple stones[46].

Further results indicating the importance of biliary proteins on stone formation have been reported recently. IgG was markedly increased in gallstone patients going up to a 12-fold increase in the high-risk Chilean population[47]. Concanavalin A-binding glycoproteins seemed to affect cholesterol crystallization only in fast-nucleating biles inducing higher crystal numbers and shorter detection times, but not in slow nucleators[48]. Increased levels of α_1-acid glycoprotein were found in 50% of gallbladder biles with multiple cholesterol gallstones, all of which were associated with very rapid nucleation times, but not in biles with other types of gallstones[49]. Apolipoprotein A-I, an antinucleator, was shown to be associated to biliary vesicles, suggesting that interaction of effector proteins with vesicular lipids does not determine promotion or inhibition of cholesterol crystallization[50].

Mixed gallstones were found to contain a pigmented core rich in calcium, upon which alternate rings of cholesterol and pigmented zones formed. Mucin was found in the core, as a meshwork interlacing among crystals in the cholesterol zones and surrounding the pigment zones. Calcium-binding protein (CBP) and aminopeptidase N were present in the pigmented core and rings, but not in the cholesterol zones. Immunoglobulin A was present in all stones and diffusely scattered throughout all regions[51].

CONCLUSIONS

Human bile contains antagonistic protein factors promoting or inhibiting cholesterol crystallization, thus playing an important role in cholesterol gallstone formation. Evidence has been provided that promoter proteins target biliary vesicles by interfering with their formation, aggregation[52] and stability[45]. On the other hand, identification of a new subgroup of crystal-binding proteins among the lectin-bound biliary proteins suggests that inhibiting activity is mediated via protein–crystal interaction[41].

Besides cholesterol crystallization, biliary proteins seem to be also involved in succeeding steps of stone formation in bile[14,51]. The protein effect probably reflects a general concept in biomineralization: proteins were identified to prevent formation of calcium oxalate nephrolithiasis in healthy persons[53], and inhibit calcium carbonate precipitation in pancreatic[54] and gallstone[33] formation.

Regarding the protein effect on cholesterol crystallization and stone formation in bile, further investigations are needed to identify the relevant growth factors. An important factor should meet most of the following criteria:

1. A quantitative or qualitative difference of the factor should exist between normal and abnormal biles.
2. Removal of the factor from bile should accelerate crystallization in the case of an inhibitor, or retard kinetic if it is a promoter.
3. Addition of the factor to native bile should retard (inhibitor) or accelerate (promoter) crystallization.
4. A significant protein effect should be detectable below or at physiological concentrations.
5. Morphology and numbers of crystals/stones should be altered.

It should be noted that these experiments, although necessary, are difficult to perform since any manipulation of the bile sample might influence the metastable ternary system, thus inducing heterogeneous nucleation. It should also be mentioned that, besides apolipoproteins and mucin, investigators are currently focusing their efforts on lectin-binding glycoproteins, thereby possibly overlooking other important kinetic protein factors in bile.

The current concepts of cholesterol gallstone pathogenesis[1,55] are summarized in Figure 2. Interactions of biliary cholesterol carriers lead to formation of multilamellar structures from which, by processes still under investigation[56], finally cholesterol monohydrate crystals are formed. Except by calcium ions, these processes are most importantly accelerated by biliary promoter proteins. On the other hand, cholesterol crystal nucleation and growth are impeded by inhibitor proteins in bile, interacting probably with cholesterol microcrystals. It has been suggested that these reactions take place in the mucin gel coating the gallbladder epithelium. In this gel, the reacting molecules are immobilized and concentrated due to solvent drag following resorption of water by the epithelium. Accumulation of mucin, crystals, pigment, proteins and precipitates of calcium and its sensitive ions is facilitated by gallbladder dysmotility. From this sludge, mature gallstones are formed by mechanisms still under investigation. The agglomeration is probably aided by mucin glycoproteins and calcium-binding proteins.

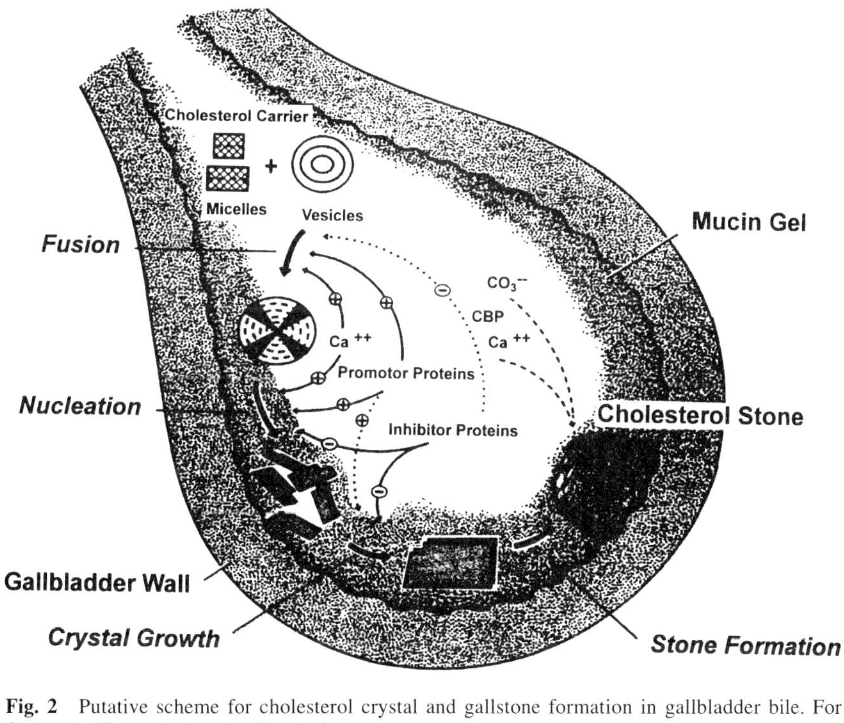

Fig. 2 Putative scheme for cholesterol crystal and gallstone formation in gallbladder bile. For further details, see text under Conclusions

Acknowledgement

This work was supported by grants Bu 822/1-1 and He 906/18-1 of the Deutsche Forschungsgemeinschaft.

References

1. Busch N, Matern S. Current concepts in cholesterol gallstone pathogenesis. Eur J Clin Invest. 1991; 21: 453–60.
2. Small DM, Bourges M, Dervichian DG. Ternary and quaternary aqueous systems containing bile salt, lecithin and cholesterol. Nature. 1966;211:816–18.
3. Carey MC, Small DM. The physical chemistry of cholesterol solubility in bile. Relationship to gallstone formation and dissolution in man. J Clin Invest. 1978;61:988–1036.
4. Admiral WH, Small DM. The physicochemical basis of cholesterol gallstone formation in man. J Clin Invest. 1968;47:1043–52.
5. Small DM. Cholesterol nucleation and growth in gallstone formation. N Engl J Med. 1980;302:1305–7.
6. Bèhar J, Lee KY, Thompson WR, Biancani P. Gallbladder contraction in patients with pigment and cholesterol stones. Gastroenterology. 1989;97:1479–84.
7. Van der Werf SDJ, van Berge Henegouwen GP, Palsma DMH, Ruben AT. Motor function of the gallbladder and saturation of duodenal bile. Neth J Med. 1987;30:160–71.
8. Holan KR, Holzbach RT, Hermann RE, Cooperman AM, Claffey WJ. Nucleation time: a key factor in the pathogenesis of cholesterol gallstone disease. Gastroenterology. 1979;77:611–17.
9. Holzbach, RT, Marsh M, Olszewski M, Holan KR. Cholesterol solubility in bile. Evidence that supersaturated bile is frequent in healthy man. J Clin Invest. 1973;52:1467–79.
10. Holzbach, RT, Kibe A, Thiel E, Howel LH, Marsh M, Hermann RE. Biliary proteins: Unique inhibitors of cholesterol crystal nucleation in human gallbladder bile. J Clin Invest. 1984;73:35–45.
11. Burnstein, JM, Ilson RG, Petrunka CN, Strasberg SM. Evidence for a potent nucleation factor in gallbladder bile of patients with cholesterol gallstones. Gastroenterology. 1984;85:801–7.
12. Levy, PF, Smith BF, LaMont JT. Human gallbladder mucin accelerates nucleation of cholesterol in artificial bile. Gastroenterology. 1984;87:270–5.
13. Lee SP, LaMont JT, Carey MC. Role of gallbladder mucus hypersecretion in the evolution of cholesterol gallstones. J Clin Invest. 1981;67:1712–23.
14. Smith BF. Human gallbladder mucin binds biliary lipids and promotes cholesterol crystal nucleation in model bile. J Lipid Res. 1987;28:1088–97.
15. Gallinger S, Taylor RD, Harvey PRC, Strasberg SM. Effect of mucous glycoprotein on nucleation time of human bile. Gastroenterology. 1985;89:648–58.
16. Gallinger S, Harvey PRC, Petrunka CN, Ilson RG, Strasberg SM. Biliary proteins and the nucleation defect in cholesterol cholelithiasis. Gastroenterology. 1987;92:867–75.
17. Groen AK, Noordam C, Drapers JAG, Egbers P, Jansen PLM, Tytgat GNJ. Isolation of a potent cholesterol nucleation promoting activity from human gallbladder bile. Hepatology. 1990;11:525–33.
18. Busch N, Matiuck N, Sahlin S, Holzbach RT. Inhibition and promotion of cholesterol crystallization by protein fractions from normal human gallbladder bile. J Lipid Res. 1991;32:695–702.
19. Holzbach RT, Busch N. Nucleation and growth of cholesterol crystals. Kinetic determinants in supersaturated bile. Gastroenterol Clin N Am. 1991;20:67–83.
20. Busch N, Tokumo H, Holzbach RT. A sensitive method for determination of cholesterol crystal growth using model solutions of supersaturated bile. J Lipid Res. 1990;31:1903–9.
21. Halpern Z, Dudley MA, Lynn MP, Nader JM, Breuer AC, Holzbach RT. Vesicle aggregation in model systems of supersaturated bile: Relation to crystal nucleation and lipid composition of the vesicular phase. J Lipid Res. 1986;27:295–306.
22. Halpern Z, Dudley MA, Kibe A, Lynn MP, Breuer AC, Holzbach RT. Rapid vesicle formation and aggregation in abnormal human bile. A time-lapse video-enhanced contrast microscopy study. Gastroenterology. 1986;90:875–85.
23. Kibe A, Dudley MA, Halpern Z, Lynn MP, Breuer AC, Holzbach RT. Factors affecting cholesterol monohydrate crystal nucleation time in model systems of supersaturated bile. J Lipid Res. 1985;26:1102–11.

24. Donovan JM, Carey MC. Physical–chemical basis of gallstone formation. Gastroenterol Clin N Am. 1991;20:47–66.
25. Cabral DJ, Small DM. Physical chemistry of bile. In: Schulz SG, Forte JG, Rauner BB, eds. Handbook of physiology – The gastrointestinal system III, Section 6. Baltimore: American Physiological Society;1989:621–62.
26. Sedaghat A, Grundy SM. Cholesterol crystals and the formation of cholesterol gallstones. N Engl J Med. 1980;302:1274–7.
27. Jüngst DT, Lang C, von Ritter C, Paumgartner G. Role of high total protein in gallbladder bile in formation of cholesterol gallstones. Gastroenterology. 1991;100:1724–9.
28. Lee SP, Maher K, Nichols JF. Origin and fate of biliary sludge. Gastroenterology. 1988;94:170–8.
29. Offner GD, Gong D, Afdhal NH. Identification of a 130-kilodalton human biliary Concanavalin A binding protein as aminopeptidase N. Gastroenterology. 1994;106:755 -62.
30. Harvey PRC, Upadhya GA, Strasberg SM. Immunoglobulins as nucleating proteins in the gallbladder bile of patients with cholesterol gallstones. J Biol Chem. 1991;266:13996–4003.
31. Pattinson NR, Willis KE. Effect of phospholipase C on cholesterol solubilization in model bile. A Concanavalin A-binding nucleation-promoting factor from human gallbladder bile. Gastroenterology. 1991;101:1339–44.
32. Abei M, Kawczak P, Nuutinen H, Langnas A, Svanvik J, Holzbach RT. Isolation and characterization of a cholesterol crystallization promoter from human bile. Gastroenterology. 1993;104:539–48.
33. Shimizu S, Sabsay B, Veis A, Ostrow JD, Rege RV, Dawes LG. Isolation of an acidic protein from cholesterol gallstones, which inhibits precipitation of calcium carbonate in vitro. J Clin Invest. 1989;84:1990–6.
34. Okido M, Shimizu S, Ostrow JD, Nakayama F. Isolation of a calcium-regulatory protein from black pigment gallstones: Similarity with a protein from cholesterol gallstones. Hepatology. 1992;15:1079–85.
35. Domingo N, Grosclaude J, Bekaert ED, Mege D, Chapman MJ, Shimizu S, Ayrault-Jarrier M, Ostrow JD, Lafont H. Epitope mapping of the human biliary amphiphatic, anionic polypeptide: similarity with a calcium-binding protein isolated from gallstones and bile, and immunologic cross-reactivity with apolipoprotein A-I. J Lipid Res. 1992;33:1419–30.
36. Kibe A, Holzbach RT, LaRusso NF, Mao SJT. Inhibition of cholesterol crystal formation by apolipoproteins in supersaturated model bile. Science (Wash. DC). 1984;225:514–16.
37. Sewell RB, Mao SJ, Kawamoto T, LaRusso NF. Apolipoproteins of high, low, and very low density lipoproteins in human bile. J Lipid Res. 1983;24:391–401.
38. Ohya T, Schwarzendrube J, Busch N, Gresky S, Chandler K, Takabayashi A, Igimi H, Egami K, Holzbach RT. Isolation of a human biliary glycoprotein inhibitor of cholesterol crystallization. Gastroenterology. 1993;104:527–38.
39. Paumgartner G, Sauerbruch T. Gallstones–Pathogenesis. Lancet. 1991;338:1117–21.
40. Busch N, Holzbach RT. Crystal growth-inhibiting proteins in bile. Hepatology. 1990;12:195S–8S.
41. Busch N, Lammert F, Matern S. A subgroup of lectin bound biliary proteins attaches to cholesterol crystals and modifies crystal morphology. Hepatology. 1992;16:124A.
42. Busch N, Lammert F, Schwarzendrube J, Marschall H-U, Matern S. Evidence for the 74 kD inhibitor protein of cholesterol crystallization to be the secretory component of human biliary immunoglobulin A. Hepatology. 1994;20:116A.
43. Busch N, Lammert F, Franz I, Schwarzendrube J, Marschall H-U, Matern S. The 63 kD and 28kD crystal binding protein fractions represent the heavy and light chains of human biliary immunoglobulin A. Gastroenterology. 1995;108:A407.
44. Miquel JF, Nunez L, Rigotti A, Amigo L, Brandan E, Nervi F. Isolation and partial characterization of cholesterol pronucleating hydrophobic glycoproteins associated to have native biliary vesicles. FEBS. 1993;318:45–9.
45. de Brujin MA, Goldhorn G, Zilstra AIM, Tytgat GNJ, Groen AK. Interaction of cholesterol crystallization-promoting proteins with vesicles. Biochem J. 1995;305:93–6.
46. Wolpers C, Blaschke R. Electron microscopy of human gallstones. In: Arceneaux CJ, ed. 29th Annual Proceedings Electron Microscopy Society America, Boston. 1971:296–7.
47. Nunez L, Amigo L, Miquel JF, Rigotti A, Puglielli L, Raddatz A, Piment F, Strasberg SM, Harvey PRC, Nervi F. Role of biliary immunoglobulins on cholesterol gallstone disease:

Marked increase of IgG in gallbladder bile of gallstone patients. Gastroenterology. 1995;108:A1135.

48. Keulemans JCA, Mok KS, Gouma DJ, Groen AK. The role of Concanavalin A-binding glycoprotein in cholesterol crystallization in native human bile. Gastroenterology. 1995;108:A1096.
49. Abei M, Tanaka N, Tomita S, Shoda J, Yamaguchi T, Matsuzaki Y, Osuga T. α_1-Acid glycoprotein in increased and associated with rapid nucleation in gallbladder bile with multiple cholesterol gallstones but not with solitary cholesterol or pigment gallstones. Gastroenterology. 1995;108:A1022.
50. Secknus R, Yamashita G, Ginanni Corradini S, Chernosky A, Krivacic K, Holzbach RT. Immobilized artificial membrane chromatography for analysis of biliary vesicle-associated proteins. Gastroenterology. 1995;108:A1165.
51. Lechene de la Porte P, Domingo N, van Wijland MJA, Groen AK, Ostrow JD, LaFont H. Localization of biliary proteins, Ca, Cu, P, S, in the pigment zones of mixed gallstones. Gastroenterology. 1995;108:A1107.
52. Groen AK, Ottenhoff R, Jansen PLM, van Marle J, Tytgat GNJ. Effect of cholesterol nucleation-promoting activity on cholesterol solubilization in model bile. J Lipid Res. 1989;30:51–8.
53. Nakagawa Y, Ahmed M, Hall SL, Deganello S, Coe FL. Isolation from human calcium oxalate renal stones of nephrocalcin, a glycoprotein inhibitor of calcium oxalate crystal growth: Evidence that nephrocalcin from patients with calcium oxalate nephrolithiasis is deficient in gamma-carboxyglutamic acid. J Clin Invest. 1987;79:1782–7.
54. Montalto G, Bonice J, Multigner L, Rovery M, Sarles H, De Caro A. Partial amino acid sequence of human pancreatic stone protein, a novel pancreatic secretory protein. Biochem J. 1986;238:227–32.
55. LaMont JT, Carey MC. Cholesterol gallstone formation. 2. Pathobiology and pathomechanics. Prog Liver Dis. 1992;10:165 -91.
56. Konikoff FM, Chung DS, Donovan JM, Small DM, Carey MC. Filamentous, helical, and tubular microstructures during cholesterol crystallization from bile: Evidence that cholesterol does not nucleate classic monohydrate plates. J Clin Invest. 1992;90:1155–61.

Section V
Management of Cholelithiasis

16
Therapeutic options and choice of appropriate treatment

G. PAUMGARTNER

Gallstones represent a considerable health problem in industrialized countries. The prevalence of gallstone disease in a population aged 18–65 years in a study performed in Italy[1] was 11%. It increases with age and is about twice as high in women as in men. In women aged 50–65 years, it reached 27%. Seventy-eight per cent of subjects with gallstones had no specific biliary symptoms and 82% were not aware of their disease[1].

During recent decades, considerable advances in the treatment of gallstone disease have been made and the physician is increasingly faced with the following two questions;

1. For which patients with gallstone disease are therapeutic interventions necessary?
2. Which therapeutic interventions are applicable to individual patients?

The decision for or against a therapeutic intervention must take into account the balance between the risks of the disease and the risks of therapy and between the patient's complaints and the discomfort from therapy, as well as between the expected benefits and the costs of therapy (Table 1).

SPECTRUM OF SYMPTOMS

There may be *no symptoms* at all or only *unspecific abdominal pain* (Table 2). As has already been pointed out, about 80% of patients with gallstones have no symptoms or only unspecific abdominal pain, often assessed as dyspeptic symp-

Table 1 Determinants of therapeutic decisions

• Risks of disease	• Risks of therapy
• Patient's complaints	• Discomfort from therapy
• Expected benefits	• Costs

Table 2 Spectrum of symptoms of gallstone disease

- No symptoms
- Unspecific abdominal pain
- Biliary colic
- Symptoms from complications (acute cholecystitis, biliary pancreatitis etc.)

toms[1]. These unspecific symptoms have been found to be equally frequent in patients with and without gallstones[2].

Acute biliary pain, usually called biliary colic, has been defined as one or more attacks of pain located in the epigastrium or right upper quadrant, with or without radiation to the back or right shoulder, usually lasting more than 15–30 min but less than five hours. These attacks of pain are usually well remembered by the patient, occur irregularly, with a peak incidence at night, and are separated by symptom-free intervals of weeks or even years. Causes of abdominal pain other than gallstones must be excluded.

Finally, gallstone disease can present with the symptoms of well-known *complications*, such as acute cholecystitis, biliary pancreatitis or others. Pain lasting for more than five hours always raises the suspicion that complications such as acute cholecystitis are developing.

NATURAL HISTORY

The natural history is quite different in patients with asymptomatic and those with symptomatic gallstone disease. Several large studies with a follow-up of 10–20 years, which have been reviewed by Ransohoff and Gracie[3], show that asymptomatic gallstone disease is a rather benign disease. In the study by Gracie and Ransohoff[4], the average risk of developing biliary pain was about 2% per year during the first 5 years of follow-up and then decreased to about 0.5% during the third 5-year period. A biliary complication occurred in only 3 of 123 asymptomatic persons, and, in all three, an episode of pain preceded the complication, thus providing a 'warning' symptom. This study, however, has the shortcoming that mainly male subjects were included.

Recently, the results of a large population study by the GREPCO group in Italy[5] became available. This prospective study in a free-living population used ultrasonography for the detection of gallstones. It showed that the cumulative probability of developing symptoms was 26% after 10 years. The cumulative probability of developing complications after 10 years was only 3%. The annual incidence of complications (0.3%) in this study was somewhat higher than in the study by Gracie and Ransohoff[4] but lower than that reported by Friedman *et al.*[6] (1%).

The available studies show that neither sex nor age, nor size, number and composition of the stones or non-visualization of the gallbladder have a clear predictive value for the development of symptoms. Furthermore, it is important that, in general, patients develop biliary symptoms prior to complications. The study by the GREPCO group[5] reported no deaths due to gallstone disease except for one asymptomatic patient who died of gallbladder carcinoma.

Taking into account the total number of approximately 6500 person-years of follow-up included in published cohort studies, the calculated incidence of gallbladder carcinoma in asymptomatic subjects can be estimated as about 0.015% per year[5]. Ransohoff and Gracie[3] estimated that the incidence of gallbladder cancer in an asymptomatic gallstone subject aged 50 years or older is about 0.02% per year. Incidence rates in certain ethnic groups (Pima Indians and other New World Indians) and in subgroups of gallstone patients (porcelain gallbladder, stones with a diameter >3 cm), however, may be considerably higher[7].

The natural history of gallstone patients with biliary pain is different from that of asymptomatic gallstones. Although most of the information is fragmentary and anecdotal, several studies show that the percentage of patients with *symptomatic gallstones* who experience recurrent pain or develop complications is high. Between 5 and 30 years of follow-up, 66% had recurrent biliary pain or complications and 28% developed complications[8]. A study in Sirmione has recently confirmed that persistence or recurrence of pain in previously symptomatic subjects is frequent and occurs in about 50% of patients[8]. However, about 30% of patients who have had one attack of biliary pain do not experience further attacks of pain[3]. The risk of developing complications is higher in patients who have frequent and severe symptoms[9].

MANAGEMENT

Decision analysis tells us that, with the low risks of asymptomatic gallstone disease, even a perfect prophylactic therapy with no morbidity and no mortality would result in only a very small gain in life expectancy in asymptomatic subjects with gallstones, namely of the order of about 1–2 weeks[3]. From the data on the natural history of gallstones, it may, therefore, be concluded that asymptomatic gallstones, in general, should be managed expectantly[3,7,10]. Exceptions are patients with porcelain gallbladder, American Indians and possibly patients with very large gallstones because of an increased risk of gallbladder cancer[3,7].

On the basis of the natural history of patients with symptomatic gallstones, therapeutic intervention should be recommended for most patients with symptomatic gallstones. However, if a patient with a first attack of biliary pain wants to try a period of watchful waiting to see if pain recurs, this is acceptable[3].

CHOICE OF TREATMENT

Table 3 lists the various treatment options for symptomatic gallstones according to their invasiveness, oral bile acid dissolution therapy being the least, open cholecystectomy the most, invasive procedure.

Laparoscopic or *open cholecystectomy* must be regarded as the standard treatments for patients with symptomatic gallstones[7,10]. The stones can be removed regardless of their type, number and size and regardless of gallbladder function. Moreover, cholecystectomy is the treatment of choice in acute cholecystitis.

Table 3 Treatment options for symptomatic gallstones according to increasing invasiveness

1. Oral bile acid dissolution therapy
2. Extracorporeal shockwave lithotripsy
3. Topical dissolution therapy
4. Laparoscopic cholecystectomy
5. Open cholecystectomy

In a subset of patients without complications of their gallstone disease, non-surgical treatments are possible, such as *oral bile acid dissolution therapy, extracorporeal shockwave lithotripsy* or *topical dissolution therapy*.

There are a number of common requirements of non-surgical gallstone treatments. They include certain stone characteristics, such as the presence of cholesterol stones without calcification. Stone size should be limited to <5 mm (optimal) to 10 mm (acceptable) for oral bile acid dissolution therapy, and to <20 mm (optimal) to 30 mm (acceptable) for extracorporeal shockwave lithotripsy[7,11,12]. The number of the stones should be limited to one (optimal) to three (acceptable) for shockwave lithotripsy[11–13]. All non-surgical gallstone treatments require a functioning gallbladder that ideally empties at least 60% of its contents after a standard test meal.

The non-surgical treatments, such as oral bile acid dissolution therapy and extracorporeal shockwave lithotripsy, have the advantage of being non-invasive procedures with low morbidity and no or negligible mortality. Common problems of these therapies are delayed clearance of stones[12,13] and recurrence of stones[14,15]. Cumulative stone recurrence after four years has been 12% after dissolution of single stones and 45% after dissolution of multiple stones[14]. It was 20% after extracorporeal shockwave lithotripsy of mainly solitary stones[15].

Laparoscopic cholecystectomy has the advantage of immediate stone clearance but the disadvantages of an invasive procedure with anaesthesia, the risk of

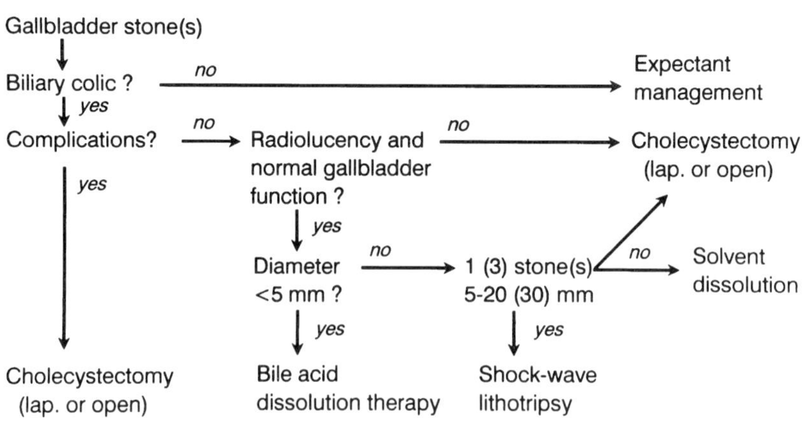

Fig. 1 Algorithm for the treatment of gallbladder stones when the least invasive procedure is to be chosen

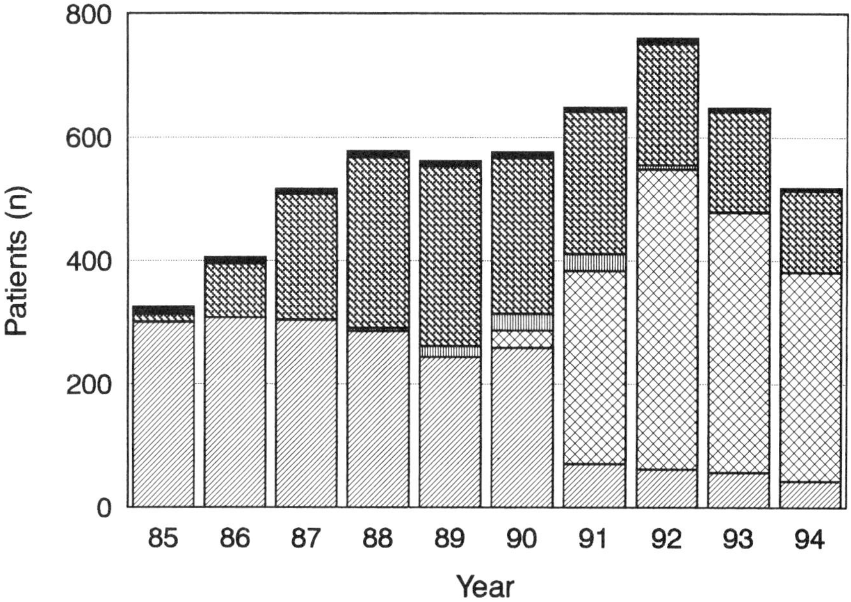

Fig. 2 Utilization of gallstone treatments at Klinikum Grosshadern from 1985–1994. ■ Bile acid dissolution therapy; extracoporeal shockwave lithotripsy; topical dissolution with methyl tert-butyl ether; laparoscopic cholecystectomy; open cholecystectomy

bile duct injury[16] and a low mortality rate[17]. Many patients are reluctant to undergo surgery or general anaesthesia despite the low risks of morbidity and mortality and they opt for the least invasive treatment that can be justified on medical grounds. For these patients, we have developed the algorithm shown in Figure 1. The utilization of the various gallstone treatments in our hospital, the Grosshadern Clinic, in the years 1985–1994 is shown in Figure 2.

References

1. Barbara L, Sama C, Morselli Labate AM *et al.* A population study on the prevalence of gallstone disease: The Sirmione study. Hepatology, 1987;7:913–17.
2. Schoenfield LJ, Carulli N, Dowling RH, Ransohoff D, Sama C, Wolpers C. Asymptomatic gallstones. Definition and treatment. Gastroenterol Int. 1989;2:25–9.
3. Ransohoff DF, Gracie WA. Treatment of gallstones. Ann Intern Med. 1993;11:606–19.
4. Gracie WA, Ransohoff DF. The natural history of silent gallstones: The innocent gallstone is not a myth. N Engl J Med. 1982;307:798–803.
5. Attili AF, De Santis A, Capri R, Recipe AM, Maselli S and the GREPCO Group. The natural history of gallstones: The GREPCO Experience. Hepatology. 1995;21:656–60.
6. Friedman GD, Ravioli CA, Fireman B. Prognosis of gallstones with mild or no symptoms: 25 years of follow-up in health maintenance organization. J Chronic Dis. 1989;42:127.
7. Paumgartner G. Nonoperative management of gallstone disease. In: Sleisenger KH, Fordtran JS, eds. Gastrointestinal disease: Pathophysiology/diagnosis/managment. Philadelphia: WB Saunder, Co.; 1994:1844–57.
8. Sama C, Morselli Labate AM, Taroni F, Barbara L. Epidemiology and natural history of gallstone disease. Semin Liver Dis. 1990;10:149–58.

9. Lund J. Surgical indications in cholelithiasis: Prophylactic cholecystectomy elucidated on the basis of long-term follow up on 526 nonoperated cases. Ann Surg. 1960;151:153.
10. Paumgartner G, Carr-Locke DL, Dubois F, Roda E, Thistle JL. Strategies in the treatment of gallstone disease. Gastroenterol Int. 1993;6:65–75.
11. Paumgartner G. Extracoporeal shock-wave lithotripsy. Eur J Gastroenterol Hepatol. 1994;6:867–72.
12. Paumgartner G, Pauletzki J, Sackmann M. Ursodeoxycholic acid treatment of cholesterol gallstone disease. Scand J Gastroenterol. 1994;29(Suppl 204):27–31.
13. Sackmann M, Pauletzki J, Sauerbruch T, Holl J, Schelling G, Paumgartner G. The Munich gallbladder lithotripsy study: Results of the first 5 years with 711 patients. Ann Intern Med. 1991;114:290–6.
14. Villanova N, Bazzoli F, Taroni F. Gallstone recurrence after successful oral bile acid treatment. Gastroenterology. 1989;97:726.
15. Sackmann M, Niller, H, Klueppelberg U *et al.* Gallstone recurrence after shock-wave therapy. Gastroenterology. 1994;106:225–30.
16. Strasberg SM, Hertl M, Soper NJ. An analysis of the problem of biliary injury during laparoscopic cholecystectomy. J Am Coll Surg. 1995;180:101–25.
17. The Southern Surgeons Club. A prospective analysis of 1518 laparoscopic cholecystectomies N Engl J Med. 1991;324:1072–8.

17
Indications for expectant management

C. SAMA, M. MALAVOLTI, A. M. MORSELLI-LABATE, G. POLLINI, G. DANESI, A. MASTROIANNI and L. BARBARA

For more than 100 years, cholecystectomy was the management option for gallstone patients.

Now patients with cholecystolithiasis have three options:

1. Expectant management;
2. Non-surgical treatment;
3. Surgical treatment (open or laparoscopic cholecystectomy).

The choice depends on the presence or absence of biliary symptoms, and on the characteristics of the patient, the gallstones and the gallbladder.

The purpose of this paper is to describe the indications for expectant management in gallstone patients. Expectant management is a strategy that recommends treatment only when specific indications arise during the course of the disease. Expectant management has been proposed for asymptomatic patients[1] and more recently for patients with mild or moderate symptoms[2]. In the following pages, we will examine the consequences of expectant management in relation to the natural history of asymptomatic and symptomatic gallstone patients.

ASYMPTOMATIC GALLSTONE PATIENTS

Knowledge of the natural history of gallstones in people without biliary symptoms is mandatory to decide whether silent gallstones should be treated or not.

In the past, many textbooks indicated that up to 50% of people with silent gallstones would develop biliary symptoms or complications. We know now that asymptomatic gallstones have a more benign course than symptomatic ones. Our improved knowledge of the disease depends on a more correct definition of biliary symptoms. In many instances in the past, dyspeptic symptoms were defined as mild or sometimes 'non-specific' biliary symptoms when defining the population at risk and the rate of appearance of symptoms. It is now widely recognized that gallstones do not cause dyspeptic symptoms[3–7]. The definition of true biliary symptoms, namely biliary colic, deserves some comment. Considering several epidemiological studies, we find different definitions of symptomatic gallstones. In one study[6], symptomatic gallstone disease was defined as a disease in which there was a history of pain in the upper abdomen; others[7] stated that biliary pain is an episode of upper abdominal pain that does not have another cause. In the two Italian epidemiological studies, the GREPCO and the Sirmione study[3–5], biliary colic was defined as "pain in the right hypocondrium or epigastrium that lasted for more than half an hour". According to this definition, more than two thirds of gallstones detected in epidemiological studies are asymptomatic.

Therefore, the correct definition of an asymptomatic gallstone patient is: 'a patient who has never had specific biliary symptoms'.

If we look at the natural history of asymptomatic patients, we find that, unfortunately, most of the studies performed during the last 40 years do not fulfil the criteria for correct natural history study, i.e. careful definition of the population at risk, large cohort of subjects, a prolonged period of surveillance and unequivocal characterization of what is being measured. Nevertheless, all these studies can provide important information. The most important point is that the natural history of silent gallstones seems to be benign (Table 1).

In the available studies, over a time period ranging from 4 to 30 years, the yearly incidence of biliary pain ranged from 0.5% to 4%. The probability of complications (acute cholecystitis, acute pancreatitis or obstructive jaundice) is less than 0.5% per year, and the mortality from gallstone disease is <1% for the entire lifetime.

Examining these studies in more detail, the studies of Comfort *et al.*[8] and of Ralston and Smith[9] were based on retrospective evaluation of cases, whereas, in the study of Newman *et al.*[10] there is lack of information on the characteristics of the patients; the study of Gracie and Ransohoff[7] reported on 123 faculty members at the University of Michigan with asymptomatic gallstones followed for 11–24 years, but the study group consisted almost entirely of white

Table 1 Natural history of asymptomatic gallstone disease

Authors	*No. of cases*	*Duration of follow-up (y)*	*Overall incidence (%)* Colic or complications	*Overall incidence (%)* Complications
Comfort *et al.*[8]	112	10–20	19	4.4
Ralston and Smith[9]	14	15–30	29	NR
Newman *et al.*[10]	191	2–22	10	NR
Gracie and Ransohoff[7]	123	11–24	16	1
McSherry *et al.*[11]	135	mean 3.8	10.4	2
Friedman *et al.*[17]	123	5–20	18.7	5.7
Sama *et al.*[12]	103	10	20.2	1.3
Attili *et al.*[13]	118	10	25.8	3

NR = not reported

American males, only 13 of the 123 subjects being female. McSherry *et al.*[11] reviewed the records of 135 patients with silent gallstones, who were subscribers of the Health Insurance Plan of Greater New York and who were followed for a variable period of time (median 46.3 months) from the time of diagnosis. In the Sirmione Study, a 10-year follow-up study of gallstone patients detected during the cross-sectional study[5] has been completed[12]. Results indicate a relatively high rate of development of symptoms in previously asymptomatic subjects (20.2% in 10 years); however, most symptoms were observed during the first 5 years of observation (yearly incidence 2.9%) and a much lower rate was observed thereafter (1.1%). A recent paper from GREPCO confirmed these results[13].

Cancer of the gallbladder was detected in only two patients in all follow-up studies. It was estimated that, in the United States, the yearly risk for gallbladder cancer in patients with silent stones may be 0.01%[14].

A possible question arising from studies on the natural history of silent stones, is whether the difference in outcome for patients with gallstone disease might be related to predictive factors, either demographic or related to the characteristics of gallstones or the gallbladder. The available studies show that patient sex and age, size, number and composition of stones and non-visualization of the gallbladder do not have a clear predictive value for the occurrence of symptoms. The question has been raised whether some concomitant disease, like diabetes, could modify the natural history of gallstones. Two studies in the last few years have addressed this question[15,16]. In both studies (Table 2), it was demonstrated that the natural history of diabetic gallstone patients is similar to that of non-diabetic gallstone subjects.

Another important problem is the mode of presentation of symptoms in terms of biliary colic or biliary complications. Few studies addressed this important issue. One showed that 10% of patients without symptoms presented initially with biliary complications[10], whereas, in another study[7], there was biliary pain in 16 persons and complications in none. In the Sirmione study[12], nobody with asymptomatic stones become symptomatic with biliary complications during 10 years follow-up. Slightly worse results came from a recent article[17] that described the prognosis of 123 patients with asymptomatic gallstones followed up for 25 years in the setting of a health maintenance organization: seven patients (5.7%) had a severe event (acute cholecystitis, biliary acute pancreatitis or extrahepatic obstructive jaundice).

For all these reasons, expectant management is the treatment of choice for patients with asymptomatic gallstones. There are some exceptions:

Table 2 Natural history of diabetic patients with asymptomatic gallstones

Authors	*No. of cases*	*Duration of follow-up (y)*	*Overall incidence (%)*	
			Colic or complications	*Complications*
Sama *et al.*[15]	72	2–8	13.9	—
Del Favero *et al.*[16]	47	5	14.9	4.2

1. Patients who voluntarily ask for treatment, assuming they have been correctly informed by their doctor.
2. The presence of microlithiasis that, in case of cholesterol stones, can be safely cured in a short period of time with oral bile acids and has been claimed to carry a high risk of complications (such as pancreatitis).
3. The presence of a 'porcelain gallbladder' (a condition known to have a high risk of cancer).

PATIENTS WITH MILD TO MODERATE SYMPTOMS

Patients with mild to moderate symptoms are patients with 'uncomplicated symptomatic gallstone disease'[18].

Information concerning the natural history of patients with biliary symptoms who have not been operated on is, for the most part, fragmentary and anecdotal. From the published studies (Table 3), we can see that most of the patients have a recurrence of symptoms and that many have biliary complications[9,17,19–21]. Studies involving non-hospitalized patients indicate a more benign natural history as far as complications are concerned[13,19,21]. However, the yearly incidence of biliary symptoms is very high in these series, being 41% in the National Cooperative Gallstone Study[21] and 12% in the Sirmione study[12].

Although it was claimed that gallstone disease is a risk factor for the occurrence of gallbladder cancer, little is known about the probability of cancer in a person with symptomatic stones. The risk of gallbladder cancer occurring in a person with symptomatic stones is roughly 0.04 per year[14]. A cohort study[22] reported a rate of 9 instances per 10 000 person-years of follow-up study.

Recently, a quantitative analysis study[2] addressed the issue of correct management of patients with mild to moderate symptoms considering the possibility of expectant management. Using life-table techniques, they calculated the risk of death in patients with symptomatic gallstones treated immediately with cholecystectomy or managed expectantly until pain recurred or a biliary complication occurred. They found that, with expectant management, the cumulative lifetime probability of death from gallstone disease in a 30-year-old patient was about

Table 3 Natural history of symptomatic gallstone disease

			Overall incidence (%)	
Authors	*No. of cases*	*Duration of follow-up (y)*	*Colic or complications*	*Complications*
Lund[19]	201	5–20	58	27
Ralston and Smith[9]	71	15–30	68	NR
Wenckert and Robertson[20]	781	1–11	33	18
Gomand *et al.*[23]	40	8–17	72	28
Friedman *et al.*[17]	289*	25	25	9
Thistle *et al.*[21]	112*	2	69	6

NR = not reported; * outpatients

2% and that most death occurred after the age of 65. In comparison, elective cholecystectomy had only a 0.1% rate of gallstone death, but all death occurred at age 30 years. They concluded that, for persons with symptomatic gallstones, the life expectancy gain of immediate cholecystectomy is relatively small. However, the risk of developing pain in this study is assumed to be 40% per year, and the risk of developing complications is 3% per year.

The indications for expectant management in patients with mild to moderate symptoms still seems to be controversial in our opinion. In any case it should depend on:

1. The clinical picture and the age of the patient;
2. Composition, number and size of the gallstones;
3. Function and condition of the gallbladder;
4. The patient's choice when correctly informed by the doctor.

References

1. Ransohoff DF, Gracie WA, Wolfenson LB, Neuhauser D. Prophylactic cholecystectomy or expectant management for silent gallstones. Ann Int Med. 1983;99:199–204.
2. Ransohoff DF, Gracie WA. Management of patients with symptomatic gallstones: a quantitative analysis. Am J Med. 1990;88:154.
3. Rome Group for the Epidemiology and Prevention of Cholelithiasis. Prevalence of gallstone disease in an Italian adult female population. Am J Epidemiol. 1984;119:796.
4. Rome Group for the Epidemiology and Prevention of Cholelithiasis. The epidemiology of gallstone disease in Rome, Italy: Part I. Prevalence data in men: Part II. The epidemiology of gallstone disease in Rome, Italy. Hepatology. 1988;8:904.
5. Barbara L, Sama C, Morselli Labate AM *et al.* A population study on the prevalence of gallstone disease: the Sirmione study. Hepatology. 1987;7:913.
6. Bainton D, Davies GT, Evans KT *et al.* Gallbladder disease: prevalence in a South Wales industrial town. N Engl J Med. 1976;294:1147.
7. Gracie WA, Ransohoff DF. The natural history of gallstones: the innocent gallstone is not a myth. N Engl J Med. 1982;307:798.
8. Comfort MW, Gray HK, Wilson JM. The silent gallstone: a ten to twenty year follow-up study of 112 cases. Ann Surg. 1948;128:913.
9. Ralston DE, Smith LA. The natural history of cholelithiasis: a 15 to 30-year follow up of 116 patients. Minn Med. 1965;48:327.
10. Newman HF, Northup JD, Rosenblum M *et al.* Complications of cholelithiasis. Am J Gastroenterol. 1968;50:476.
11. McSherry CK, Ferstenberg H, Calhoum WF *et al.* The natural history of diagnosed gallstone disease in symptomatic and asymptomatic patients. Ann Surg. 1985;202:59.
12. Sama C, Morselli Labate AM, Venturoli N *et al.* The natural history of asymptomatic and symptomatic gallstones: 10-years follow-up Sirmione study. Hepatology. 1992;16:86a.
13. Attili AF, De Santis A, Capri R, Repice AM, Maselli S, and the GREPCO GROUP. The natural history of gallstones: the GREPCO experience. Hepatology. 1995;21:656–60.
14. Gracie WA, Ransohoff DF. Natural history and expectant management of gallstone disease. In: Cohen S, Soloway RD, eds. Contemporary issue in gastroenterology: Gallstones. New York: Churchill Livingstone; 1985;27.
15. Sama C, Morselli Labate AM, Venturoli N *et al.* Gallstone and diabetes. Hepatology. 1993;18:98A.
16. Del Favero G, Caroli A, Meggiato T *et al.* Natural history of gallstones in non-insulin dependent diabetes mellitus. A prospective five-year follow-up. Dig Dis Sci. 1994;39:1704–7.
17. Friedman GD, Raviola CA, Fireman B. Prognosis of gallstones with mild or no symptoms: 25 years of follow-up in a health maintenance organization. J Clin Epidemiol. 1989;42:127.
18. Paumgartner G, Carr-Locke DL, Roda E, Thistle JL. Biliary stones: non-surgical therapeutic approach. Gastroenterol. Int. 1988;1:17–24.

19. Lund J. Surgical indications in cholelithiasis. Ann Surg. 1960;151:153.
20. Wenckert A, Robertson B. The natural course of gallstone disease: Eleven-year review of 871 non-operated cases. Gastroenterology. 1966;50:376.
21. Thistle JL, Cleary PA, Lachin JM, Malcom PT, Hersh T, the Sterin Committee and the National Cooperative Gallstone Study Group. The natural history of cholelithiasis: the National Cooperative Gallstone Study. Ann Int Med. 1984;101:171–5.
22. Maringhini A, Moreau J, Meltom LJ III *et al.* Gallstones, gallbladder cancer, and other gastrointestinal malignancies. Ann Int Med. 1987;107:30.
23. Gomand L, Vandenbroncke J, De Groote J. De natuurlijke evolutie van colelithiase. Tydschrift Gastro-Enterologie. 1966;9:594.

18 Indications for oral bile acid dissolution therapy

H. FROMM

BACKGROUND

In spite of the wide use of laparoscopic cholecystectomy for the treatment of cholelithiasis, bile acid dissolution therapy remains an important option in the management of selected gallstone patients[1,2]. Indeed, the increasing realization that laparoscopic cholecystectomy is associated with significant complications in a significant number of patients[3,4] has refocused attention to non-surgical treatment modalities and provided a special impetus for reviewing the criteria for oral bile acid dissolution therapy. Although both ursodeoxycholic acid (UDCA) and combinations of UDCA and chenodeoxycholic acid (CDCA) are used for gallstone dissolution[5,6], treatment with UDCA alone finds the widest clinical application. A major advantage of UDCA treatment is its unique safety[7]. In addition to its safety, UDCA has a number of other remarkable features. It has hepatoprotective qualities and finds increasing use for the treatment of chronic liver diseases[8–10]. UDCA also has favourable effects on cholesterol metabolism[11]. It increases cholesterol catabolism, presumably due to both decreased bile acid absorption and direct stimulation of the LDL receptor[12–14].

Finally, there is evidence that UDCA improves symptoms in gallstone patients. This effect is to be considered in symptomatic patients with non-dissolvable gallbladder stones who either refuse surgery or present a major operative risk.

RATIONALE FOR MEDICAL VERSUS SURGICAL TREATMENT

Surgery, i.e. laparoscopic cholecystectomy, represents the mainstay of treatment for patients with symptomatic gallbladder stones. In the hand of a well-trained and experienced surgeon, laparoscopic cholecystectomy results in the eradication of the main site of gallstone formation in all patients and in the improvement of abdominal pain in approximately 80%, with a low rate of morbidity and mortality[15]. However, complications from laparoscopic cholecystectomy are significant. Bile duct injury is reported to occur about twice as often with the laparoscopic procedure than with open cholecystectomy. In a recent national survey in The Netherlands the incidence rates of bile duct injuries has been reported to be 1.09% for laparoscopic cholecystectomy versus 0.51% for open cholecystectomy[16]. Not only the incidence rate, but also the severity, of bile duct injuries is increased with the laparoscopic cholecystectomy[17]. However, in spite of these complications, laparoscopic cholecystectomy is now considered the treatment of choice for symptomatic gallstones, because it is associated with low postoperative morbidity and fast recovery. Gallstone patients with biliary pain who present no significant surgical risk should be given the option of laparoscopic cholecystectomy as the first choice versus one of the medical treatment methods. If the patient is unwilling to undergo the operation, a non-surgical treatment option should be considered and discussed with the patient. However, it appears reasonable to advise a patient with one episode of biliary pain without complication to wait with treatment until the pain recurs. About half of the patients have no recurrence of biliary pain in 1 year, and about one-third of the patients remain free of biliary pain for at least 10 years, i.e. may never have a recurrence of biliary pain.

INDICATIONS FOR ORAL BILE ACID DISSOLUTION THERAPY

Only non-calcified cholesterol stones located in a gallbladder that communicates with the common bile duct through a patent cystic duct can be dissolved by UDCA treatment. The ideal case for UDCA dissolution treatment has small, i.e. less than 0.5 cm, radiolucent gallstones. Up to 90% success rates are observed in these small stones[6]. Gallstones that are larger than 1.0 cm in diameter have little chance (generally less than 10–20%) to dissolve. Patients with single gallbladder stones in the 1.0–2.0 cm size category benefit most from extracorporeal shockwave lithotripsy and adjuvant UDCA treatment.

UDCA is particularly successful in patients with so-called floating stones, which dissolve in 70–80% of the cases[1]. The floating quality is detectable by oral cholecystography, and indicates the presence of relatively pure cholesterol stones. However, an oral cholecystogram is usually not required since, in the absence of clinical or laboratory signs of pancreatico-biliary complications, the cystic bile duct is virtually always patent. An ultrasonogram of the gallbladder, as well as a plain X-ray film of the abdomen, to exclude gallstone calcifications, are sufficient to determine the eligibility of patients for oral bile acid dissolution therapy. Ultrasound is more sensitive than an oral cholecystogram in the detection of gallstones. However, occasionally, gallstones are found by oral cholecystography in spite of a normal ultrasound examination. Although CT scan is more sensitive than a plain X-ray film in the detection of gallstone calcifications, in most instances it does not seem either cost-effective or practical to include CT routinely in the diagnostic work-up of gallstone patients for cholelitholytic therapy.

SAFETY AND CONTRAINDICATIONS TO ORAL BILE ACID DISSOLUTION THERAPY

As mentioned above, UDCA is an extremely safe compound; therefore, few contraindications to its use exist. If a patient takes both UDCA and cholestyramine, the two drugs should not be given together. A time interval of 2 hours should suffice to minimize binding of UDCA to cholestyramine.

DOSE OF UDCA

UDCA has been found to be effective over a relatively wide range of doses. The usually recommended dose is 8–10 mg per kg body weight. Although the optimal number of doses – once a day versus twice a day – has not been established by carefully controlled studies, twice-a-day dosing may be superior to the once-a-day bedtime dose. This may be related to the absorptive capacity of the intestine.

CONCLUSIONS

Oral bile acid dissolution therapy offers a safe and successful alternative to surgery in appropriately selected patients. Small, non-calcified gallbladder stones show the best success rate. Symptomatic improvement is an additional benefit of the treatment in many patients.

References

1. Fromm H, Roat JW, Gonzalez V, Sarva RP, Farivar S. Comparative efficacy and side effects of ursodeoxycholic and chenodeoxycholic acids in dissolving gallstones: a double blind controlled study. Gastroenterology. 1983;85:1257–64.
2. Yoon PJ, Fromm H. Medical dissolution therapy of gallstones. In Braasch JW, Tompkins RK, editors: Surgical disease of the biliary tract and pancreas: multidisciplinary management. St Louis, MO: Mosby;1984:207–19.
3. Lee VS, Chari FS, Cucchiaro G, Meyers WC. Complications of laparoscopic cholecystectomy. Am J Surg. 1993;165:420–6.
4. Steiner CA, Bass EB, Talamini MA, Pitt HA, Steinberg EP. Surgical rates and mortality for open and laparoscopic cholecystectomy in Maryland. N Engl J Med. 1994;330:403–8.
5. Roehrkasse R, Fromm H, Malavolti M. Gallstone dissolution treatment with a combination of chenodeoxycholic and ursodeoxycholic acids. Studies of the safety, efficacy and effects on bile lithogenicity, bile acid pool, and serum lipids. Dig Dis Sci. 1986;31:1032–40.
6. Podda M, Zuin M, Battezzati PM. Efficacy and safety of a combination of chenodeoxycholic acid and ursodeoxycholic acid for gallstone dissolution: a comparison with ursodeoxycholic acid alone. Gastroenterology. 1989;96:222–39.
7. Leuschner U, Fischer H, Kurtz W. Ursodeoxycholic acid in primary biliary cirrhosis. Results of a controlled double-blind trial. Gastroenterology. 1989;97:1268–74.
8. Poupon RE, Balkau B, Eschwege E. A multicenter controlled trial of ursodiol for the treatment of primary biliary cirrhosis. N Engl J Med. 1991;324:1548–54.
9. Lindor KD, Dickson ER, Baldus W. Ursodeoxycholic acid in the treatment of primary biliary cirrhosis. Gastroenterology. 1994;106:1284–90.
10. Bachrach WH, Hofmann AF. Ursodeoxycholic acid in the treatment of cholesterol cholelithiasis. Dig Dis Sci. 1982;27:773–856.
11. Fromm H. Gallstone dissolution and the cholesterol-bile acid-lipoprotein axis. Propitious effects of ursodeoxycholic acid. Gastroenterology. 1984;87:229–33.

12. Malavolti M, Fromm H, Ceryak S, Roberts IM. Modulation of low density lipoprotein receptor activity by bile acids: differential effects of chenodeoxycholic and ursodeoxycholic acids in the hamster. J Lipid Res. 1987;28:1281–95.
13. Bouscarel B, Fromm H, Ceryak S, Cassidy MM. Ursodeoxycholic acid increases low density lipoprotein binding, uptake and degradation in isolated hamster hepatocytes. Biochem J. 1991;280:589–98.
14. Bouscarel B, Ceryak S, Robins SJ, Fromm H. Studies on the mechanism of the ursodeoxycholic acid-induced increase in hepatic low density lipoprotein binding. Lipids. 1995 (In press).
15. Vander Velpen GC, Shimi SM, Cuschieri A. Outcome after cholecystectomy for symptomatic gall stone disease and effect of surgical access: laparoscopic v open approach. Gut. 1993;34:1448–51.
16. Gouma DJ, Go PM. Bile duct injury during laparoscopic and conventional cholecystectomy. J Am Coll Surg. 1994;178:229–33.
17. Madariaga JR, Dodson SF, Selby R, Todo S, Iwatsuki, Starzl TE. Corrective treatment and anatomic considerations for laparoscopic cholecystectomy injuries. J Am Coll Surg. 1994;179:321–5.

19
Indications for shockwave lithotripsy

T. SAUERBRUCH

INTRODUCTION

Shockwave lithotripsy of gallstones (ESWL) was performed in humans for the first time about 10 years ago. This report[1] underlined two possibilities: first, a broadening of the indication of oral litholytic therapy for gallbladder stones and second, a facilitation of non-surgical treatment of bile duct stones, primarily not amenable to endoscopic extraction. Meanwhile, numerous studies have confirmed the feasibility of gallstone-ESWL. It remained an important adjuvant procedure for the treatment of bile duct stones[2]. However, with regard to gallbladder stones the application of ESWL is now being discussed controversially, especially after the introduction of newly modified surgery, namely laparoscopic cholecystectomy.

It is now well established that it does not matter whether an electrohydraulic, piezoceramic or electromagnetic device to generate shockwaves is used, provided the acoustic shockwave energy that hits the stone remains constant. Nevertheless, technical features (such as the shockwave focal size, the imaging system for stone localization, the monitoring of the procedure or the shockwave coupling device) may influence the ease and success of treatment. More important, however, are patients and stone characteristics that predict long-term therapeutic success. An important achievement of the past 10 years has been to define these parameters by carefully conducted clinical trials, and to assess the optimal candidate for ESWL.

Relevant criteria that determine the indication for shockwave therapy of gallbladder stones are defined by the patient's symptoms, imaging of the gallstones, stone number and stone size as well as gallbladder motor function.

PATIENT'S SYMPTOMS

Gallbladder stones are a benign disease. Less than 3% of patients will die from their stones and only about 30% will suffer symptoms or complications[3]. After an occurrence of gallstone-related symptoms the chance of developing further symptoms or even complications is doubled; therefore there is a general consensus that patients should have had at least one episode of biliary pain or a complication prior to the initiation of any type of treatment. In this context it is important that physicians adhere to the definition of biliary pain[4], otherwise a lot of patients with non-biliary pain will receive inadequate therapy and continue to suffer from abdominal discomfort. As to ESWL, only symptomatic but uncomplicated stones should be treated. Patients should be informed that, following ESWL (mainly within the first post-treatment months), the chance of suffering recurrent biliary pain, mostly from passing fragments, is in the range of 30–40%[5]. The patient should also know that this pain is accompanied by mild pancreatitis or cholestasis in 1–2% of all treatments, and will require endoscopic sphincterotomy in one out of 100 patients. Furthermore, the patient should be told that, even if the gallbladder stones are not completely cleared from the gallbladder, cholecystectomy is not essential. Only every fourth patient not rendered stone-free underwent cholecystectomy in the clinical trials with a mean follow-up time of 1–2 years. Symptoms arising after ESWL – according to one study – reflect the natural history of the patient's stone disease more than aggravation through lithotripsy[6]. In summary, symptomatic gallbladder stone disease is adequately influenced by ESWL only when the gallbladder has been rendered stone-free. However, ESWL is probably not harmful for the patient, even when fragments remain in the gallbladder.

STONE CHARACTERISTICS

Radiolucency

ESWL of gallbladder stones was introduced as a treatment in combination with oral litholytic therapy, which means it is recommended for patients with radiolucent stones that suggest high cholesterol content of the calculi. Fragments of these stones may be attacked by drugs that lower the biliary cholesterol content. Within the past few years the need for bile salts adjuvant to ESWL has been debated[7]. Stones can be pulverized by shockwaves and may therefore not require additional litholytic therapy[6–8]. This is achieved, however, only by several ESWL sessions with subsequent spontaneous fragment clearance into the intestine. This new treatment approach in patients with solitary stones had a clearance rate of 90% within 6 months when sludge-like disintegration was achieved[8]. On the other hand the success rate in patients with stones with a calcified rim[9] is lower (about 40% after 5–8 months). In addition, a low CT-density of the stones[10], at least according to one trial, predicts a higher stone clearance rate. Therefore, radiolucent stones are the preferred stones for ESWL, whether with or without adjuvant litholytic therapy. Exceptionally radiopaque stones may be treated if they are small, and if there is sufficient gallbladder contraction (>60%), and if reasonable arguments advising against cholecystectomy exist.

Ultrasound

Several attempts have been made to correlate physical and chemical stone properties with their fragmentation under shockwave treatment. None of the factors studied (e.g. radiolucency, CT-density, cholesterol content) was of significant importance for the prediction of stone disintegration[11]. This disintegration process is almost exclusively determined by the amount of applied acoustic energy per stone volume[12,13]. As to ultrasounding gallbladder stones, there is evidence from one *in-vitro* study[12], and from a clinical study[8], that a certain echo pattern of the stone, namely homogeneously distributed internal echoes extending behind the stone, predicts a high cholesterol content (>90) on one hand, and improved disintegration behaviour on the other. The latter finding, however, is not corroborated by *in-vitro* studies which have found the echo pattern not to be a major determinant of fragmentation[12]. This may, nevertheless, be an additional finding in favour of lithotripsy.

STONE SIZE AND STONE NUMBER

There are numerous trials showing that radiolucent solitary stones with a diameter up to 2 cm are most easily crushed, and show the best long-term results[5]. About 70% of patients with these stones are rendered stone-free within 6 months (versus 40% in patients with large solitary stones between 2 and 3 cm and 30% in patients with two or three stones). This difference in outcome also holds true for treatment strategies that use repeated shockwave application[7]. It is unknown whether patients with very small multiple stones are an exception to the rule that multiple stones are bad candidates for ESWL. In case of multiple stones, debris caused by disintegrated stones may attenuate the shockwaves directed to the still-intact stones[13]. As to long-term results, stone recurrence is probably lower in patients with solitary stones than in those with multiple stones[14]. Sackman and co-workers found a recurrence rate of 30% after 5 years in patients of whom nearly 90% had solitary stones.

GALLBLADDER FUNCTION

ESWL should be performed only in patients with a functioning gallbladder, e.g. at least a patent cystic duct and no signs of alteration in the gallbladder wall. Within recent years the influence of gallbladder motility has been further investigated. It was shown that, on average, gallstone patients have a higher fasting gallbladder volume and a higher residual volume than controls, facilitating the formation of stones[15,16].

Gallbladder stone patients can be divided into so-called contractors and non-contractors. Those with adequate gallbladder contraction fare considerably better. Patients with an ejection fraction higher than 60% had a complete clearance rate for gallbladder stones of 66% at 3 months vs. only 29% in those with a contraction of less than 60%, suggesting that the capability to empty the gallbladder is an important determinant of early gallstone clearance after ESWL[17]. This finding is supported by the observation that patients who do not clear the fragments have more than a doubled residual gallbladder volume as compared to patients who were rendered stone-free[18]. These data suggest that only patients with adequate gallbladder contraction should be treated. Patients with intact gallbladder motor function are probably also less prone to stone recurrence[16].

SUMMARY

Ten years after its introduction ESWL of gallbladder stones has found its proper place. Patients with symptomatic radiolucent solitary stones and an adequate gallbladder contraction are ideal candidates. They can be advised to undergo ESWL with or without adjuvant bile acid treatment, especially when they are reluctant to receive open surgery. These patients, however, comprise no more than 5–10% of those with symptomatic radiolucent stones.

References

1. Sauerbruch T, Delius M, Paumgartner G *et al.* Fragmentation of gallstones by extracorporeal shock waves. N Engl J Med. 1986;314:818–22.
2. Sauerbruch T, Holl J, Sackmann M, Paumgartner G. Fragmentation of bile duct stones by extracorporeal shockwave lithotripsy. A five-year experience. Hepatology. 1992;15:208–214.
3. Ransohoff DF, Gracie WA. Treatment of gallstones. Ann Intern Med. 1993;119:606–19.
4. Paumgartner G, Carr-Locke DL, Dubois F, Roda E, Thistle JL. Strategies in the treatment of gallstone disease. Gastroenterol Int. 1993;6:65–75.
5. Sackmann M, Pauletzki J, Sauerbruch T, Holl J, Schelling G, Paumgartner G. The Munich gallbladder lithotripsy study – results of the first 5 years with 711 patients. Ann Intern Med. 1991;114:290–6.
6. Boscaini M, Piccinni-Leopardi M, Andreotti F, Montori A. Gallstone pulverisation strategy in patients treated with extracorporeal lithotripsy and follow up results of maintenance treatment with ursodeoxycholic acid. Gut. 1994;35:117–21.
7. Soehendra N, Nam V-C, Binmoeller KF, Koch H, Bohnacker S, Schreiber HW. Pulverisation of calcified and non-calcified gallbladder stones: extracorporeal shock wave lithotripsy used alone. Gut. 1994;35:417–22.
8. Tsuchiya Y, Takanashi H, Haniya K *et al.* An early gallstone clearance following repeat piezoelectric lithotripsy. J Gastroenterol Hepatol. 1994;9:597–603.
9. Sackmann M, Pauletzki J, Delius M *et al.* Noninvasive therapy of gallbladder calculi with a radiopaque rim. Gastroenterology. 1992;102:988–93.
10. Ell Ch, Schneider HT, Benninger J *et al.* Significance of computed tomography for shock-wave therapy of radiolucent gallstones. Gastroenterology. 1991;101:1409–16.
11. Sauerbruch T, Neubrand M. Lithotripsy of gallbladder stones. Eur J Clin Invest. 1994;24:20–1.
12. Neubrand M, Greinwald I, Lobentanzer H, Paumgartner G, Hermeking H, Sauerbruch T. The physical laws governing the fragmentation of human gallbladder stones and their clinical relevance. (submitted)
13. Lobentanzer H, Neubrand M, Hermeking H, Sauerbruch T. *In vitro* study to elucidate the physical laws concerning the fragmentation of both solitary and multiple artificial stones. Clin Invest. 1993;71:882–7.
14. Sackmann M, Niller H, Klüppelberg U *et al.* Gallstone recurrence after shock-wave therapy. Gastroenterology. 1994;106:225–30.
15. Pauletzki J, Cicala M, Holl J, Sauerbruch T, Schafmayer A, Paumgartner G. Correlation between gallbladder fasting volume and postprandial emptying in patients with gallstones and healthy controls. Gut. 1993;34:1443–7.
16. Berr F, Mayer M, Sackmann M, Sauerbruch T, Holl J, Paumgartner G. Pathogenic factors in early recurrence of cholesterol gallstones. Gastroenterology. 1994;106:215–24.
17. Pauletzki J, Sailer Ch, Klüppelberg U *et al.* Gallbladder emptying determines early gallstone clearance after shock-wave lithotripsy. Gastroenterology. 1994;107:1496–502.
18. Sackmann M, Eder H, Spengler U *et al.* Gallbladder emptying is an important factor in fragment disappearance after shock wave lithotripsy. J Hepatol. 1993;17:62–6.

20
ESWL – the Charité experience

K. WENGLER

INTRODUCTION

In the last 10 years, external shockwave lithotripsy has gained an established and also clearly defined position in the treatment of gallstones. The further technical development of lithotripters, the growing and widespread use of endoscopic methods and progress in the operative treatment of gallstone disease have led to a clear and restricted indication decision for the conservative treatment of cholelithiasis.

Sonography plays a decisive role in diagnosis in the area of cholecystolithiasis and in the recognition of complications of this disease. The same is increasingly true with regard to choledocho- and cholangiolithiasis, whereby the sensitivity and accuracy of the diagnosis depends even more on the level of knowledge of the examiner (Wermke).

The aim of any conservative treatment of gallstones is the most complete fragmentation possible of the concretions, irrespective of whether these are situated in the gallbladder, in the intrahepatic bile ducts or in the common bile ducts. The aim of shockwave treatment is to achieve fragments which can be eliminated spontaneously whereby adjuvant oral litholysis can accelerate stone elimination. With regard to choledocholithiasis, shockwave treatment can create the conditions for endoscopic stone extraction and this fact is also the basis for the treatment of pancreaticolithiasis.

METHODS

Since December 1990, 1297 treatments have been carried out on 616 patients at the Charité Clinic of Internal Medicine (now the IVth Medical Clinic). The predominant reason for treatment was cholecystolithiasis. ESWL was carried out in only 52 patients (8.4%) suffering from choledocholithiasis ($n =$) who could not be treated by endoscopy, and the shockwave treatment was carried out in individual cases for an intrahepatic cholangiolithiasis or pancreaticolithiasis ($n =$).

Most (68%) of the patients were women, with middle-aged patients predominating for both sexes (mean age 50.1 years). However, in the case of choledocholithiasis, the patients were older, with a mean age of 68.4 years.

The central means of diagnosis in all cases was upper abdominal sonography. Before the initial gallstone consultation, a plain X-ray was taken of the gallbladder region in order to be able to recognize without delay patients with complete stone calcification – these patients usually underwent immediate surgical treatment.

Apart from the anamnesis (symptoms would have to be present), clinical examination and sonography, a contraction test was carried out on the gallbladder, whereby the gallbladder volume was compared by sonography before and after a rice meal. A volume reduction of at least 33% was a requirement.

Oesophagogastroscopy was only carried out in cases of imprecise upper abdominal symptoms.

Exclusion criteria for ESWL were all forms of cholecystitis, pregnancy, coagulation disorders, focal liver lesions in the shockwave field and florid ventricular and duodenal ulcers. Similarly, the latter contraindications also apply in treatment of cholangio and pancreaticolithiasis.

ESWL PROCEDURE AND SIDE-EFFECTS

ESWL was carried out mostly on in-patients. Normally, we administered midazolam as a sedative and Afentanil as an analgesic. The ESWL was carried out in the prone position with a mean energy of 19.5 kV, usually consisting of 2000 shockwave impulses. The siting was carried out by sonography except in two cases of choledocholithiasis.

Premature discontinuation of treatment was only necessary in certain cases because of cardiological symptoms in the form of rhythm disorders ($n =$), transitory respiratory depression resulting from the sedoanalgesia ($n =$) and failure to locate the stone ($n =$).

Two per cent of patients suffered from colic-type problems during the first 24 h following ESWL; micro- or macrohaematuria was observed in 15% of cases; and a sonographic picture of an oedematous gallbladder wall thickening (maximum 5 mm) was present in 4% of patients.

RESULTS

Table 1 shows the percentage of stone-free patients, separated according to single stones and multiple concretions. The number of treatments and the timing of the second or repeated treatments had no influence on the results. The first shockwave treatment was regarded as the start of treatment.

After a two-year observation period, 4.8% of patients with a single concretion and 11.2% of patients with multiple concretions suffered a recurrence.

In the case of choledocholithiasis, ESWL was only used when endoscopic stone extraction was not successful. Fifty-two patients were treated externally by shockwave treatment; in one patient with a 5-cm concretion, 6 treatments were required before complete stone extraction was achieved.

Table 1 Percentage of stone-free patients at certain times following ESWL

	Percentage of stone-free patients after ESWL		
	6 weeks	6 months	12 months
Patients with a sinlge stone	18	47	84
Patients with multiple stones	9	30	75

Effective fragmentation of concretions removable by endoscopy was possible in 42 patients (81%); in 4 patients, endoprosthesis was the final solution for the common bile duct and 5 patients underwent surgery.

The cases of intrahepatic cholangiolithiasis were not easily treated by simple stone siting. Successful treatment here lay in clinical improvement and avoidance of cholestasis, which was possible in all cases.

With regard to pancreaticolithiasis, ESWL was carried out as a preparatory measure for further endoscopic interventions. In one case, the treatment had to be discontinued because of the large number of stones and the hardness of the concretions.

DISCUSSION

With clear confirmation of indication and preference given to ideally suited patients, the external shockwave treatment of cholecystolithiasis is shown to be an efficient and, above all, well-tolerated treatment possibility, even with the current range of therapeutic possibilities. The essential point of treatment is effective fragmentation. Rapid stone reduction and few side-effects are observed with fragments which, according to sonographic criteria, do not exceed 2 mm, or, even better, complete pulverization of the concretions.

Based on our experience, adjuvant oral litholysis has been shown to be useful, particularly in protracted procedures. However, it does not significantly influence the rapid elimination of stones – more data on this will be available in the future.

It has been shown that ESWL is a possible treatment of choledocholithiasis, which is easy to carry out and can be used as preparation for endoscopic treatment, particularly in cases with large concretions.

The treatment of intrahepatic cholangiolithiasis is only successful in certain cases but the technical procedure is not very costly.

With regard to pancreaticolithiasis, we do not have sufficient treatment experience in our clinic to reach any conclusions.

Overall, ESWL is shown to be a treatment which: is successful after accurate confirmation of indication, is not costly to carry out, and is extremely well tolerated by the patients.

21 Indications for topical dissolution therapy

A. HELLSTERN

In 1985, contact dissolution with methyl tert-butyl ether (MTBE) applied through a transhepatic catheter has been established as a safe and effective treatment option for patients with cholesterol gallbladder stones[1]. In the same year, extracorporeal shockwave lithotripsy (ESWL)[2] and soon thereafter laparoscopic cholecystectomy[3] were introduced into treatment of gallstone disease.

Since then, laparoscopic cholecystectomy has become a widely accepted minimally invasive surgery technique, leading to a re-evaluation of the role of all other forms of gallstone therapy.

In order to assess the status of contact dissolution with MTBE, we performed a survey in 21 European hospitals, asking about the technical procedure, the results of litholysis, the indications and contraindications, occurence of complications and lethality. We also calculated gallstone recurrence of all patients treated in our hospital and we asked patients to rate the procedure.

PATIENTS AND METHODS

The access to the gallbladder was performed either by radiology or by ultrasonography as previously described[4]. MTBE was instilled into the gallbladder either manually with a glass syringe or else using an automatic pump[5–7]. Treatment was continued until the stones dissolved or until the lytic process reached a standstill.

The recurrence rate following stone dissolution was examined in 173/264 patients from Frankfurt during a follow-up period of 5 years. The recurrence rate was related to stone number and to left-over sludge in the gallbladder. The probability of recurrence of stone formation was determined using the Kaplan–Meier estimator with Hall–Wellner confidence bands of 95% confidence. Kaplan–Meier curves of the different groups were compared by the log-rank test.

One hundred and eight patients treated in Frankfurt were asked to indicate on an analogue scale whether they found contact litholysis to be painful and distressing (grade 0) or not distressing at all (grade 10).

RESULTS

A total of 803 patients with cholesterol gallbladder stones were selected for MTBE treatment (Table 1). In all the patients, one or more episodes of biliary colic or relapsing severe pain had occurred.

In 95% of the patients, the introduction and proper placement of the perfusion catheter was achieved in an average time of 32 min. The success rate for radiological or ultrasonographic guidance was the same (Table 2).

Some minor side-effects which required no therapeutic intervention are listed in Table 3. After removal of the catheter bile leakage occured in 39 patients (Table 4). Twelve patients then underwent cholecystectomy. In 4 patients, the gallbladder was punctured anew, the bile drained externally, and the catheter then removed a few days later without any complications. In 23 patients with leakage, further treatment was not required.

Table 1 Results of topical dissolution therapy data of 21 European centres

Patients scheduled for therapy	803
Solitary stones	26%
Multiple stones	74%
Placement of catheter successful	95%
Stone dissolution*	95%
Sludge in the gallbladder	43%
30-day mortality	0.4%

*>90% of stone burden

Table 2 Catheter placement and success

	Total (*n* = 803)	*Sonographic technique* (*n* = 312)	*Radiological technique* (*n* = 491)
Successful			
n	761	296	467
%	94.8	94.9	95.1
Time for placement (min)			
Mean	32	30	35
Range	12–62	18–40	12–62

Table 3 Side-effects not requiring therapeutic intervention

	20 Centres	Frankfurt
Leucocytosis	7.8	8.2
Fever	5.6	1.5
Transaminases	8.0	4.1
Lipase	0.4	0
Haematobilia	0.7	1.5

All figures are percentages

Table 4 Side-effects requiring therapeutic intervention

Bile leak after catheter removal	39/761 (5.1%)
Cholecystectomy	12
Repuncture	4
No further treatment	23

One hundred and eight patients were asked to assess the procedure after removal of the catheter and 13 (12%) rated the method as being distressing and painful (grades 0–2), whereas 76 (70.4%) described it as not distressing (grades 8–10).

Pregnancy and stone density above 100 Hounsfield units are general accepted exclusion criteria for contact dissolution with MTBE. Over half of all centres excluded patients with gallbladder anomalies (Table 5).

Of the 253/264 successfully treated patients in Frankfurt, 173 (68.4%) were followed up for a further period of 5 years. The probability of the different patient groups forming recurrent stones within 5 years is shown in Figures 1–3. These show that, in patients with multiple stones, the risk of forming recurrent stones is statistically significantly greater ($p<0.001$) than in those with solitary stones, whereas the probability in patients with residual sludge after litholysis is not higher than in those without sludge ($p = 0.156$).

DISCUSSION

Gallstone disease, which means that gallstone carriers suffer from pain, colic or even complications, is one of the most common diseases of the Western world[8,9] and therefore represents a tremendous financial burden for any health system. Since, at the same time, many patients wish to avoid undergoing surgery, it was sensible to search for non-surgical procedures that are safe, successful and cost-effective. The results of litholysis with MTBE were favourable. However, the numerous reports from single sources, often with only small patient numbers, did not allow a reasonable assessment of the procedure[10–12]. Therefore, we have

Table 5 Exclusion criteria for topical dissolution with MTBE. Opinions of 21 European centres

Contraindication	*Number of Centres*
Pregnancy	21/21
Hounsfield units >100	17/21
Gallbladder anomalies*	15/21
Extreme overweight	6/21
Too many stones	5/21
Stones >2 cm	5/21
Floating stones	4/21
Age below 18 years	3/21
Age below 25 years	1/21
Age above 65 years	1/21

*Marked gallbladder septation, large diverticulae, distorted gallbladder, mobile gallbladder

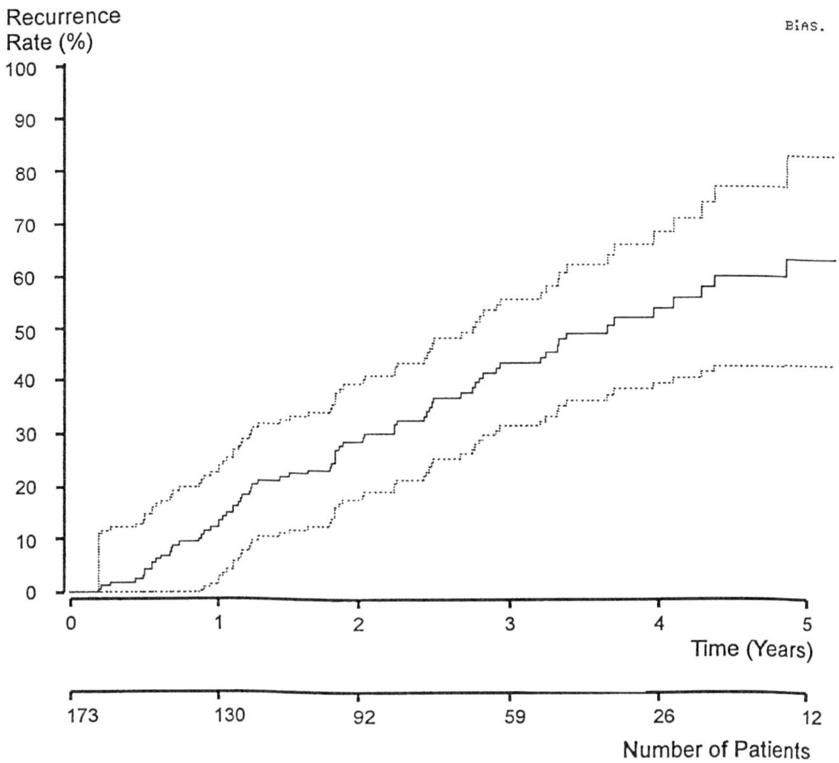

Fig. 1 Probability of stone recurrence in patients after topical dissolution therapy with MTBE (Kaplan–Meier estimator with Hall–Wellner confidence bands of 95% confidence; $n = 173$)

performed a survey in 21 European hospitals in order to estimate the day-to-day practicability of topical dissolution therapy with MTBE.

Only about 44–45% of patients remain stone free after MTBE, since about 50% develop recurrent stones during the following 5 years. This recurrence rate corresponds approximately to that of oral litholysis[13,14] but is 3 times higher than after ESWL[14]. However, with ESWL, most patients treated had solitary stones, and therefore a priori a lower recurrence rate can be expected. Thus, if we compare the probability of recurrent stone formation in patients with solitary stones after MTBE with that in patients with solitary stones after ESWL over a period of 3 years[15], the values of 22–27% (42 patients at risk) for MTBE compared with 12% (29 patients at risk) for ESWL do not differ fundamentally.

The recurrence rate following MTBE may not only depend on stone number[16], which probably correlates with the occurrence of nucleating factors in bile[17], but is also believed to depend on residual sludge after removal of the catheter[1,10]. Sludge was left in the gallbladder more often in patients with multiple stones than in those with solitary stones. The probability of patients with and without sludge developing new stones over a period of 5 years, then statistically the chances are not significantly different. The reason for this could

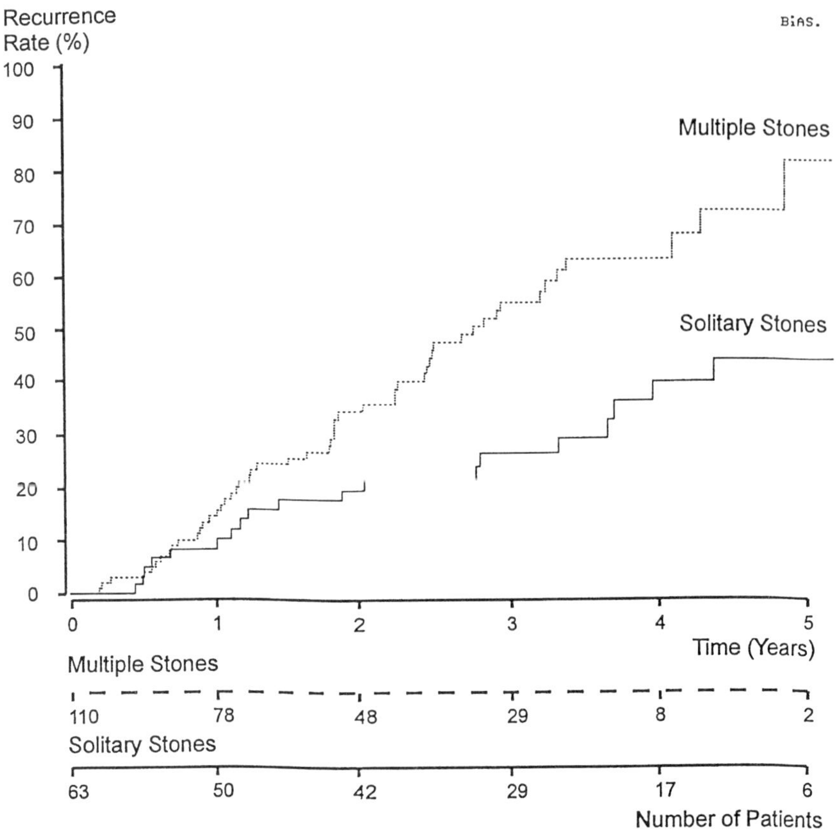

Fig. 2 Probability of stone recurrence in patients with solitary or multiple stones ($p<0.001$)

be that the sludge left after MTBE treatment, besides a mixture of lecithin and cholesterol, predominantly consists of non-soluble pigment remnants[18] which do not cluster to form new stones.

Although topical dissolution therapy with MTBE is an invasive method, the rate of therapy-related complications is low: 1.6% of all patients treated had to undergo elective cholecystectomy. If patients with bile leaks are not operated on, but drained externally after renewed puncture or a nasobiliary catheter is placed, the number of surgical patients can be further reduced. All other side-effects, such as a rise in transaminases or a rise in lipase, were transitory and did not require treatment. Haemolysis or kidney failure did not occur as complications in our relatively large survey, but a few single cases have been reported in the literature[19]. The concentrations of MTBE and its metabolites in blood, urine and mother's milk after contact litholysis are, however, very low[20], and animal experiments imply only negligible toxicity[21–26]. Haemorrhage (haematobilia) into the gallbladder occurred in 8 cases, but this prevented therapy only for a short time. The low complication rate and the absence of a method-related mor-

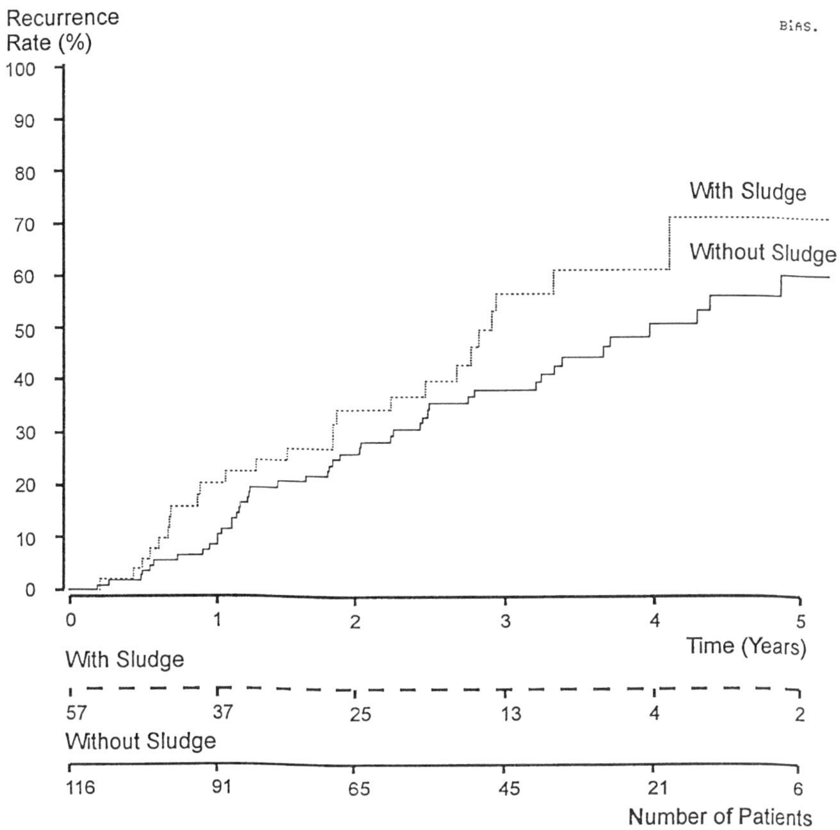

Fig. 3 Probability of stone recurrence in patients with or without sludge in the gallbladder (p=0.156)

tality in 21 European centres show that topical dissolution therapy with MTBE, when scrupulously performed, is a safe procedure.

Based on the data derived from 803 patients in 21 European centres, we are able to give the following recommendations for contact litholysis with MTBE. The method is suitable for all symptomatic patients over 18 years and there is no upper age limit. As with other conservative procedures, it is only suitable for patients with radiolucent non-calcified cholesterol stones. The gallbladder must be functioning. If bile duct stones are simultaneously present, these can be endoscopically removed prior to gallbladder puncture. Stone burden and stone size are not limiting factors according to most centres. However, floating stones can present problems as these stones do move around the gallbladder during MTBE injection and thus preclude rapid dissolution. But, when the gallbladder is kept collapsed to keep the stones trapped within the pigtail, the stones dissolve rapidly. Marked gallbladder anomalies are a contraindication[27], as they may lead to rapid stone recurrence (however, this has not yet been confirmed) and puncture of the gallbladder is more difficult but, in general, not impossible. Extreme obesity could be a contraindication; however, in some countries, longer introduction sheaths are available. Also, obese persons usually have a fatty liver which could predispose to bile leakage[11]. As for other procedures, pregnancy, acute or chronic hepatitis, cholecystitis, and hepatic cirrhosis are contraindications.

In conclusion, contact dissolution therapy with MTBE is a safe and successful procedure for the treatment of cholesterol stones in a functioning gallbladder. This is especially evident if we consider that most centres have not yet completed their training phase, yet their results correspond to those of a centre experienced in using this treatment in a large number of patients. The advantages of MTBE treatment compared with other non-surgical procedures are that patients with any stone burden and stone size can be treated at 30–45% lower costs compared with oral litholysis, shock wave lithotripsy and surgery (for Germany[28]), the technical expenditure of the procedure is minor and the hospital stay for the patient is kept short. In addition, it is worthwhile noting that all patients who are at high risk for anaesthesia and surgery can be treated successfully and safely in spite of most of the exclusion factors listed in Table 5. A disadvantage is the 5-year relapse rate, which is comparable to that for oral litholysis of multiple stones, and to that for extracorporeal shock wave lithotripsy for solitary stones. The greatest problem is the staffing situation, although this can be overcome by a trained physician and a trained nurse. Whether the combination of extracorporeal shock wave lithotripsy with contact litholysis in patients with slightly calcified gallbladder stones[12,29] is superior to MTBE alone has to be investigated.

References

1. Allen MJ, Borody TJ, Bugliosi TF, May GR, LaRusso NF, Thistle JL. Rapid dissolution of gallstones by methyl tert-butyl ether. Preliminary observations. N Engl J Med. 1985;312:217–20.
2. Sauerbruch T, Delius M, Paumgartner G *et al.* Fragmentation of gallstones by extracorporeal shockwaves. N Engl J Med. 1986;314:8181–22.
3. Perissat J, Collet DR, Belliard R. Gallstones: Laparoscopic treatment, intracorporeal lithotripsy followed by cholecystostomy or cholecystectomy – a personal technique. Endoscopy. 1988;21:373–4.
4. Hellstern A, Leuschner U. Percutaneous transhepatic dissolution of gall-bladder stones using methyl tertiary butyl ether. Min Invas Ther. 1992;1:125–9.
5. Zakko S, Hofmann AF. Microprocessor-assisted solvent-transfer system for gallstone dissolution. *In vitro* and *in vivo* validation. Gastroenterology. 1990;99:1807–13.
6. Leuschner U, Hellstern A, Ansell A, Gatzen M, Güldütuna S, Leuschner M. Manual and automatic gallstone dissolution with methyl tert-butyl ether. Dig Dis Sci. 1994;39:1302–8.
7. Sanden H v, Schmitt W, Burlefinger R, Ottenjann R. Pumpengestützte perkutan-transhepatische Litholyse von Gallensteinen. Dtsch Med Wschr. 1989;114:481.
8. Sama C, Labate AMM, Taroni F, Barbara L. Epidemiology and natural history of gallstone disease. Semin Liver Dis. 1990;3:149–58.
9. GREPCO (Rome Group for the Epidemiology and Prevention of Cholelithiasis). Prevalence of gallstone disease in an adult female population. Am J Epidemiol. 1984;119:796–805.
10. Thistle JL, May GR, Bender CE *et al.* Dissolution of cholesterol gallbladder stones by methyl tert-butyl ether administered by percutaneous transhepatic catheter. N Engl J Med. 1989;320:633–9.
11. Hellstern A, Leuschner M, Frenk H, Dillinger W, Caspary W, Leuschner U. Gallstone dissolution with methyl tert-butyl ether: How to avoid complications. Gut. 1990;331:922–5.
12. Neubrand M, Holl J, Sackmann M *et al.* Combination of extracorporeal shock-wave lithotripsy and dissolution of gallbladder stones with methyl tert-butyl ether: a randomized study. Hepatology. 1994;19:133–7.

13. O'Donnell LD, Heaton KW. Recurrence and re-recurrence of gall stones after medical dissolution: A longterm follow up. Gut. 1988;29:655–8.
14. Hood KA, Gleeson D, Ruppin DC, Dowling RH, and the British–Belgian Gall Stone Study Group. Gall stone recurrence and its prevention: the British/Belgian Gall Stone Study Group's post dissolution trial. Gut. 1993;34:1277–88.
15. Sackmann M, Ippisch E, Sauerbruch T, Holl J, Brendel W, Paumgartner G. Early gallstone recurrence rate after successful shock-wave therapy. Gastroenterology. 1990;98:392–6.
16. Villanova N, Bazzoli F, Taroni F *et al.* Gallstone recurrence after successful oral bile acid treatment. A 12-year follow-up study and evaluation of long-term postdissolution treatment. Gastroenterology. 1989;97:726–31.
17. Groen AK, Noordam C, Drapers JAG, Ottenhoff R. Isolation of potent cholesterol nucleation-promoting activity from human gallbladder bile; role in the pathogenesis of gallstone disease. Hepatology. 1990;11:525–33.
18. Lee SP, Maher K, Nicholls JF. Origin and fate of biliary sludge. Gastroenterology. 1988;94:170–6.
19. Ponchon T, Baroud J, Pujol B, Valette PJ, Perrot D. Renal failure during dissolution of gallstones by methyl tert-butly ether. Lancet. 1988;2:276–7.
20. Leuschner U, Hellstern A, Schmidt K *et al.* Gallstone dissolution with methyl tert-butyl ether in 120 patients – Efficacy and safety. Dig Dis Sci. 1991;36:193–9.
21. Hofmann AF, Schteingart CD, van Sonnenberg E, Esch O, Zakko SF. Contact dissolution of cholesterol gallstones with organic solvents. Gastroenterol Clin N Am. 1991;20:183–99.
22. Akimoto R, Rieger E, Moossa AR, Hofmann AF, Wahlstrom HE. Systemic and local toxicity in the rat and methyl tert-butyl ether: A gallstone dissolution agent. J Surg Res. 1992;53:527–77.
23. Esch O, Spinosa JC, Hamilton RL *et al.* Acute effects of topical methyl tert-butyl ether or ethyl propionate on gallbladder histology in animals: A comparison of two solvents for contact dissolution of cholesterol gallstones. Hepatology. 1992;16:984–91.
24. Esch O, Schteingart CD, Pappert D, Kirby D, Streich R, Hofmann AF. Increased blood levels of methyl tert-butyl ether but not of ethyl propionate during instillation with contact gallstone dissolution agents in the pig. Hepatology. 1993;18:373–9.
25. Savolainen H, Pfäffi P, Elovaara E. Biochemical effects of methyl tertiary-butyl ether in extended vapor exposure of rats. Arch Toxicol. 1985;57:285–8.
26. Conaway CC, Schroeder RE, Snyder NK. Teratology evaluation of methyl tertiary butyl ether in rats and mice. J Toxicol Environ Health. 1985;16:797–809.
27. Hellstern A, Rübesam D, Leuschner M, Wendt T, Fuchs H, Leuschner U. Percutaneous transhepatic gallstone dissolution with methyl tert-butyl ether in complicated stone diagnosis and gallbladder anomalies. Endoscopy. 1990;22:254–8.
28. Leuschner U. Effektivität und Wirtschaftlichkeit heutiger Therapieverfahren bei Cholezystolithiasis. Gastro-Liga Rep. 1994;5:11–4.
29. Lu SDK, Ho C-S, Allen LC. Gallstone dissolution in methyl tert-butyl ether after mechanical fragmentation: In vitro study. JR. 1990;155:67–72.

22
Laparoscopic cholecystectomy – achievements and problems, 1995

S. M. STRASBERG, N. J. SOPER and M. P. CALLERY

INTRODUCTION

Laparoscopic cholecystectomy, was introduced widely in 1989 and quickly changed the treatment of cholelithiasis. Now, several years later, it is acknowledged as the new standard of treatment. However, laparoscopic cholecystectomy is associated with an increased incidence of biliary injury. Laparoscopic cholecystectomy stimulated the development of other laparoscopic hepatobiliary procedures, most importantly laparoscopic common bile duct exploration. This review will describe and evaluate these and other less well-developed aspects of the subject.

TREATMENT OF GALLSTONES BY LAPAROSCOPIC SURGERY

Results of laparoscopic cholecystectomy

Laparoscopic cholecystectomy vs other forms of treatment

As regards laparoscopic cholecystectomy vs ESWL and bile salt dissolution, no randomized trials comparing these procedures exist. A review of case series examining clinical effectiveness, cost-effectiveness and patient satisfaction criteria suggested that bile salt therapy and ESWL have the advantage of safety, but recurrence and prolonged treatment periods are offsetting disadvantages[1]. This analysis predicted that ESWL was competitive with laparoscopic cholecystectomy in about 7% of patients with stones, while dissolution therapy would be competitive in about 10% patients[1].

Two randomized trials have documented the superiority of laparoscopic cholecystectomy over open cholecystectomy. In the study of Barkun *et al.* hospital stay was shorter in the laparoscopic group, as was the duration of convalescence and time to resume a normal diet[2]. McMahon *et al.* studied 302 patients; this trial demonstrated that patients treated by laparoscopic cholecystectomy had a lower pain score, returned to work earlier, and were more satisfied with the cosmetic result of the procedure[3]. Direct costs of laparoscopic cholecystectomy were higher than open cholecystectomy in one English study[3]; conversely McIntyre *et al.* of Denver reported that the mean charge for laparoscopic cholecystectomy was more than $2000 less than open cholecystectomy[4]. A lower direct cost was predicted in an analytical cost-effectiveness evaluation[5], provided the incidence of biliary injury could be held at 0.5%. Indirect costs are much lower, since patients return to normal activities much earlier[3].

Laparoscopic cholecystectomy and overall cholecystectomy rates

There has been a large increase (33–66%) in the number of cholecystectomies performed since the introduction of the laparoscopic technique[6–8]. Consequently, although mortality and cost have fallen on a per-procedure basis, the total number of cholecystectomy-related deaths and cost of treating gallstones by cholecystectomy[7,8] have remained steady. Two possible causes of the increase in cholecystectomies are treatment of symptomatic patients who would have refused open cholecystectomy or treatment of symptomatic patients referred at an earlier stage of disease. Inappropriate therapy might also be contributing; for instance, treatment of asymptomatic patients or treatment of patients with minimal or questionable symptoms of cholelithiasis. More studies are required to determine whether laparoscopic cholecystectomy is being used for incorrect indications.

Metabolic and pulmonary effects of laparoscopic cholecystectomy vs open cholecystectomy

Pneumoperitoneum creates venous stasis in the lower extremities, an effect that can be reduced by compression stockings. There is an improvement in postoperative pulmonary function in patients having laparoscopic cholecystectomy over open cholecystectomy, as shown in randomized trials[9,10].

Special situations in laparoscopic cholecystectomy

Pregnancy

Pregnant patients are preferably managed conservatively until delivery, but sometimes patients require operation[11] for worsening biliary colic[11], acute cholecystitis, non-response to medical management[12], and in some cases of choledocholithiasis and gallstone pancreatitis[13]. Several recent reports indicate that laparoscopic cholecystectomy can be performed safely in pregnancy. The safest time for laparoscopic cholecystectomy is the second timester.

Obesity

Morbid obesity is not a contraindication to laparoscopic cholecystectomy; pulmonary, thromboembolic, wound and cardiovascular complications[14] are less frequent than with open cholecystectomy. Extra-long trocars and other instruments, and occasional use of additional ports for retraction and exposure, are helpful. By avoiding large incisions, the morbidly obese patient returns to normal activity sooner.

Previous abdominal surgery

Laparoscopic access is complicated by prior abdominal surgery, especially in the upper abdomen. Although laparoscopic adhesiolysis may be safely performed, conversion is more common under these circumstances. Factors leading to conversion are extensive adhesions, adhesions involving viscera in such a way that safe dissection is questionable, and anatomical uncertainty or bleeding during dissection. Despite these problems, with experience, laparoscopic cholecystectomy can be performed in most patients with previous upper abdominal surgery.

Other intercurrent conditions

Cardiopulmonary disease occasionally contraindicates use of a general anaesthetic[15], especially when cardiac ejection fractions are less than 20%. Patients with pre-existing obstructive lung disease may retain CO_2 disproportionately during laparoscopic cholecystectomy under CO_2 pneumoperitoneum. Cirrhosis is a relative contraindication to laparoscopic cholecystectomy[15], due to the danger of operating in the face of portal hypertension and coagulopathy. Other patients with severe coagulopathies (haemophilia, etc.) should not undergo laparoscopic cholecystectomy. The laparoscopic approach is suitable for Jehovah's witnesses, but meticulous haemostasis is critical. In patients with generalized peritonitis of uncertain aetiology, laparoscopic cholecystectomy may limit a thorough evaluation of the abdominal cavity. Standard open laparotomy is preferred for both diagnosis and therapy.

Laparoscopic cholecystectomy in children. Laparoscopic cholecystectomy in children is quite successful, although understandably the series are small[16–19]. Vinograd *et al.*[16] summarized their experience with laparoscopic cholecystectomy in 14 children aged 4–15. The gallbladder was successfully removed in 13 patients. The times to discharge and return to normal activities were brief. In another series of uncomplicated laparoscopic cholecystectomies in 12 children, Davidoff *et al.*[17] demonstrated decreased pain and ileus after surgery, improved cosmesis, shortened hospitalization, and faster return to activity as compared to open cholecystectomy for the same age group. We have managed choledocholithiasis and biliary pancreatitis in children with laparoscopic techniques similar to those used in adults[18]. Although choledocholithiasis is very rare in children, paediatricians must be aware of the minimally invasive options available. ERCP with stone retrieval is effective in children, but requires expert paediatric endoscopists.

Complications of laparoscopic cholecystectomy

Biliary injuries

This is the most important problem in laparoscopic cholecystectomy. We recently reviewed this subject[20]. Biliary injury causes great morbidity and cost. Four reliable reports[6, 21–23] suggest that the major bile duct injury rate is between 0.3% and 0.6%. If all biliary injuries are considered the injury rate ranges from 0.6% to 1.5%. This is three to four times higher than reported rates for open cholecystectomy.

Most reports include both major bile duct injuries and 'bilomas' or 'bile leaks'. The latter are more common during laparoscopic cholecystectomy than in open cholecystectomy. To deal with this development we proposed a classification more appropriate for the laparoscopic era[20] (Fig. 1). Type A injuries are injuries to minor ducts without loss of continuity of the biliary tree. Almost all such injuries are due to failure to properly occlude the cystic duct, or are due to an injury to a small bile duct in the liver bed. Type B and C injuries are injuries to aberrant right hepatic bile ducts. Although aberrant right bile ducts are present in only 2% of patients, it seems they are very susceptible to injury during laparoscopic surgery. In Type B injuries the ducts are occluded, while in Type C transection is the problem; both have the common feature of discontinuity of the biliary tree, but have different clinical presentations. Type D injuries, like type A injuries, are lateral injuries, but are more serious because they involve the main ducts and can progress to Type E injuries. Type E injuries are also injuries to the main bile ducts; there are five types, and these are grouped according to the Bismuth classification of major ductal injuries produced at open cholecystectomy. Type A and E injuries predominate in reports from referral centres[20]. However, it is likely that Type D and A injuries are really the most common, since most of these injuries can be treated locally without referral to a tertiary centre.

Risk factors include experience of the surgeon, local operative risk factors such as acute and chronic inflammation, and aberrant anatomy, especially of the right duct. Direct causes of injury are misidentification of ductal anatomy or technical errors. Misidentification of the common duct as the cystic duct leads to Type D or E injuries, and misidentification of an aberrant right duct as the cystic duct leads to Type B or C type injuries (Fig. 2). Misidentification tends to occur in the presence of acute or chronic inflammation. The technical causes of biliary injury are injudicious use of cautery, improper closure of the cystic duct, and too deep a plane of dissection on the liver bed. Prevention of injury requires that the operation be performed by trained surgeons who avoid difficult situations such as acute cholecystitis until experience is gained. The key to avoiding injury due to misidentification is conclusive identification of the cystic duct and artery, since these are the structures to be divided[20]. Routine operative cholangiography has not lessened injury in published series, although it may lessen the extent of injury, by providing early diagnosis[24]. The most serious technical problem is cautery injury. This may be avoided by either not using cautery in the portal dissection or using it on low settings, and only on small pieces of tissue that are lifted off underlying structures.

Biliary injuries are best managed by a team of biliary endoscopists, interventional radiologists and hepatobiliary–pancreatic (HPB) surgeons. The clinical presentations of Type A and Type E injury tend to be distinct[20]. Type A injuries are usually recognized in the early postoperative period. Type E injuries are more often recognized during the first week after surgery also, but some are also recognized intraoperatively and a few (5%) present more than 1 month after surgery. Type A injuries usually present with pain and sepsis, due to an intraperitoneal collection of bile. In some cases the presentation is a bile fistula. Patients with Type A injuries are almost never jaundiced; conversely most patients with Type E injuries appear with painless jaundice.

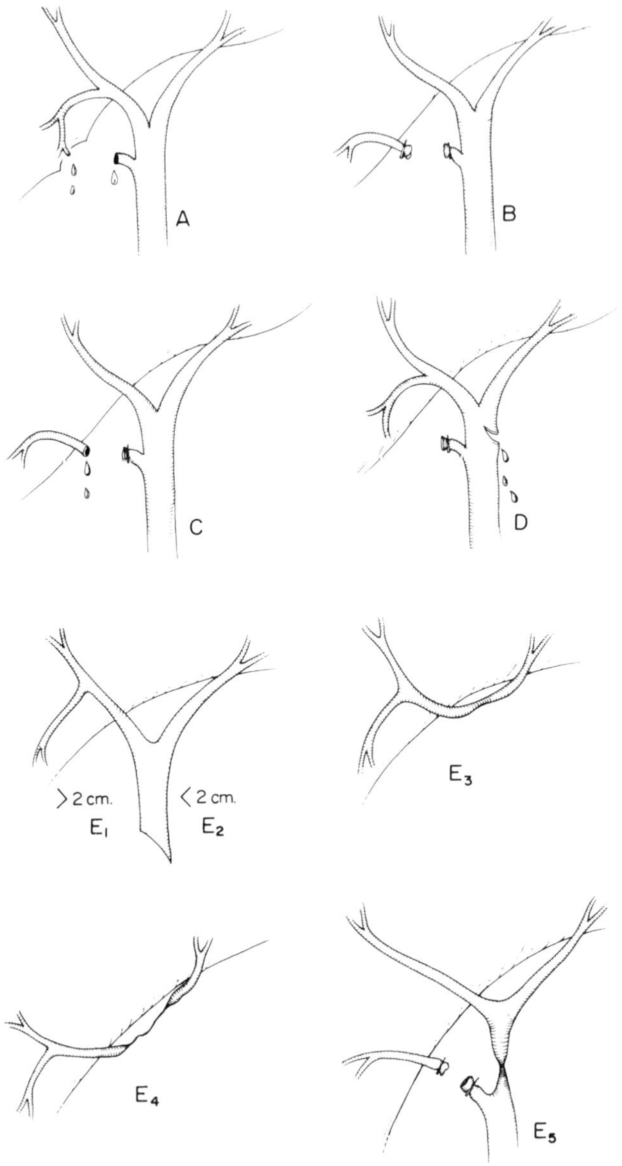

Fig. 1 Classification of laparoscopic injuries to the biliary tract. Injuries Type A to E are illustrated. Type E injuries are subdivided according to the Bismuth classification. Type A injuries originate from small bile ducts that are entered in the liver bed or from the cystic duct. Type B and C injuries almost always involve aberrant right hepatic ducts. Type A, C, D, and some E injuries may cause bilomas or fistulas. Type B and other type E injuries occlude the biliary tree and bilomas do not occur. (From ref. 20)

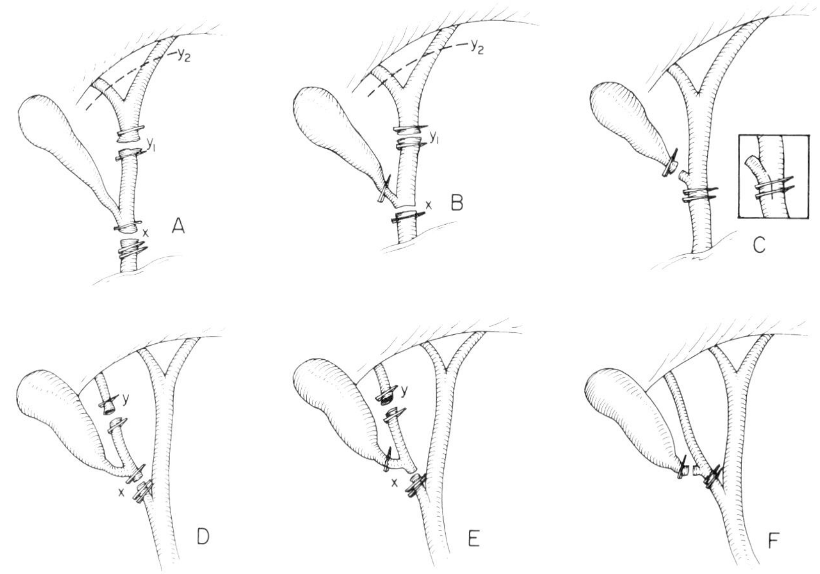

Fig. 2 Patterns of biliary injury due to misidentification. **A** 'classical' Type E injury in which the common duct is divided between clips (point X). The ductal system is later divided again to remove the gallbladder (point Y1, E1 and E2 injuries, or Y2, E3 or E4 injuries). **B and C**: variants of the injury to common bile duct. **D, E, F** represent variants of injury to aberrant right hepatic duct, producing Type B and C injuries. (From ref. 20)

If a biliary injury is diagnosed intraoperatively conversion and immediate repair are almost always mandatory. For patients first presenting in the postoperative period investigation depends on the mode of presentation, i.e. pain/sepsis, jaundice, or fistula. With pain/sepsis, ultrasound or CT is used to search for intraperitoneal fluid collections. Collections are drained percutaneously to determine if they contain bile and, if so, scintigraphy is performed to determine if the leak is continuing. If there is a continuing bile leakage, diagnostic ERCP is performed. In almost all Type A injuries, some Type D injuries and a few Type E injuries, treatment occurs during the same ERCP procedure. Type A injuries are treated by endoscopic sphincterotomy and an internal stent or a nasobiliary catheter. In patients presenting with jaundice ERCP is the first investigation. The distal duct will usually be found to be occluded or transected, and continuity to the proximal duct lost. In these cases PTC is needed to outline the proximal ducts and to provide bile drainage. Stenting may be performed at this time by ERCP or PTC if the problem is a stenosis. In our experience stenting usually fails unless the stenotic segment is short, less than 1 cm, mild, or the problem presents late, i.e. months or years after cholecystectomy. With an external bile fistula the first investigation should be a fistulagram. Subsequent management depends upon results.

Surgery is required in Type A and D injuries that have failed closed treatment, Type B injuries that need treatment, all Type C injuries, and most Type E injuries. Hepaticojejunostomy is the treatment of choice for Type B, C and E injuries[20]. Percutaneous stents are useful guides to the position of the ducts. The timing of surgery must take into account the degree of inflammation present, and often it is wise to delay surgery until acute inflammation has subsided. The principles of repair are to recognize all injured ducts and establish a wide mucosa-to-mucosa anastomosis without tension, with good blood supply. Most severe injuries are best treated at specialized HPB surgery units. There has been no long-term follow-up of laparoscopic biliary injuries. It is likely that the long-term recurrence will be in the order of 20%, most recurrences presenting in the first 3 years after repair.

Other complications of laparoscopic cholecystectomy. Cardiopulmonary complications are less common after laparoscopic surgery than after open surgery[1]. This is probably due to reduction in postoperative upper abdominal pain and resulting improvement in pulmonary function. The commonest complication is wound infection, occurring in 1–2% of patients; this is a minor problem compared to infection of a laparotomy incision. There have been other major, but rare complications, such as bowel or vascular injuries[25], which may almost always be avoided by open pneumoperitoneum using the Hasson technique[26]. There are reports of hernias at the umbilical trocar site[27]; these are avoidable by suture of this incision when the trocar is removed. Spillage of stones during laparoscopic cholecystectomy is not a rare event, occurring in about 10% of operations, Leaving stones in the peritoneal cavity may result in intra-abdominal abscess, subcutaneous abscess and later discharge of stones through the abdominal wall, or through the lung and trachea[28–30].

CHOLEDOCHOLITHIASIS

This section will focus on choledocholithiasis when it is present, or potentially present, in a patient who has an indication for laparoscopic cholecystectomy. The main issues in these patients are the following. What are the indications for preoperative removal of stones by ERCP and how are such stones to be detected? How are stones detected intraoperatively and what are the laparoscopic techniques for managing these stones? How should stones be managed when laparoscopic methods of removal fail? The prevalence of choledocholithiasis was 8–20% in patients having elective cholecystectomy during the era of open surgery[31], but it seems to be lower in the laparoscopic era, i.e. 3–10% in recent series[32,33]. Suggested explanations include earlier referral for laparoscopic surgery, selection of patients with less advanced disease for laparoscopic cholecystectomy, and perhaps missed stones.

Preoperative detection of bile duct stones

Liver function tests, ultrasonography and clinical criteria

Jaundice, cholangitis, prior pancreatitis, and age are the usual criteria for predicting choledocholithiasis preoperatively. Jaundice is obviously a good predictor, but recent pancreatitis is not[34], presumably because the small stones associated with this problem usually pass. Ultrasonography is much less sensitive for choledocholithiasis than cholelithiasis. The sonographic indicators of choledocholithiasis are duct dilation (>6 mm) and visualization of echogenic foci in the duct[35,36]. If the common bile duct (CBD) is not dilated, stones are more difficult to detect.

Barkun *et al.* examined clinical parameters, and found that only four independently predicted the presence of CBD stones, i.e. age, bilirubin level and sonographic evidence of CBD dilatation or stones[34]. A predictive model based on serum bilirubin and alkaline phosphatase concentration, and CBD size measured by imaging, was described by Onken *et al.*[37]. Montariol *et al.*[38] evaluated a scoring system based on age, CBD diameter, diameter of the smallest stones, and history of biliary colic and acute cholecystitis. Such scoring systems tend to have a high negative predictive value, but as about one-half of patients predicted to have stones actually do not have stones. Many negative ERCPs would be performed if predictive scores were relied on to make the decision for preoperative ERCP.

Preoperative intravenous cholangiography

There has been a resurgence of interest in intravenous cholangiography (IVC) for detection of CBD stones. Adequate imaging has been obtained in 95% of cases, with an incidence of mild reactions in <1%[39]. However, CBD stones were missed in 16% of cases.

Routine preoperative endoscopic retrograde cholangiopancreatography (ERCP)

ERCP produces excellent imaging of the bile ducts in almost all patients[40]. Routine ERCP for detection and treatment of stones has been used, but is associated with a high rate of negative studies[41], and the rate of complications approximates the incidence of unsuspected stones. In addition there are cost considerations; thus, routine preoperative ERCP before laparoscopic cholecystectomy is contraindicated.

Preoperative treatment of bile duct stones

Patient selection for preoperative ERCP

Patient selection for preoperative ERCP has become a keenly discussed issue. Preoperative ERCP had been compared to open exploration of the duct, before the advent of laparoscopic cholecystectomy. It resulted in slightly reduced length of hospital stay, but preoperative ERCP and sphincterotomy was associated with increased morbidity. There have been no trials comparing preoperative ERCP to laparoscopic CBD exploration (LCBDE). The indications may be described as a hierarchy, at the bottom of which is routine ERCP; at the top is preoperative ERCP for 'jaundice', which is an absolute indication, since without it malignancy of the bile duct or surrounding structures cannot be ruled out[42]. Between the indications 'routine ERCP' and 'ERCP for jaundice' lie the controversial indications, ones which depend upon the available level of expertise of laparoscopic surgeon and biliary endoscopist.

The most compelling indication, next to jaundice, is 'difficult' choledocholithiasis. 'Difficult' choledocholithiaisis includes large stones (>8 mm), multiple stones and intrahepatic stones. Laparoscopic methods for dealing with difficult choledocholithiasis are evolving, but are unproven, and very few surgeons are adept at them at the present time. Therefore, presently difficult choledocholithiasis is an indication for preoperative ERCP. Choledocholithiasis which is not difficult is not an indication for preoperative ERCP, in centres proficient in LCBDE and ERCP. Great proficiency in ERCP is needed because the team must have confidence that, when LCBDE fails, postoperative ERCP will work. The alternatives are to perform preoperative ERCP, or open CBDE, if LCBDE fails. A final level of indication for preoperative ERCP is based on probability scores. As noted, this will result in treatment removal of almost all choledocholithiasis preoperatively, because of the excellent sensitivity of these indices, but will also result in about 40% of the studies being negative due to the low specificity. The preceding data refer to patients with symptomatic cholecystolithiasis in which elective laparoscopic cholecystectomy is intended. There are other instances in which the value of preoperative ERCP is indisputable, as in patients with acute cholangitis and severe gallstone pancreatitis.

Results of preoperative ERCP

Many series have been reported. The indications generally included elevations of serum liver function tests, clinical history suggesting choledocholithiasis or sonographic evidence of CBD stones. ERCP was performed preoperatively in 4–11% and choledocholithiasis was demonstrated in 40–60% of the examinations[32,33,39,43–45]. Thus 40–60% of patients had an 'unnecessary' ERCP prior to laparoscopic cholecystectomy. The fundamental question is where to set the indication for preoperative ERCP, and this question can be settled only by comparative trials with LCBDE. Even then the results may apply only to centres that are expert in the techniques. At present our practice is to perform preoperative ERCP only for jaundice and 'difficult' stone disease. Other stones are removed by LCBDE or postoperative ERCP.

Intraoperative detection of bile duct stones

Intraoperative contrast cholangiography

There is debate as to whether cholangiography should be performed routinely or selectively. Proponents of routine cholangiography cite the following purposes and advantages: to obtain a 'road map' of the biliary ductal system and thereby prevent or minimize the severity of bile duct injury; to diagnose concomitant biliary anomalies or pathological conditions; to develop technical proficiency in cholangiography and to teach it; to develop skills which are essential for transcystic ductal exploration. The success rate of laparoscopic intraoperative cholangiography varies from 60% to 98% with false-positive and false-negative rates of less than 5%. Opponents cite many of the same arguments as in the era of open surgery, and the issue of selective versus routine cholangiography has not been successfully resolved.

Digital fluoroscopic imaging is very desirable for intraoperative cholangiography. A standard C-arm connected to a digital image processor allows enhancement and magnification achieving resolution of defects as small as 1 mm[46,47].

Laparoscopic intracorporeal ultrasonographic cholangiography

High-frequency transducers are used. Ultrasonography may be used to map the extrahepatic ductal system, identify anomalies of ductal and vascular structures, quantify ductal diameter and visualize CBD stones casting sharp acoustic shadows (Fig. 3). In experienced hands, laparoscopic intracorporeal ultrasonography appears to be as accurate and rapid as contrast cholangiography for demonstrating choledocholithiasis and abnormal anatomy[48–50], but comparative trials with contrast cholangiography are not yet available.

Intraoperative management of CBD stones

Observation of small asymptomatic stones

Many CBD stones discovered during the course of treatment of cholecystolithiasis are asymptomatic and small. Small CBD stones often pass through the ampulla of Vater, as demonstrated by stool analysis in patients with acute pancreatitis[51] and from following patients who have been treated with ESWL. However, one cannot define a stone size that is safe to leave behind, since size is not the only determinant of complications. Small stones may lodge at a critical point; therefore, one must recommend treating all stones in patients who have had gallstone pancreatitis. In other patients the risk of treating stones smaller than 3 mm that are seen on cholangiograms must be balanced against the risk of complications from the stone, particularly since some of these very small 'stones' are artefacts such as air bubbles.

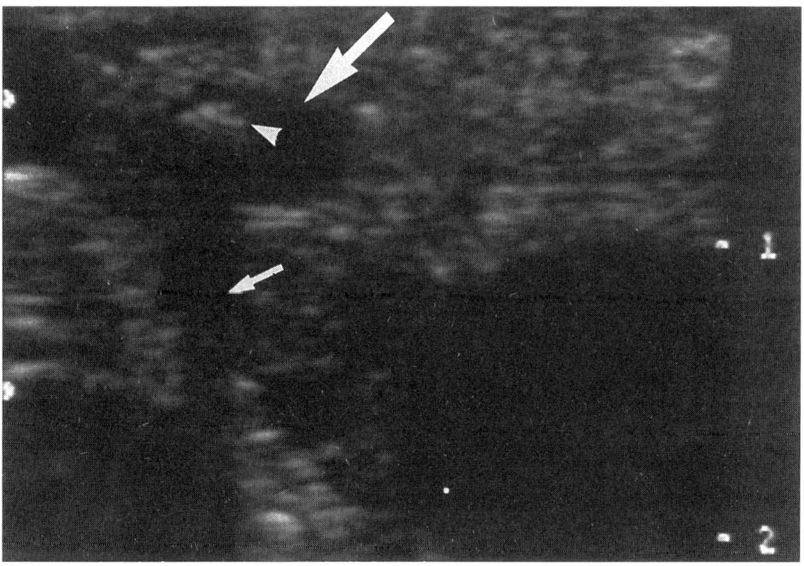

Fig. 3 Laparoscopic ultrasound demonstrating a stone (arrowhead) in the bile duct (large arrow) with acoustic shadowing posterior to the stone (small arrow). The echo-poor circular object below and to the right is the portal vein, and the one below to the left is the inferior vena cava. (From ref. 69)

Laparoscopic treatment of CBD stones

'Transcystic' exploration. Intraoperative fluorocholangiography is needed. Cholangiography, is used to determine the size and location of the CBD stone(s) and thus the best method for extraction. Stones smaller than 4 mm in size can often be flushed through the ampulla into the duodenum, a technique that is facilitated by relaxing the sphincter of Oddi by sublingual nitroglycerine or intravenous glucagon (1–2 mg). When this simple method fails, a guide wire is inserted through the cholangiogram catheter into the bile duct, and helical stone baskets are passed over the guidewire into the CBD to extract stones under fluoroscopic guidance[52]. If basket extraction fails, a choledochoscope is passed through the cystic duct into the CBD for removal of the stones under direct vision. Large or impacted stones contained within the distal CBD that cannot be extracted with a basket may be fragmented using either pulsed dye laser or electrohydraulic lithotripsy prior to removal[53].

Results of laparoscopic transcystic duct stone extraction are very good[52–62]. Successful extraction has been reported in 67–96% of cases. Complications, primarily infectious or due to self-limited pancreatitis, were reported in 5–10% of patients with a mortality rate of 1–2%. Duration of hospitalization following an uncomplicated transcystic duct stone extraction is the same as that for laparoscopic cholecystectomy alone, averaging 1–2 days.

Laparoscopic choledochotomy. Experience with this technique is limited. It is used when duct stones are multiple, large, or contained within the proximal bile ducts, and in patients in whom the common bile duct is larger than 10 mm in diameter[59,60]. It requires direct incision with subsequent suture closure of the CBD and placement of a T-tube. Many surgeons have not mastered the laparoscopic suturing techniques required for this procedure. A longitudinal choledochotomy is made on the anterior wall of the distal CBD and a standard size (15 Fr) choledochoscope inserted. Stones are removed under endoscopic visualization and a 14 Fr latex T-tube is placed in the duct. The ductotomy is closed with fine absorbable sutures using intracorporeal suturing techniques, and the T-tube is exteriorized through a lateral port site. In early results this technique is successful in more than 90% of patients with a minor morbidity rate of 5–10% and a mortality rate of 1–2%. Direct complications of laparoscopic choledochotomy include laceration of the CBD, bile leakage, sewn-in T-tubes and postoperative strictures. Minor postoperative strictures were reported in two of the 38 patients (5%) reported by Dion *et al.*[60].

Open choledochotomy. This technique remains a reasonable option for managing choledocholithiasis. It has low morbidity (<1%) in young patients, but in the elderly it carries a higher risk. Postoperative hospitalization and duration of disability are significantly longer. Laparotomy with open choledochotomy is now reserved for the rare patient with contraindications to laparoscopy, and patients in whom laparoscopic CBD therapy fails, and who have relative contraindications to postoperative endoscopic management, e.g. previous gastrectomy with Roux-en-Y or Billroth II reconstruction.

Postoperative ERCP

When CBD stones cannot be removed using laparoscopic techniques, the choices are postoperative endoscopic sphincterotomy or conversion to open exploration. It is very important to explain to patients preoperatively the possibility of finding CBD stones and the means by which they can be treated, so that patients can indicate preferences. Patients should be informed of the small risk of pancreatitis occurring in the short interval between cholecystectomy and postoperative ERCP. In practice, except for instances in which postoperative ERCP would be difficult, most surgeons do choose postoperative ERCP. In experienced hands ERCP with sphincterotomy has a 5–10% chance of failure[40]. Leaving a catheter in the CBD at the time of laparoscopic cholecystectomy may further diminish the likelihood of failure. Postoperative ERCP is the procedure of choice when endoscopic expertise is high, whereas an open choledochotomy should be strongly considered in its absence[40].

Gallstone pancreatitis

Over the past two decades several studies have shown that cholecystectomy should be performed during the initial admission for gallstone pancreatitis, in order to avoid a second and possibly more severe attack in the interval between the initial attack and cholecystectomy. Cholecystectomy is performed after the acute phase of the disease resolves. In the presence of concomitant cholangitis[63] or severe acute biliary pancreatitis[64], early ERCP with sphincterotomy and stone extraction is beneficial.

Based on historical data, and these recent reports, the following conclusions and recommendations for the current management of acute gallstone pancreatitis are suggested:

1. Urgent ERCP with sphincterotomy, if necessary, is indicated for those patients with severe ongoing pancreatitis, cholangitis, or CBD stones demonstrated by sonographic examination.
2. Laparoscopic cholecystectomy may be performed in most patients during the index admission without preoperative ERCP; intraoperative cholangiography should be performed routinely, with laparoscopic extraction of CBD stones, if demonstrated. Postoperative ERCP should be used for residual stones where endoscopic expertise is high.
3. As effective debridement of necrotic pancreas is presently not feasible laparoscopically, clinical evidence of necrotizing pancreatitis should prompt a CT scan; if infected necrosis is identified, open operative debridement combined with cholecystectomy is the procedure of choice.

ACUTE CHOLECYSTITIS

At the advent of laparoscopic cholecystectomy acute cholecystitis was considered to be a contraindication to this procedure. It has become clear that laparoscopic cholecystectomy can be performed safely during the phase of acute inflammation, although the procedure is more difficult, takes longer to perform and is associated with an increased rate of conversion[65–67]. Patients enjoy the same benefits as in elective laparoscopic cholecystectomy. Several studies have commented on the relationship between biliary injury and performance of laparoscopic cholecystectomy during the acute phase of inflammation. Laparoscopic cholecystectomy should not be attempted once the inflammation has been present for more than 72 hours, because of increased vascularity and tissue oedema. The surgeon should be experienced in elective laparoscopic cholecystectomy before operating in the presence of acute inflammation. In circumstances in which conservative treatment of acute cholecystitis fails we perform percutaneous cholecystostomy[68] followed by interval laparoscopic cholecystectomy rather than open cholecystectomy in the acute phase. The former preserves the minimally invasive nature of the treatment.

References

1. Strasberg SM, Clavien PA. Cholecystolithiasis. Lithotherapy for the 1990s. Hepatology. 1992;16:820–39.
2. Barkun JS, Barkun AN, Sampalis JS *et al.* Randomized controlled trial of laparoscopic versus mini cholecystectomy. Lancet. 1992;350:1116–19.
3. McMahon AJ, Russel IT, Baxter JN *et al.* Laparoscopic versus minilaparotomy cholecystectomy: a randomized controlled trial. Lancet. 1994;343:135–8.
4. McIntyre RC Jr, Zoeter MZA, Weil KC, Cohen MM. A comparison of outcome and cost of open vs. laparoscopic cholecystectomy. J Laparoend Surg. 1992;2:143–7.
5. Bass EB, Pitt HA, Lillimoe KD. Cost-effectiveness of laparoscopic cholecystectomy versus open cholecystectomy. Am J Surg. 1993;165:466–71.
6. Orlando III R, Russell JC, Lynch J, Mattie A. Laparoscopic cholecystectomy, a statewide experience. Arch Surg. 1993;128:494–9.
7. Steiner CA, Bass EB Talamini MA, Pitt HA, Steinberg EP. Surgical rates and operative mortality for open and laparoscopic cholecystectomy in Maryland. N Engl J Med. 1994;330:403–8.
8. Lagoretta AP, Silber JH, Constantino GN, Kobylinski RW, Zatz SL. Increased cholecystectomy rate after the introduction of laparoscopic cholecystectomy. JAMA. 1993;270:1429–32.
9. Coelho JC, de Araujo RP, Marchesini JB, Coelho IC, de Araujo LR. Pulmonary function after cholecystectomy performed through Kocher's incision, a mini-incision and laparoscopy. World J Surg. 1993;17:544–6.
10. McMahon AJ, Russel IT, Ramsy G *et al.* Laparoscopic and minilaparostomy cholecystectomy: a randomized trial comparing postoperative pain and pulmonary function. Surgery. 1994;115:533–9.
11. Hiatt JR, Hiatt JCG, Williams RA *et al.* Biliary disease in pregnancy: strategy for surgical management. Am J Surg. 1986;150:263–5.
12. Dixon NP, Faddis DM, Silberman H. Aggressive management of cholecystitis during pregnancy. Am J Surg. 1987;154:292–4.
13. Block P, Kelly TR. Management of gallstone pancreatitis during pregnancy and the postpartum period. Surg Gynecol Obstet. 1989;168:426–8.
14. Schirmer BD, Dix J, Edge SB, Hyser MJ, Hanks JB, Aguilar M. Laparoscopic cholecystectomy in the obese patient. Ann Surg. 1992;216:146–52.
15. Soper NJ. Effect of nonbiliary problems on laparoscopic cholecystectomy. Am J Surg. 1993;165:522–6.
16. Vinograd I, Halevy A, Klin B *et al.* Laparoscopic cholecystectomy: treatment of choice for cholelithiasis in children. World J Surg. 1993;17:263–6.
17. Davidoff AM, Branum GD, Murray EA *et al.* The technique of laparoscopic cholecystectomy in children. Ann Surg. 1992;215:186–91.
18. Callery MP, Soper NJ. Laparoscopic management of complicated biliary tract disease in children. Surg Laparosc Endosc. 1995 (In press).
19. Ware RE, Kinney TR, Casey JR *et al.* Laparoscopic cholecystectomy in young patients with sickle hemoglobinopathies. J Pediatr. 1992;120:58–61.

20. Strasberg SM, Hertl M, Soper NJ. An analysis of the problem of biliary injury during laparoscopic cholecystectomy. J Am Coll Surg. 1995;180:101–25.
21. Bernard HR, Hartman TW. Complications after laparoscopic cholecystectomy. Am J Surg. 1993;165:533–5.
22. Wherry DC, Rog CG, Marohn MR, Rich NM. An external audit of laparoscopic cholecystectomy performed in medical treatment facilities of the Department of Defense. Ann Surg. 1994;220:626–34.
23. Adamsen S, Hansen OH, Jensen PF *et al.* Bile duct injury in laparoscopic cholecystectomy in Denmark. Gastroenterology. 1995 (In press).
24. Woods MS, Traverso LW, Kozarek RA *et al.* Characteristics of biliary tract complications during laparoscopic cholecystectomy: a multi-institutional study. Am J Surg. 1994;167:27–34.
25. Alpegren KN, Scheeres DE. Aortic injury. A catastrophic complication of laparoscopic cholecystectomy. Surg Endosc. 1994;8:689–91.
26. Strasberg SM, Sanabria JR Clavien P-A. Complications of laparoscopic cholecystectomy. Can J Surg. 1992;35:275–80.
27. Plaus WJ. Laparoscopic trocar site hernias. J Laparoend Surg. 1993;3:567–70.
28. Leslie KA, Rankin RN, Duff JH. Lost gallstones during laparoscopic cholecystectomy: are they really benign? Can J Surg. 1994;37:240–2.
29. Cacdac RG, Lakra YP. Abdominal wall sinus tract secondary to gallstones: a complication of laparoscopic cholecystectomy. J Laparoend Surg. 1993;3:509–11.
30. Downie GH, Robbins MK, Sousa JJ, Paradowski LJ. Cholelithoptysis: a complication following laparoscopic cholecystectomy. Chest. 1993;103:616–17.
31. DenBesten L, Berci G. The current status of biliary tract surgery: an international study of 1,072 consecutive patients. World J Surg. 1986;10:116–22.
32. Aliperti G, Edmundowicz SA, Soper NJ, Ashley SW. Combined endoscopic sphincterotomy and laparoscopic cholecystectomy in patients with choledocholithiasis and cholecystolithiasis. Ann Intern Med. 1991;115:783–5.
33. Graham SM, Flowers JL, Scott TR *et al.* Laparoscopic cholecystectomy and common bile duct stones. The utility of planned perioperative endoscopic retrograde cholangiography and sphincterotomy: experience with 63 patients. Ann Surg. 1993;218:61–7.
34. Barkun AN, Barkun JS, Fried GM and the McGill Gallstone Treatment Group. Useful predictors of bile duct stones in patients undergoing laparoscopic cholecystectomy. Ann Surg. 1994;220:32–9.
35. Gross BH, Harter LP, Laing FC *et al.* Ultrasonic evaluation of common bile duct stones: prospective comparison with endoscopic retrograde cholangiopancreatography. Radiology. 1983;146:471–4.
36. Joyce WP, Keane R, Burke GJ *et al.* Identification of bile duct stones in patients undergoing laparoscopic cholecystectomy. Br J Surg. 1991;78:1174–6.
37. Onken J, Brazer S, Eisen G *et al.* Accurate prediction of choledocholithiasis Gastroenterology. 1994;106:A20.
38. Montariol T, Rey C, Charlier A *et al.* Preoperative evaluation of the probability of common duct stones. J Am Coll Surg. 1995;180:293–6.
39. Salky B, Bauer J. Intravenous cholangiography, ERCP, and selective operative cholangiography in the performance of laparoscopic cholecystectomy. Surg Endosc. 1994;8:289–91.
40. Cotton PB. Endoscopic retrograde cholangiopancreatography and laparoscopic cholecystectomy. Am J Surg. 1993;165:474–8.
41. Neuhaus H, Feussner H, Ungeheuer A *et al.* Prospective evaluation of the use of ERCP prior to laparoscopic cholecystectomy. Endoscopy. 1992;24;745–9.
42. Kullman E, Borch K, Tarpila E *et al.* Endoscopic retrograde cholangiopancreatography (ERCP) in patients with jaundice and suspected biliary obstruction. Acta Chir Scand. 1984;150:657–63.
43. Barkun JS, Fried GM, Barkun AN *et al.* Cholecystectomy without operative cholangiography. Implications for common bile duct injury and retained common bile duct stones. Ann Surg. 1993;218:371–9.
44. Frazee RC, Roberts J, Symmonds R *et al.* Combined laparoscopic and endoscopic management of cholelithiasis and choledocholithiasis. Am J Surg. 1993;166:702–6.
45. Rieger R. Sulzbacher H, Woisetschläger R, Schrenk P, Wayand W. Selective use of ERCP in patients undergoing laparoscopic cholecystectomy. World J Surg. 1994;18:900–5.
46. Soper NJ, Dunnegan DL. Routine versus selective intra-operative cholangiography during laparoscopic cholecystectomy. World J Surg. 1992;16:113–140.

47. Handy JE, Rose SC, Nieves AS, Johnson RL, Hunter JG, Miller FJ. Intraoperative cholangiography: use of portable fluoroscopy and transmitted images. Radiology. 1991;181:205–7.
48. Machi J, Sigel B, Zaren HA *et al.* Operative ultrasonography during hepato-biliary and pancreatic surgery. World J Surg. 1993;17:640–6.
49. Orda R, Saygan J, Levy Y. Routine laparoscopic ultrasonography in biliary surgery. Surg Endosc. 1994;8:1239–42.
50. Machi J, Sigel B, Zaren A *et al.* Technique of ultrasound examination during laparoscopic cholecystectomy. Surg Endosc. 1993;7:545–9.
51. Acosta JM, Ledesma CL. Gallstone migration as a cause of acute pancreatitis. N Engl J Med. 1974;290:484–7.
52. Hunter JG. Laparoscopic transcystic common bile duct exploration. Am J Surg. 1992;163:53–8.
53. Shapiro SJ, Gordon LA, Daykhovsky L, Grundfest W. Laparoscopic exploration of the common bile duct: experience in 16 selected patients. J Laparoendosc Surg. 1991;1:333–41.
54. Petellin JB. Laparoscopic approach to common duct pathology. Am J Surg. 1993;165:487–91.
55. Fielding GA, O'Rourke NA. Laparoscopic common bile duct exploration. Aust NZ J Surg. 1993;63:113–15.
56. Fletcher DR. Common bile duct calculi at laparoscopic cholecystectomy: a technique for management. Aust NZ J Surg. 1993;63:710–14.
57. Bagnato VJ. Laparoscopic choledochoscopy and choledocholithotomy. Surg Laparosc Endosc. 1993;3:164–6.
58. DePaula AL, Hashiba K, Bafutto M. Laparoscopic management of choledocholithiasis. Surg Endosc. 1994;8:11399–403.
59. Phillips EH, Rosenthal RJ, Carroll BJ, Fallas MJ. Laparoscopic trans-cystic-duct common-bile-duct exploration. Surg Endosc. 1994;8:1389–94.
60. Dion Y-M, Ratelle R, Morin J, Gravel D. Common bile duct exploration: the place of laparoscopic choledochotomy. Surg Laparosc Endosc. 1994;4:419–24.
61. Ferzli GS, Massaad A, Kiel T, Worth MH Jr. The utility of laparoscopic common bile duct exploration in the treatment of choledocholithiasis. Surg Endosc. 1994;8:296–8.
62. Franklin ME, Pharand D, Rosenthal D. Laparoscopic common bile duct exploration. Surg Laparosc Endosc. 1994;4:119–24.
63. Lai ECS, Mok FPT, Tan ESY *et al.* Endoscopic biliary drainage for severe acute cholangitis. N Engl J Med. 1992;326:1582–6.
64. Fan S-T, Lai ECS, Mok FPT, Lo C-M, Zheng S-S, Wong J. Early treatment of acute biliary pancreatitis by endoscopic papillotomy. N Engl J Med. 1993;328:228–32.
65. Zucker KA, Flowers JL, Bailey RW, Graham SM, Bueli J, Imbembo AL. Laparoscopic management of acute cholecystitis. Am J Surg. 1993;165:508–14.
66. Cox MR, Wilson TG, Luck AJ, Jeans PL, Padbury RTA, Toouli J. Laparoscopic cholecystectomy for acute inflammation of the gallbladder. Ann Surg. 1993;218:630–4.
67. Wilson RG, Macintyre IM, Nixon SJ, Saunders JH, Varma JS, King PM. Laparoscopic cholecystectomy as a safe and effective treatment for severe acute cholecystitis. Br Med J. 1992;305:394–5.
68. Picus D, Hicks ME, Darcy MD *et al.* Percutaneous cholecystolithotomy: analysis of results and complications in 58 consecutive patients. Radiology. 1992;183:779–84.
69. Strasberg CM, Callery MP, Soper NJ. Laparoscopic hepatobiliary surgery. In: Boyer JL, Ockner RK, eds. Progress in liver disease. Philadelphia: WB Saunders; 1995 (In press).

Section VI
Management of Bile Duct Stones

23
Pathogenesis of biliary tract stones

R. D. SOLOWAY

GEOGRAPHICAL DIFFERENCES

The presence of stones within the biliary tract raises distinctly independent connotations in different parts of the world. In western countries, secondary bile-duct stones are found at cholecystectomy due to passage from the gallbladder and are predominantly cholesterol or black pigment stones which form only in the gallbladder[1]. Primary bile duct stones are detected years after cholecystectomy and are predominantly brown pigment stones[2]. In eastern countries, predominantly in East Asia, common duct stones are predominantly brown pigment stones and may occur in the absence of gallbladder stones. They frequently occur as part of the syndrome of cholangiohepatitis and co-exist with variable numbers of intrahepatic gallstones[3].

Brown pigment stone disease occurs with variable frequency throughout Asia[4] and predominates in areas which consume a low-protein, low-calorie, rice, vegetable and fish diet. In countries throughout Asia, as the standard of living increases and a westernized high-calorie high-protein high-fat diet is consumed, cholesterol stones become the primary form of stone within the gallbladder and therefore they contribute to the predominance of secondary cholesterol common bile duct stones[5].

In Japan, some patients may have congenital differences in biliary secretion or in bile duct structure and/or physiology since primary cholesterol intrahepatic lithiasis is now being identified in a few patients[5]. When Asians move to areas where western diets are consumed, they may still form primary brown pigment common duct stones and may be grossly mismanaged because western physicians have had little personal experience with the disease. In contrast, surgeons throughout Asia are expert in the surgery and management of intrahepatic lithiasis since this is the predominant type of stone disease in many parts of Asia. This is not predominantly a genetic condition since children born in a new environment assume the gallstone disease of the new area. However, intrahepatic cholesterol lithiasis is now being recognized in Japan[5], with the implication that a duct structural abnormality, such as choledochal cysts or Caroli's disease (intrahepatic cystic dilatation of the biliary tree), or a unique metabolic abormality, could now be expressing itself in the formation of cholesterol rather than brown pigment stones because bile composition had changed and more cholesterol was being secreted into hepatic bile.

STONE TYPES FORMED PRIMARILY WITHIN THE BILIARY TRACT

Brown pigment stones

These contain alternating layers, primarily composed of calcium salts of bilirubin and/or fatty acids with a variable amount of protein and cholesterol. These stones are associated with significant infection of the bulk phase of bile[6], usually more than 10^5 bacterial colony forming units (cfu ml^{-1})[7]. The factors determining which type of calcium salt is deposited and the start and stop signals for precipitation are, at present, unknown. Due to the significant concomitant infection, either bacterial or tissue glucuronidase or phospholipase cleave bilirubin mono- or diglucuronides or lecithin, respectively, it is believed that the resultant stones form and grow through rapid precipitation of calcium bilirubinate or calcium salts of fatty acids. At times during stone growth either calcium salt can be precipitated almost exclusively. The pathogenesis of the layered pattern which results from this alternation is unknown.

Black pigment stones

These are composed of calcium salts of bilirubinate, carbonates and/or hydroxyapatite with virtually no cholesterol and a variable, but significant, proportion of protein[1]. A portion of the calcium bilirubinate reacts with molecular oxygen producing the black colour[8]. These stones contain microcrystalline calcium salts and are thought to be the result of slow precipitation of these salts[9] on a protein matrix containing an amino acid template for formation of these crystals. In an otherwise normal biliary tree, these stones do not form again after cholecystectomy. The pathogenesis of these stones has been related to the formation of dental calculus[10,11] and has been associated with less than 10^5 cfu ml^{-1} bacteria in the gallbladder, a level thought to be clinically unimportant for infection. Nonetheless, this concentration of bacteria might promote the formation of bacterial biofilm and calcium salts. Perhaps, in the presence of stasis without clinical infection, bacteria not ordinarily active in forming calcium salts could proliferate and produce sufficient biofilm to provide an adequate template for proper calcium spacing and crystal nidation. This may be the pathogenesis involved in the formation of small black stones behind strictures in patients with primary sclerosing cholangitis.

SCANNING ELECTRON MICROSCOPY (SEM) CAN DIFFERENTIATE BETWEEN CALCIUM BILIRUBINATE IN BROWN AND BLACK PIGMENT STONES

For this experiment, we chose a stone that contained 96% of calcium salts as calcium bilirubinate and more than 90% of stone weight as calcium bilirubinate[9]. The stone presented a chonchoidal (glass-like) appearance on fractured section, in marked contrast to the rough surface of a pigmented layer from a brown pigment stone. After 15 min exposure of the stone surface to an argon beam in the vacuum of a scanning electron microscope, in which the argon atoms bombarded the surface without chemical interaction, the softer (non-crystalline) components of surface, such as protein, are etched away leaving rod-like microcrystals of calcium bilirubinate behind[9]. Since electron scanning for chemical analysis (ESCA) spectroscopy, which only measures the outer 5 nm of the surface, demonstrates progressive enrichment in calcium, it is clear that microcrystalline calcium bilirubinate has been demonstrated. In contrast, exposure of brown stones to the argon beam for the same length of time produces no visible change and demonstrates no microcrystals[9]. We concluded that calcium bilirubinate is present in a microcrystalline form in black stones but is present in non-crystalline amorphous form in brown pigment stones, reflecting the more rapid precipitation of this latter group.

EFFECTS OF AGE ON THE INCIDENCE AND TYPE OF CBD STONE

Age is a factor in determining what type of stone forms in the biliary tract. In a multihospital series of several thousand patients from Japan, the peak age for cholesterol stones, accounting for 70% of patients was 40–50 years[12]. In contrast, among 856 patients with primary brown stones, accounting for 21% of the series, the incidence of stones rose geometrically with increasing age up through the 9th decade[12]. In the western hemisphere, many of the causes of biliary dysmotility, such as paravaterian diverticulae, which are associated with primary common bile duct stones, are also associated with aging[13]. The most common situation in which primary common duct stones are identified is following cholecystectomy for cholesterol or black pigment stones. For the first two years after operation, the majority of stones were these same types with only a very few brown stones (12%)[2]. Even so, the presence of a few patients with brown stones in the common bile duct at cholecystectomy indicates that factors leading to infection and stasis in the common bile duct differed from the factors that concomitantly led to cholesterol and black stone formation in the gallbladder. Among common duct stones which are detected more than two years after cholecystectomy, the majority are brown pigment stones[2], suggesting that dysmotility of the biliary tract may develop in 5–10% of patients requiring a cholecystectomy.

EXAMINATION OF GALLSTONE COMPOSITION MAY PROVIDE CLUES TO PATHOGENESIS

Calcium salts of bilirubinates

The three-dimensional model of protonated bilirubin[14] explains why this dicarboxylic acid molecule is so unusually insoluble in water. This model, developed by X-ray diffraction analysis of a single crystal of bilirubin, indicates that each carboxyl group forms three hydrogen bonds with the pyrrole NH and the lactam NH and C=O from the other half of the molecule. These multiple intramolecular (hydrogen) H bonds are much stronger than single isolated H bonds. Only one set of three H bonds is severed at a time, allowing the acid salt of bilirubin to form much of the time. In *in-vitro* conditions, salts can be formed containing 3–12% calcium[15]. At 3% calcium, the bilirubinate carboxylates are incompletely neutralized and the acid salt is present[15]. At 6% calcium, the acid salt is still present but to a smaller extent as noted by the height of the infrared (IR) peak at 1700 cm^{-1} due to the carboxyl carbonyl (C=O) group. The pyrrole NH, a bond at 3400 cm^{-1} decreased in intensity in parallel, suggesting donation of the H^+ from the pyrrole NH as well as from the carboxyl hydroxyl group. If only the carboxyl hydroxyl groups were donating protons, no carboxyl carbonyl peak should be seen. In fact, it takes twice as much calcium (12%) as bilirubin to eliminate the carbonyl peak, indicating that both the carbonyl and the pyrrole groups are donating hydrogens simultaneously. Thus, protonated bilirubin is capable of donating up to four hydrogen atoms per molecule with each molecule able to bind as many as two calciums[15]. This does not happen *in vivo* and, thus, the acid salt of bilirubinate is the most common finding in stones. We have examined pigment stones and found a series of bilirubinates of somewhat varying stoichiometry[15], perhaps reflecting a range of pH during salt formation.

Calcium salts of fatty acids

We have recently made mixtures of calcium palmitate, the most common fatty acid salt, and palmitic acid to examine the potential to measure a range of the pH at which precipitation of these salt might have taken place. Examination of the IR spectra of these mixtures and of brown pigment stones indicates that some palmitic acid, as well as calcium palmitate, might be present in these stones. This has been suggested previously, using X-ray diffraction, by Sutor[16] and suggests that acid salts of fatty acids may also be formed during precipitation. Thus, the formation of acid salts in these stones should be considered a more generalized phenomenon in nidation and stone growth.

Figure 1 summarizes the effects of stasis and infection on the activation of tissue or bacterial glucuronidases and/or phospholipases on glucuronidated bilirubin and the biliary phospholipid lecithin to produce unconjugated bilirubin and/or fatty acids which quickly exceed their solubility in bile and precipitate as calcium salts. Lysolecithin can cause additional membrane injury with further release of tissue glucuronidases and phospholipases. In formation of black pigment gallstones, bilirubin, in protecting against free-radical oxidation of phospholipids, can form soluble black complexes containing molecular oxygen with copper and calcium. If calcium is in excess, the complexes will be less soluble and will precipitate. The mechanisms initiating and controlling these events need further study.

References

1. Soloway RD, Wu J-G. Analysis of Gallstones. In: Muraca M, ed. Methods in biliary research. Boca Raton, Fl: CRC Press; 1995:167–90.
2. Malet PF, Dabezies MA, Huang GH, Long WB, Gadacz TR, Soloway RD. Quantitative infrared spectroscopy of common duct gallstones. Gastroenterology. 1988;94:1217–21.
3. Nagase M, Hikasa Y, Soloway RD, Tanimura H, Setoyama M, Kato H. Gallstones in Western Japan. Factors affecting the prevalence of intrahepatic gallstones. Gastroenterology. 1980;78:684–90.

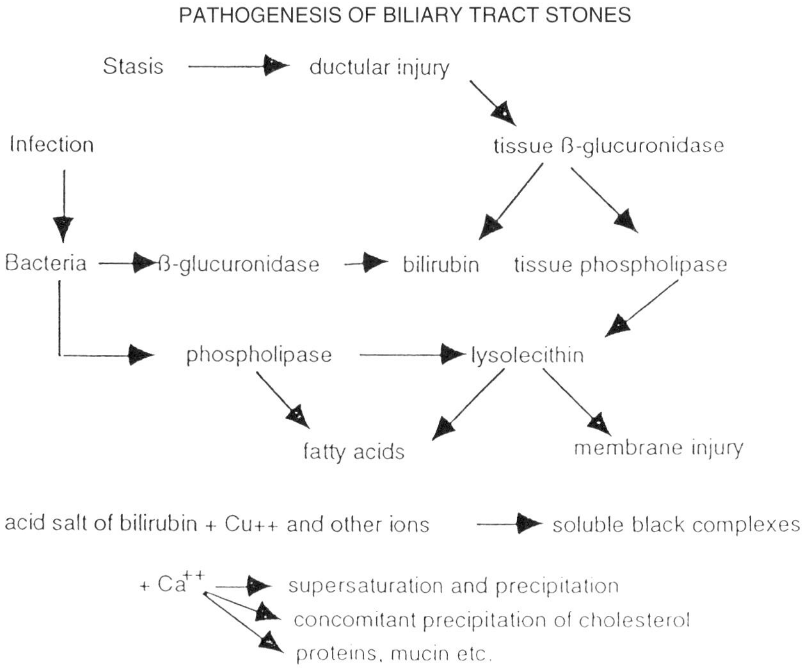

Fig. 1 Pathogenesis of brown and black pigment gallstones

4. Nakayama F, Soloway RD, Nakama T *et al.* Hepatolithiasis in East Asia: retrospective study. Dig Dis Sci. 1986;31:21–6.
5. Soloway RD. Editorial. Primary cholesterol hepatolithiasis – a disease with a different pathogenesis. Hepatology. 1993;17:737–8.
6. Maki T. Pathogenesis of calcium bilirubinate gallstone: role of E. coli, glucuronidase and coagulation by inorganic ions, polyelectrolytes and agitation. Ann Surg. 1966;164:90.
7. Goodhart GL, Levison ME, Trotman BW, Soloway RD. Pigment vs cholesterol cholelithiasis. Bacteriology of gallbladder stone, bile and tissue correlated with biliary lipid analysis. Am J Dig Dis. 1978;23:877–82.
8. Shen G-R, Li W-H, Soloway RD, Wen J, Wu J-G. Cu^{++} increases solubility of black Ca-bilirubinate complexes in vitro: possible protection against gallstones. Clin Res. 1993;41:159A.
9. Malet PF, Takabayashi A, Trotman BW, Soloway RD, Weston NS. Black and brown pigment gallstones differ in microstructure and microcomposition. Hepatology. 1984;4:227–34.
10. Hou R-Z, Wu J-G, Soloway RD *et al.* Fourier transform infrared photoacoustic spectroscopy of dental calculus. Presented at the 6th International Conference on Transform Spectroscopy, Vienna, Austria, 1987, 2.8. Microchim Acta Suppl. 1987.
11. Crowther RS, Soloway RD. Pigment gallstone pathogenesis: From man to molecules. Semin Liver Dis. 1990;10:171–180.
12. Hikasa Y, Nagase M, Soloway RD, Tanimura H, Setoyama M, Kato H. Gallstones in Western Japan. 1. Epidemiologic factors affecting the type and location of gallstones. Arch Jpn Surg. 1981;50:272–88.
13. Loveit T, Osnes M. Duodenal diverticula. Scand J Gastroenterol. 1984;19:579–81.
14. Bonett R, Davies JE, Hursthouse MB. The structure of bilirubin. Proc R Soc Lond. 1978;202:249.
15. Soloway RD, Wu J-G, Yang Y-L *et al.* Why does Ca^{++} vary from 3 to 12% in non-stoichiometric calcium bilirubinates? Gastroenterology. 1994;106:A359.
16. Sutor DJ. Calcium palmitate and α-palmitic acid in gallstones. Gut. 1970;11:618–19.

24 New techniques in the treatment of common bile duct stones

C. ELL

About 90% of all common bile duct (CBD) stones can be removed endoscopically following endoscopic sphincterotomy of the papilla of Vater. Stone removal is performed with the aid of baskets, balloons and mechanical lithotripsy. Promising new or essentially improved techniques for managing the difficult 10% of CBD stones include intracorporeal and extracorporeal lithotripsy (ISWL and ESWL). Both techniques are expensive and require endoscopic pre- and post-treatment. ISWL and ESWL represent auxiliary techniques in those cases where transpapillary conventional endoscopy is unsuccessful. In consequence, ISWL and ESWL should be performed only in centres where a high level of experience and frequency of biliary endoscopy exists. This should also include competence in the percutaneous approach to the biliary tract.

In recent years, essential improvements were achieved both in ESWL and in ISWL techniques: for example, ESWL procedures based on third-generation modalities are now more convenient for the patient and the relationship between 'power and pain' is better balanced. On the other hand, a new dye laser system with an integrated stone–tissue-detection system enhances the safety of laser lithotripsy and opens up the possibility of 'blind' stone fragmentation.

NEW TECHNIQUES IN THE THERAPY OF COMMON BILE DUCT STONES

The onset of the era of non-surgical therapy of common bile duct stones was marked by the introduction of endoscopic sphincerotomy in the year 1973. In the 1980s, the medical world witnessed an intensified pace in the development of new auxiliary techniques, such as electrohydraulic lithotripsy, mechanical lithotripsy, and, by the mid-80s, the introduction of ESWL and laser lithotripsy in the field of gastroenterology. In the 1990s, a plateau appears to have been reached, even though there exists a number of further development options, including 'blind', i.e. purely radiologically controlled laser lithotripsy, papilla dilatation techniques with subsequent stone extraction, and, finally, improvements in percutaneous stone treatment techniques.

This contribution focuses on the more recent developments in the fields of ESWL, laser lithotripsy – including 'blind' applications – papilla dilatation and percutaneous techniques.

Extracorporeal shockwave lithotripsy (ESWL)

The first extracorporeal shockwave treatment in the gastrointestinal tract was performed in Munich in the mid-80s using a waterbath lithotripter[1]. In the meantime, shockwave technology has undergone considerable changes. The electrohydraulic principle of shockwave generation has been abandoned and replaced by the piezoelectric and electromagnetic principles[2,3]. The waterbath lithotripters are well on their way to becoming exhibits in museums of medical history and have been replaced by third-generation modalities (Figure 1).

Irrespective of this technical evolution, there is no doubt about the fact that ESWL represents a highly efficient method of treating difficult bile duct stones.

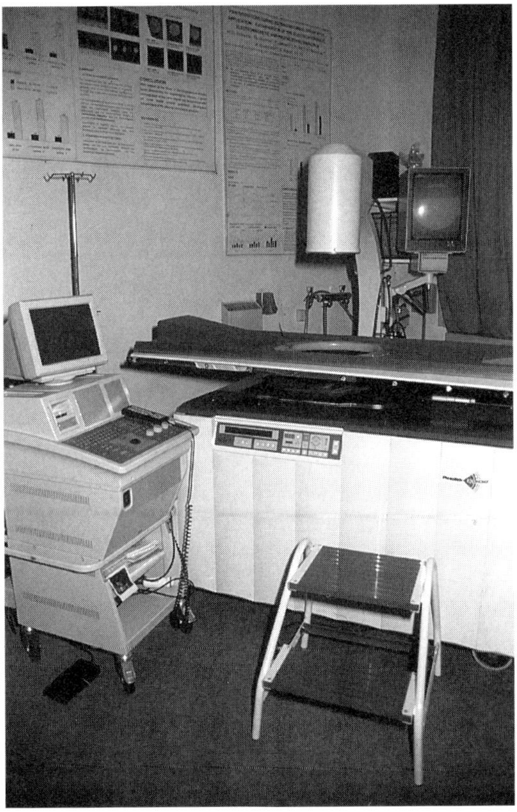

Fig. 1 A typical third-generation piezoelectric lithotripter with a combined X-ray and ultrasound targeting system

Table 1 Results of ESWL for difficult common bile duct stones

	Sauerbruch et al. *1992*[5] (n = *103*) *Electrohydraulic*	*Adamek* et al. *1993*[4] (n = *64*) *Piezoelectric*	*Van der Hul* et al. *1994*[3] (n = *90*) *Electromagnetic*
General anaesthesia	++	---	+
Intravenous sedation	+	+++	++
Treatment sessions	1–3 mean (1,4)	1–8 mean (2,3)	1–4 mean (1,8)
Complications	8% (42%)	5% (5%)	2% (4%)
Complete clearance	88%	77%	66%

In comparing standard studies with recently published data on shockwave lithotripsy, one finds that general anaesthesia has been replaced by intravenous sedation (Table 1)[3–5]. However, this improvement for the patient has been achieved in exchange for an increased number of treatment sessions. Up to 8 treatment sessions per patient have been reported, particularly when using piezoelectric lithotripters. On the other hand, with the new systems, the complication rate is distinctly lower than that experienced by the Munich group and has fallen to a level of 2–5%; the rate of minor complications is of a similar order. Nevertheless, the overall stone clearance is merely of the order of 70%, whereas, with the waterbath lithotripter in combination with general anaesthesia, the clearance rate had reached a level of almost 90%.

What tasks remain to be tackled in ESWL development during the remainder of the 90s? We need lithotripters with a lower level of pain which are nonetheless able to provide sufficient shockwave energy to attain a satisfactory degree of fragmentation. We also need improved fluoroscopic localization systems – optimum conditions would be provided by implementing specially designed nasobiliary catheters featuring metal markers and lateral holes only at the tip. It would no doubt be an advantage to combine radiographic localization methods with on-line ultrasound imaging. The measures applied should pursue the following goals: to avoid general anaesthesia altogether, to reduce the number of treatment sessions and also the radiation dose in order to increase the treatment success, and, above all, to improve patient comfort.

Laser lithotripsy

The principle of intracorporeal laser-induced shockwave lithotripsy consists of transmitting laser light to the biliary duct via a flexible fibre with a minimized loss of energy, releasing the energy locally and converting it into local shockwaves. Even though the risk of damaging tissue by exposure to laser light is considerably lower than when using the electrohydraulic probe, until the end of the 1980s, laser lithotripsy generally involved application of the mother–babyscope technique under direct endoscopic supervision. A major step forward in the technological development of laser lithotripsy was marked by the

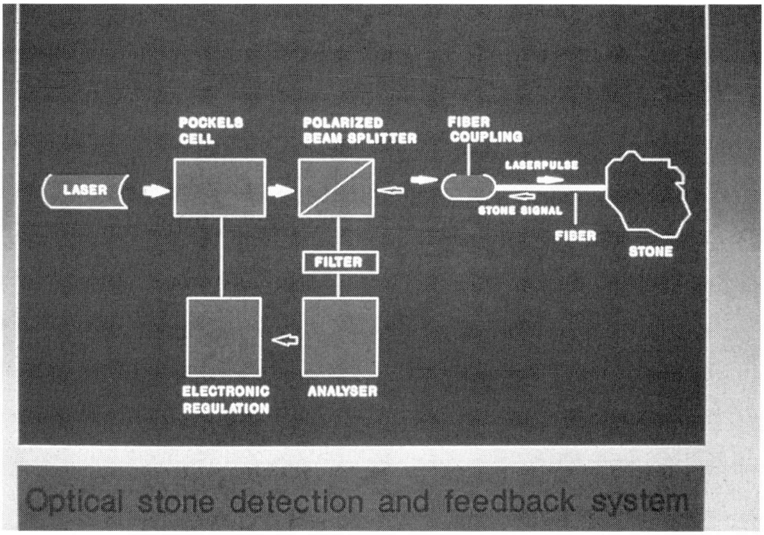

Fig. 2 Principle of the dye-laserlithotripter (Lithognost) with the integrated stone–tissue detection system allowing 'blind' laser lithotripsy

introduction of a stone–tissue-detection system. This system can discriminate between tissue and stone targets within 200 ns. Basically, a small quantity of light energy is released and focused on the target (stone or tissue). This induces fluorescence at the target site, which is transmitted back through the fibre and analysed by a detector. If the irradiated target is recognized as tissue, the laser system is automatically switched off (Figure 2). 'Blind' laser lithotripsy, i.e. laser lithotripsy applying standard duodenoscopes under fluoroscopic control only, is performed with balloon catheters, remote-controlled catheters or simple standard ERCP catheters (Figures 3–5). A number of published results (original paper, abstract) on the use of this new laser lithotripsy system, which allows 'blind' applications, have become available (see Table 2). Such 'blind' applica-

Table 2 Results of laser lithotripsy with the stone–tissue detection system for difficult common bile duct stones

	Erlangen *1993*[*6] (n = *18*)	*Neuhaus* et al. *1994*[7] (n = *38*)	*Swain* et al. *1995*[8] (n = *10*)	*Jacobs* *1995*[9] (n = *40*)
Endoscopically controlled	50%	80%	—	40%
'Blind'	50%	20%	100%	60%
Treatment sessions	1–3	1–2	1–3	1–4
Complications	1/18	—	—	2/40
Complete clearance	90%	95%	90%	75%

[*]Unpublished now 43 patients

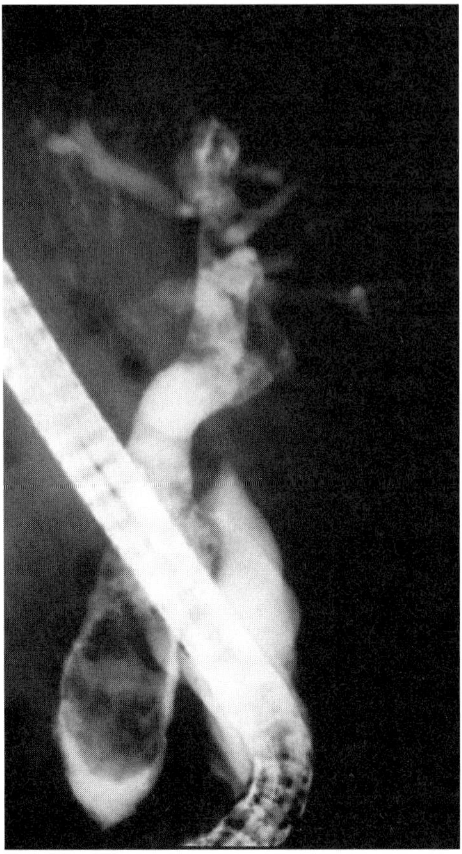

Fig. 3 Large common bile duct stone prior to 'blind' laser lithotripsy

tions using the transpapillary approach are carried out in two thirds up to 100% of all patients. When using the percutaneous approach, these figures are lower because, in this case, lithotripsy routinely involves endoscopic supervision. Complications are extremely rare and the reported stone clearance rates range from 75 to 95%.

Frequently, the question is raised whether ESWL or ISWL should be the treatment of choice in the therapy of difficult bile duct stones. The answer depends firstly on the availability of the required lithotripsy systems at the performing clinic. Secondly, the personal experience of the therapist plays a very important role. It must be emphasized that application of ESWL is much easier than that of endoscopic lithotripsy techniques which require a much higher level of expertise. Finally, the treatment decision will, of course, depend on the local pathological–anatomical situation of the patient. Basically, the best conditions are given if both treatment options (ESWL and ISWL) are available at a stone therapy centre.

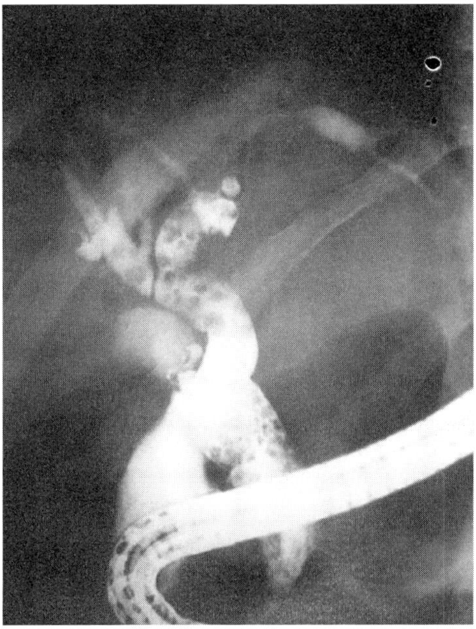

Fig. 4 Complete and fine fragmentation by means of 'blind' laser lithotripsy

Dilatation of the papilla Vateri

The method of high-pressure balloon dilatation of the papilla Vateri with subsequent stone extraction represents a new treatment option. It was above all the group of Mac Mathuna from Dublin that focused attention on this technique as early as 1993. Experience in the implementation of this technique has also been acquired in Amsterdam (Table 3)[10,11]. The current data, compiled for 100 patients in Dublin, show that stones up to 2 cm in diameter, and even up to 3 cm in Holland, could be successfully treated. The success rate is about 80%. However, the authors specified rates of complications that are similar in magnitude to those reported for endoscopic papillotomy[12].

Table 3 Results of balloon dilatation of the papilla Vateri prior to extraction of CBD stones

	Mac Mathuna et al. *1995*[11] (n = *100*)	*Bergman* et al. *1994*[10] (n = *39*)
Diameter (mm)		
Mean	10	9
Range	3–20	4–30
Complication rate (%)	5	12
Complete stone clearance (%)	82	80

Percutaneous techniques

In general, the procedure of percutaneous stone therapy comprises four steps:

1. Initially a percutaneous cholangiography or an ultrasound-guided puncture of the biliary ducts is performed.
2. A PTC-drainage catheter is inserted.
3. The third step involves the creation of a so-called sinus tract. For this purpose, a channel into the biliary ducts is created transhepatically by means of bougienage increasing with 8 French bougies up to 20 French.
4. In the final step, intracorporeal lithotripsy is carried out, at best with a laser or, alternatively, with an electrohydraulic probe.

The amount of published data available in the literature is quite scarce. Results involving larger patient series have indeed been reported by Yamakawa and other Japanese groups but they have left open a number of questions concerning complications and mortality rates[13]. A French study on 50 patients[14] reported a complication rate of 22% and a high mortality rate of 8%. An Italian research group was able to achieve distinctly lower complication rates[15]. The reported overall clearance rates appeared to be higher than those achieved by ESWL or transpapillary laser lithotripsy (Table 4). However, it can be expected that, as experience in implementing the percutaneous techniques increases, the complication rate will decline.

SUMMARY

In summarizing the status established in the therapy of common bile duct stones in the year 1955, it can be concluded that classical sphincterotomy combined with mechanical lithotripsy remains the therapy of choice for about 80% of patients treated in general hospitals. Only a subgroup of about 10% has to be referred to a stone therapy centre. Thus, nearly all patients can be successfully treated using non-invasive methods (Table 5). The application of endoprostheses as a palliative treatment strategy and also the new technique of dilatation must certainly be viewed as auxiliary methods, or as still being at the stage of clinical testing, at the present time. Local chemolitholysis has no particular clinical significance at present because of the long periods of hospitalization, the local and systemic side-effects and the rather modest results.

Table 4 Results of percutaneous techniques for difficult CBD stones

	Yamakawa *1989*[13] (n = *216*)	*Bonnel* et al. *1991*[14] (n = *50*)	*Righi* et al. *1992*[15] (n = *150*)
Complications (%)	?	22	12
Complete stone clearance (%)	93	75	91
Mortality (%)	?	8	2

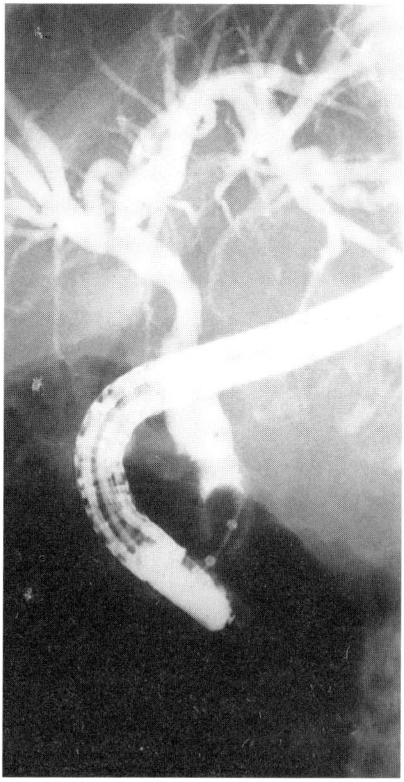

Fig. 5 Complete clearance of the bile duct documented by a balloon catheter

Table 5 Therapeutic strategy in 1995 for CBD stones

General hospital:	
Sphincterotomy + extraction	70–80%
	+
Mechanical lithotripsy	10–20%
Stone centre:	
Either	
ISWL (laser, EHL)	+
Or	
ESWL	5–10%
Either	
PTCD + ISWL	+
Or	
Operation	1–2%
Or	
Endoprosthesis/dilatation	

References

1. Sauerbruch T, Delius M, Paumgartner G *et al.* Fragmentation of gallstones by extracorporeal shock waves. N Engl J Med. 1986;314:818–22.

2. Ell C, Kerzel W, Schneider HT *et al.* Piezoelectric lithotripsy. Stone disintegration and follow-up results in patients with symptomatic gallbladder stones. Gastroenterology. 1990;99:1439.
3. von der Hul RL, Plaisier PW, van Blankenstein M, Terpstra OT, den Toom R, Bruining HA. Extracorporeal shock wave lithotripsy of common bile duct stones in patients with increased operative risk. Eur J Surg. 1994;160:31–5.
4. Adamek HE, Buttmann A, Hartmann CM, Jakobs R, Riemann JF. Extrakorporale piezoelektrische Lithotripsie von intra- und extrahepatischen Gallengangsteinen. Dtsch med Wschr. 1993;118:1053–9.
5. Sauerbruch T, Holl J, Sackmann M, Paumgartner G. Fragmentation of bile duct stones by extracorporeal shock-wave lithotripsy: A five-year experience. Hepatology. 1992;15:208–14.
6. Ell C, Hochberger J, May A *et al.* Laser lithotripsy of difficult bile duct stones by means of a rhodamine-6G laser and an integrated automatic stone–tissue detection system. Gastrointest Endosc. 1993; 39:755–62.
7. Neuhaus, H, Hoffmann, W, Gottlieb K, Classen M. Endoscopic lithotripsy of bile duct stones using a new laser with automatic stone recognition. Gastrointest Endosc. 1994;40:708–15.
8. Swain CP, Glynn M, Ainley C, van Someren N, Bewick E. Laser lithotripsy of large stones in the bile duct with a stone recognition system. DDW. 1995;A2785.
9. Jakobs R, Maier M, Kohler B, Riemann FJ. Laser lithotripsy of difficult bile duct stones – does a stone–tissue discrimination system reduce the need for cholangioscopy? DDW. 1995;A442.
10. Bergman JJGHM *et al.* A prospective randomized trial comparing endoscopic sphincterotomy (EST) with endoscopic balloon dilatation (EBD) for removal of common bile duct stones (CBDS): initial report. Gastrointest Endosc. 1994;40:99.
11. Mac Mathuna P, White P, Clarke E, Merriman R, Lennon JR, Crowe J. Endoscopic balloon sphincteroplasty (EBS) reduces the need for papillotomy: 2 year follow-up in 100 patients. DDW. 1995;A2697.
12. Ell C, Rabenstein T, Ruppert T, Förster P, Hahn EG, Demling L. 20 Jahre endoskopische Papillotomie: Analyse der Erlanger Erfahrungen bei 2752 Patienten. DMW. 1995;120:163–7.
13. Yamakawa T. Percutaneous cholangioscopy for management of retained biliary tract stones and intrahepatic stones. Endoscopy. 1889;21:333–7.
14. Bonnel DH, Liguory CE, Cornud FE, Lefebvre JFP. Common bile duct and intrahepatic stones: Results of transhepatic electrohydraulic lithotripsy in 50 patients. Radiology. 1991;180:345–8.
15. Righi D, Fonio P, Fronda GR *et al.* Trattamento percutaneo della litiasi dei botti biliari. Esperienza personale nei primi 150 casi. Radiol Med. 1992;83:526.

Section VII
Ursodeoxycholic acid treatment of chronic liver diseases

25
Treatment of primary biliary liver diseases

A. STIEHL

Primary biliary cirrhosis (PBC) and primary sclerosing cholangitis (PSC) are cholestatic liver diseases characterized by inflammation and progressive destruction of bile ducts. As a consequence, cholestasis is the most prominent feature of these disease states. The causes of PBC and PSC are still unknown. PBC is considered an autoimmune disease. Immunological mechanisms may also be involved in PSC, but, alternatively, bacterial toxins from the colon might play a role.

When cholestasis develops as a consequence of bile duct destruction, bile acids may aggravate the hepatic damage. Whether bile acids may initiate cholestatic liver diseases is unclear at present but seems less likely. The concept that bile acids play a major role in cholestatic liver diseases was recognized already in 1972 by Hans Popper and his associates[1]. In systematic studies of patients with extrahepatic cholestasis, a positive correlation between the tissue concentrations of dihydroxy bile acids in the livers and the degree of feathery degeneration was noted[1]. In rat liver, which effectively hydroxylates bile acids, such high concentrations of dihydroxy bile acids were not observed and feathery degeneration was absent[2]. Besides feathery degeneration, cholate stasis is also considered a characteristic lesion of bile-acid-induced liver damage.

THE ROLE OF URSODEOXYCHOLIC ACID IN PBC AND PSC

Treatment of patients with PBC leads to significant improvement of laboratory parameters, liver histology and survival[2–12]. The recent analysis of the data of three major studies[12] indicates that the survival rate without need for liver transplantation may be improved after 4 years of UDCA treatment from 40 to 60% which reflects an increase of 50%. Thus, UDCA treatment has become the gold standard of PBC treatment. However, the data also quite clearly indicate that UDCA does not stop disease progression completely.

The situation in PSC is quite similar[13]. In two controlled studies, UDCA treatment led to improvement of laboratory parameters and liver histology but had no effect on symptoms[14,15]. A study which was started in 1987 in our institution indicates that the survival rates in PSC patients treated with UDCA and, whenever necessary, by endoscopic balloon dilatations of major duct stenosis, are significantly improved compared with a dropout group[16]. Survival rates are also significantly improved in comparison with the predicted survival (unpublished data). However, also in PSC during UDCA treatment, progression of bile duct disease was noted in almost one third of patients.

Therefore, it seems justified to look for other substances which might improve the treatment results obtained with UDCA (see Table 1).

TREATMENT OF PBC

Penicillamine

After an initial report indicating that pencillamine improved liver function and might improve survival, further studies did not confirm this. According to the final analysis of a controlled study, penicillamine has no beneficial effect on symptoms, liver histology or survival[17].

Corticosteroids

Since PBC is thought to be an immune disease, immunosuppressive treatment should influence the course of the disease[18]. In a controlled trial in 36 patients, a beneficial effect was only observed when, not a single, but a combination of several parameters were evaluated[19]. A significant effect on histological pro-

Table 1 Treatment of primary biliary cirrhosis (aside from ursodeoxycholic acid)

Substance and author		*Effect on*			
	n	*Symptoms*	*Biochemistry*	*Liver histology*	*Survival*
Corticosteroids					
Mitchison *et al.*[18]	36	Improved	Improved	Improved	?
Mitchison *et al.*[19]	36	?	Improved	Favorable(?)	Unchanged
Azathioprine					
Heathcote *et al.*[21]	45	Unchanged	Improved	Unchanged	Unchanged
Crowe *et al.*[22]	236	Unchanged	Unchanged	Unchanged	?
Christensen *et al.*[23]	248	?	?	?	Improved*
Cyclosporin					
Minuk *et al.*[25]	12	Unchanged	Improved	Unchanged	Unchanged
Wiesner *et al.*[26]	29	Improved	Improved	Improved	Improved
Lombard *et al.*[27]	349	Unchanged	Improved	Unchanged	Improved*
Colchicine					
Kaplan *et al.*[31]	60	Unchanged	Improved	Unchanged	Improved
Bodenheimer *et al.*[32]	57	Unchanged	Improved	Unchanged	Favourable(?)
Warnes *et al.*[33]	64	?	Improved	Unchanged	Unchanged
Vuoristo *et al.*[34]	90	Improved	Improved	Unchanged	Unchanged

*Survival only improved after correction for differences in treatment groups

gression or survival was not observed when these parameters were evaluated separately[19]. Therefore, monotherapy with prednisolone should not be recommended. However, it seems possible that the addition of corticosteroids to UDCA, as was recently studied in a pilot study in the Netherlands, may improve the treatment results[20].

Corticosteroids accelerate the progression of osteoporosis and this should be taken into consideration when these substances are included in the treatment of PBC[18,20].

Azathioprine

Treatment of PBC in doses of 1–2 mg kg^{-1} d^{-1} led to some improvement in liver biochemistry but no improvement in liver histology[21,22]. The effect on survival was small and was calculated to be significant only when a correction for differences in the treatment and placebo groups was performed[23]. Overall, the beneficial effect of azathioprine in PBC was small. As a consequence, monotherapy with this substance cannot be recommended. The question of whether the addition of azathioprine to UDCA offers advantages in the treatment of PBC is under investigation at present[24].

Cyclosporin A

Despite preliminary reports that suggested that cyclosporin improved liver function in PBC[25,26], final analysis of a multicentre trial in 349 patients failed to demonstrate a defintite benefit[27]. Laboratory parameters were somewhat improved but the effect on histology and survival was small and nephrotoxicity was a problem. Since PBC should be treated in the early stages of the disease in order to prevent progression to cirrhosis, the benefit of substances which are associated with considerable side-effects is questionable.

Methotrexate

Preliminary studies on the use of methotrexate indicate that there may be improvement of symptoms, liver biochemistry and possibly liver histology[28]. In a trial in 12 patients, addition of methotrexate to UDCA in patients who had insufficiently responded to bile acid treatment was shown to improve symptoms and liver biochemistry[29]. The number of patients treated is too small to allow definite conclusions.

Colchicine

Colchicine represents a substance which might prevent collagen formation in the liver of patients with chronic liver disease since it decreases collagen synthesis and increases collagenase activity *in vitro*. It also has anti-inflammatory properties in gout and Mediterranean fever. In alcoholic and postnecrotic cirrhosis, colchicine led to clinical improvement and survival[30]. In PBC, except in one study in which pruritus decreased[34], colchicine had no effect on symptoms[31,32]. It had some effect on laboratory parameters[31–34] and had no effect on liver histology[31–34]. A beneficial effect on survival was observed in one study[31] but such an effect was not confirmed in two further trials[33,34].

In a recent study comparing colchicine, UDCA and placebo in 90 patients treated for two years, with respect to laboratory parameters, colchicine was less effective than UDCA and, in comparison with placebo, had only an effect on serum alkaline phosphatase[34]. In one controlled trial evaluating the effect of colchicine(1 mg/d) when administered in addition to UDCA to 24 patients with PBC, no effect of colchicine was noted[35]. This is in contrast to a multicentre trial in 90 patients who received 500 mg/d UDCA and 1 mg/d colchicine or placebo, in which an effect on the number of treatment failures and on the Mayo score was noted[36]. According to our current understanding, in this study, the dose of UDCA was too low. Since the study has so far only been published as an abstract, details are not available. In another small pilot study in patients insufficiently responding to UDCA, a beneficial effect of colchicine has been reported[37]. In PBC treatment, colchicine is less effective than UDCA and further studies are needed to define a possible additional effect of colchicine when administered in combination with UDCA.

TREATMENT OF PSC

Endoscopic dilatations of major duct stenosis probably represents the most important factor in treatment of PSC aside from UDCA[16,38,39]. PSC is characterized by multiple episodes of bacterial cholangitis and, besides endoscopic opening of major duct stenoses, early antibiotic treatment also seems essential. By adding antibiotics to the contrast media used at endoscopy, in our hands, the risk of bacterial infections during endoscopic procedures has become very low. Low-dose oral pulse methotrexate (15 mg/week) has been tested in a randomized study in 24 patients and has been reported to have a beneficial effect[40]. However, addition of methotrexate to UDCA had no effect. Moreover, immunosuppression may be harmful if bacterial infection of the bile ducts plays a role.

CONCLUSION AND OUTLOOK IN THE FUTURE

UDCA has become the standard of treatment of primary biliary liver diseases. It has a beneficial effect in PBC, PSC and possibly also in other liver diseases in which cholestasis plays a role. The aim is to treat patients as early as possible to prevent progression to these advanced stages of the diseases. In patients with very advanced disease, UDCA was not effective. Since UDCA treatment leads to improvement but not to cure of liver diseases, permanent treatment is necessary. Such prolonged treatment with UDCA may be recommended since, up to now, no side-effects have been reported. In PSC with stenosis of major ducts, endoscopic dilatation is highly effective. Recently, it has been shown that another 6β-hydroxylated bile acid, β-muricholic acid, has hepatoprotective effects similar to those of UDCA. It seems very likely that further molecules with a similar structure will be tested in the future. Since UDCA does not stop disease progression completely, combination treatment with other substances (colchicine, corticosteroids, azathioprine, methotrexate) is evaluated at present.

Monotherapy with these substances cannot be recommended since they are less effective than UDCA.

References

1. Greim H, Trülzsch D, Czygan P *et al.* Mechanisms of cholestasis. 6. Bile acids in human livers with and without biliary obstruction. Gastroenterology. 1972;63:846–50.
2. Greim H, Trülzsch D, Roboz LJ *et al.* Mechanisms of cholestasis. 5. Bile acids in normal rat livers and those after bile duct ligation. Gastroenterology. 1972;63:837–45.
3. Oka H, Toda Y, Ikeda Y, *et al.* A multi-center double blind controlled trial of ursodeoxycholic acid for primary biliary cirrhosis. Gastroenterol Jpn. 1990;25:774–80.
4. Poupon RE, Balkau B, Eschwege E, Poupon R. A multicenter controlled trial of ursodiol for the treatment of primary biliary cirrhosis. N Engl J Med. 1991;324:1548–54.
5. Combes B, Carithers RL, McDonald MF *et al.* Ursodeoxycholic acid therapy in patients with primary biliary cirrhosis. Abstract. Hepatology. 1991;14:91A.
6. Lindor KDL, Baldus WP, Jorgensen RA *et al.* Ursodeoxycholic acid is beneficial therapy for patients with primary biliary cirrhosis. Abstract. Hepatology. 1994;106:1284–90.
7. Heathcote EJL, Cauch-Dudek K, Walker V *et al.* The Canadian multi-center double blind randomized controlled trial of ursodeoxycholic acid in primary biliary cirrhosis. Hepatology. 1994;19:1149–56.
8. Battezzatti PM, Podda M, Bianchi FB *et al.* Ursodeoxycholic acid for symptomatic treatment of primary biliary cirrhosis. Preliminary analysis of a double-blind multicenter trial. J Hepatol. 1993;17:332–8.
9. Hwang SJ, Chan C-Y, Lee S-D *et al.* Ursodeoxycholic acid in the treatment of primary biliary cirrhosis: A short-term, randomized, double-blind controlled, cross-over study with long-term follow up. J Gastroenterol Hepatol. 1993;8:213–23.
10. Poupon RE, Chretien Y, Niard AM *et al.* Ursodiol for long-term therapy of primary biliary cirrhosis. N Engl J Med. 1994;330:1342–7.
11. Simko V, Michael S, Prego V. Effect of ursodeoxycholic acid in primary biliary cirrhosis: A meta analysis. Gastroenterology. 1993;104:A996.
12. Heathcote EJ, Lindor KD, Poupon R *et al.* Combined analysis of French, American and Canadian randomized controlled trials of ursodeoxycholic acid therapy in primary biliary cirrhosis. Gastroenterology. 1995;108:A1082.
13. Stiehl A, Raedsch R, Kommerell B. The effect of ursodeoxycholate in primary sclerosing cholangitis. A comparison to primary biliary cirrhosis. Abstract. Gastroenterology. 1988;94:595.
14. Stiehl A, Walker S, Stiehl L *et al.* Effects of ursodeoxycholic acid on liver and bile duct disease in primary sclerosing cholangitis. A 3 year pilot study with a placebo-controlled study period. J Hepatol. 1994;20:57–64.
15. Beuers U, Spengler U, Kruis W *et al.* Ursodeoxycholic acid for treatment of primary sclerosing cholangitis: a placebo controlled trial. Hepatology. 1992;16:707–14.
16. Stiehl A. Ursodeoxycholic acid therapy in treatment of primary sclerosing cholangitis. Scand J Gastroenterol. 1994;Suppl 204:59–61.
17. Dickson ER, Fleming TR, Wiesner R *et al.* Trial of penicillamine in advanced primary biliary cirrhosis. N Engl J Med. 1985;312:1011–15.
18. Mitchison HC, Bassendine MF, Malcolm AJ *et al.* A pilot, double blind, controlled 1 year trial of prednisolone treatment in primary biliary cirrhosis: hepatic improvement but greater bone loss. Hepatology. 1989;10:420–9.
19. Mitchison HC, Palmer JM, Bassendine MF *et al.* A controlled trial of prednisolone treatment in primary biliary cirrhosis. J Hepatol. 1992;15:336–44.
20. Wolfhagen FHJ, van Buren HR, Schalm SW. Combined treatment with ursodeoxycholic acid and prednisone in primary biliary cirrhosis. Neth J Med. 1994;44:84–90.
21. Heathcote J, Ross A, Sherlock S. A prospective controlled trial of azathioprine in primary biliary cirrhosis. Gastroenterology. 1976;70:656–60.
22. Crowe J, Christensen E, Smith M *et al.* Azathioprine in primary biliary cirrhosis: a preliminary report of an international trial. Gastroenterology. 1980;78:1005–10.
23. Christensen E, Neuberger J, Crowe J *et al.* Beneficial effects of azathioprine and prediction of prognosis in primary biliary cirrhosis. Gastroenterology. 1985;89;1084–91.

24. van Berge-Henegouwen GP, Wolfhagen FHJ. The Netherlands multi centre trial on ursodeoxycholic acid in PBC In: Fromm H, Leuschner U, eds. Bile Acids – Cholestasis – Gallstones. Lancaster UK: Kluwer Academic Publishers; 1995 [In press].
25. Minuk GY, Bohme CE, Burgess E *et al.* Pilot study of cyclosporin A in patients with symptomatic primary biliary cirrhosis. Gastroenterology. 1988; 95:1356–63.
26. Wiesner RH, Ludwig J, Lindor KD *et al.* A controlled trial of cyclosporine in the treatment of primary biliary cirrhosis. N Engl J Med. 1990;322:1419–24.
27. Lombard M, Portmann B, Neuberger *et al.* Cyclosporin A treatment in primary biliary cirrhosis: results of a long-term placebo controlled trial. Gastroenterology. 1993;104:519–26.
28. Kaplan NN, Knox TA. Treatment of primary biliary cirrhosis with low-dose weekly methotrexate. Gastroenterology. 1991;101:1332–8.
29. Buscher HP, Zietschmann Y, Gerok W. Positive responses to methotrexate and ursodeoxycholic acid in patients with primary biliary cirrhosis responding insufficiently to ursodeoxycholic acid. J Hepatol. 1993;18:9–14.
30. Kershenobich D, Vargas F, Garcia-Tsao G *et al.* Colchicine in the treatment of cirrhosis of the liver. N Engl J Med. 1988;318:1709–13.
31. Kaplan MM, Alling DW, Zimmermann HJ *et al.* A prospective trial of colchicine for primary biliary cirrhosis. N Engl J Med. 1986;315:1448–54.
32. Bodenheimer H, Schaffner F, Pezzulo J. Evaluation of colchicine therapy in primary biliary cirrhosis. Gastroenterology. 1988;95:124–9.
33. Warnes TW, Smith A, Lee FI *et al.* A controlled trial of colchicine in primary biliary cirrhosis. Trial design and preliminary report. J Hepatol. 1987;5:1–7.
34. Vuoristo M, Färkkila M, Karvonen AL *et al.* A placebo-controlled trial of primary biliary cirrhosis treatment with colchicine and ursodeoxycholic acid. Gastroenterology. 1995;108:1470–8.
35. Raedsch R, Stiehl A, Walker S, Scherrmann JM, Kommerell B. Ursodeoxycholic acid plus colchicine treatment in primary biliary cirrhosis: A controlled double-blind study. Z Gastroenterol. 1992;(Suppl. 1)30:55–7.
36. Almassio P, Provenzano G, Battezzati PM *et al.* The Italian multi-centre randomized controlled trial of ursodeoxycholic acid vs. ursodeoxycholic acid plus colchicine in symptomatic primary biliary cirrhosis. Abstract. Hepatology. 1994;20:267A.
37. Shibata J, Fuyjiyama S, Honda Y, Sato T. Combination therapy with ursodeoxycholic acid and colchicine for primary biliary cirrhosis. J Gastroenterol Hepatol. 1992;7:277–82.
38. Gaing AA, Geders JM, Cohen SA *et al.* Endoscopic management of primary sclerosing cholangitis: review, and report of an open series. Am J Gastroenterol. 1993;88:2000–8.
39. Lee JG, Schutz S, England RE, Leung JW, Cotton PB. Endoscopic therapy of sclerosing cholangitis. Hepatology. 1995;21:66–7.
40. Kaplan MM, Arora S, Pincus SH. Primary sclerosing cholangitis and low-dose oral pulse methotrexate: Clinical and hitologic response. Ann Intern Med. 1987;106:231–5.
41. Lindor KD, Jorgensen RA, Anderson ML *et al.* Ursodeoxycholic acid (UDCA) and methotrexate (MTX) for primary sclerosing cholangitis (PSC): A pilot study. Abstract. Hepatology. 1994;20:148A.

26
Bile acid metabolism in primary biliary cirrhosis

G. SALEN and A. K. BATTA

INTRODUCTION

Primary biliary cirrhosis (PBC) is a progressive cholestatic liver disease characterized by autoimmune destruction of interlobular bile ducts, progressive hepatocyte damage and fibrosis which leads to cirrhosis, and eventual liver failure[1]. The cause of the disease is not known, but the condition results from immunoinflammatory destruction of small and medium-sized enterohepatic bile ducts, fibrosis with disruption of the hepatic architecture and tissue damage associated with high concentrations of endogenous detergent bile acids[2–5]. It is believed that the initial bile duct damage is caused by abnormal expression of HLA antigens on bile duct epithelial cells and altered immune mechanisms. As a result of bile duct damage, hepatocyte bile acid clearance is impaired, with their retention in the liver that further aggravates tissue damage. Most patients show positive antimitochondrial antibody (AMA) titres greater than 1/64 dilution. However, a subset of patients with typical clinical findings of PBC show negative AMA tests but positive antinuclear antibody (ANA) tests. It has been suggested that these patients represent a different disease from PBC, termed immunocholangitis or autoimmune cholangitis. Histologically there is an increase in T_4- and T_8-lymphocytes. Immunosuppressive drugs such as azathioprine, corticosteroids, D-penicillamine, chlorambucil, phenobarbital or rifampicin have been used in controlled trials, with the aim of reducing portal inflammation and limiting bile duct destruction. In all cases there was a questionable benefit, and their use was limited by toxicity. Some improvement in liver biochemistries and histology has been suggested after colchicine and methotrexate therapy. However, serum bilirubin levels remained consistently high. Another drug, cyclosporin A, a fungal endecapeptide, alters lymphokine production and has been shown to modify immunological abnormalities in PBC. In a long-term placebo-controlled trial the drug appeared most beneficial in the early stages of the disease, while nephrotoxicity and hypertension developed in approximately 10% of patients. Ursodiol, the 7β-hydroxy epimer of the primary bile acid chenodeoxycholic acid, is a safe litholytic bile acid that has recently been shown to improve liver function in patients with stage I–III PBC; however, histological improvement has not been documented. Hepatic transplantation is so far the only definitive treatment for PBC, but even the transplanted liver is susceptible to autoimmune damage.

In PBC, biliary secretion of primary bile acids, cholic acid and chenodeoxycholic acid is impaired, resulting in their accumulation in hepatocytes and overflow into the blood. Reduced bile acid synthesis ensues from feedback inhibition. After administration, ursodiol becomes the major biliary bile acid, the proportion of cholic acid is reduced significantly and the chenodeoxycholic acid percentage remains virtually unchanged.

In this chapter we report on the effect of 2 years of ursodiol treatment on biliary and serum bile acid composition in 14 subjects with PBC. In addition, we examined the effect of feeding ursodiol on the conjugation pattern of biliary bile acids in these subjects.

METHODS

Clinical

Serum and bile was obtained from 14 subjects (12 females and two males) with primary biliary cirrhosis (mean age 53 years). The diagnosis was established in each subject by at least two of the following three criteria: (1) liver biopsy showing chronic non-suppurative destructive cholangitis; (2) positive antimitochondrial antibody titre greater than 1 : 40 dilution on two specimens separated by 6 months; (3) elevation of γ-glutamyl transpeptidase and/or alkaline phosphatase more than twice the upper limit of normal for more than 6 months. Most patients had previously been treated unsuccessfully with immunosuppressive drugs, cholestyramine, and colchicine.

Chemical

Bile acids in the serum and bile were measured according to the method of Batta *et al.*[6]. Briefly, free bile acids are isolated from the specimens by ion exchange chromatography on Sep-pak cartridges. After forming the methyl esters and trimethyl silyl ether derivatives, individual bile acids were determined by capillary gas–liquid chromatography on a 23 m column internally coated with CP-Sil-5 CB. When necessary, mass spectrometry data were obtained for structure identification.

RESULTS

Serum bile acids

Serum bile acid concentrations in the patients are shown in Table 2. As already noted, patients with moderate to severe primary biliary cirrhosis show increased fasting serum bile acid concentrations (Table 1). In contrast to controls, in whom chenodeoxycholic acid is the major serum bile acid, cholic acid predominated in all patients. Only small amounts of lithocholic and deoxycholic acids (the bacte-

Table 1 Effect of ursodiol treatment on serum bile acids in patients with primary biliary cirrhosis[a]

	Bile acids (μmol/l)				
		Uncommon		*Others[d]*	*Total*
	Endogenous[b]	*Hydroxylated[c]*	*Ursodiol*		
Patients					
Pretreatment[e]	46.1 ± 15.4	2.4 ± 0.4	1.4 ± 0.4	2.9 ± 0.2	52.8 ± 12.6
Placebo[f]	53.3 ± 16.2	2.4 ± 0.5	1.7 ± 0.3	3.5 ± 0.2	60.6 ± 14.3
Ursodiol[g] (6 months)	20.0 ± 4.2[h]	3.5 ± 0.6	19.8 ± 6.7[h]	5.4 ± 2.8	48.7 ± 9.4
Ursodiol[g] (12 months)	23.0 ± 4.1[h]	3.0 ± 0.4	26.7 ± 8.2[h]	6.2 ± 2.7	58.9 ± 11.2
Ursodiol[g] (24 months)	22.7 ± 3.8[h]	3.5 ± 0.4	30.9 ± 7.6[h]	3.2 ± 2.2	60.3 ± 9.8
Controls[i]					
Pretreatment	3.4 ± 0.5		0.2 ± 0.1		3.6 ± 0.2
Ursodiol (2 weeks)	0.6 ± 0.3	0.2 ± 0.1	7.2 ± 0.8	0.3 ± 0.1	8.3 ± 0.6

[a]Fasting serum bile acids were quantified by capillary gas–liquid chromatography.
[b]Chenodeoxycholic acid, cholic acid, deoxycholic acid, lithocholic acid.
[c] 1β,3α,12α-Trihydroxy-5β-cholanoic acid, 1β,3α,7β-trihydroxy-5β-cholanoic acid, 1β,3α,12α-tetrahydroxy-5β-cholanoic acid.
[d]Iso-ursodeoxycholic acid, ursocholic acid, hyocholic acid, ω-muricholic acid.
[e]Fasting serum was obtained immediately pretreatment. Values reported are mean ± SD (n = 14).
[f]Fasting serum was obtained every month from patients receiving placebo. The average of last two determinations for each patient was used to obtain mean ± SD (n = 11).
[g]Fasting serum was obtained every month from patients receiving ursodiol. The average of two determinations during months 5 and 6 (6-month effect, n = 11), months 11 and 12 (12-month effect, n = 8), or months 23 or 24 (24-month effect, n = 8) for each patient was used to obtain mean ± SD.
[h]$p<0.001$.
[i] Fasting serum was obtained from four healthy subjects, ursodiol (900 mg/day) was fed for 10 days, and serum was collected before and on the last day of bile acid feeding.

rial 7α-dehydroxylation products of chenodeoxycholic and cholic acids, respectively) were detected in the serum. Treatment with placebo did not change bile acid concentration or composition. The proportion of cholic acid declined during the administration of ursodiol, because more than 40% of the bile acids was ursodiol. Chenodeoxycholic acid also decreased in the serum, but the difference was not statistically significant.

Urinary bile acids

Urinary bile acid values in the patients are shown in Table 2. Just as in serum, the urinary bile acids were increased several-fold compared to healthy controls, and cholic acid was the major urinary bile acid. Substantial amounts of 1- and 6-hydroxlated derivatives of chenodeoxycholic acid and cholic acid were also excreted. Urinary bile acid levels remained virtually unchanged during placebo treatment; however, during ursodiol feeding the amount of bile acids excreted increased several-fold over pretreatment levels, with ursodiol as the predominant bile acid (Table 2). The excretion of endogenous bile acids did not change substantially; however, their hydroxylated derivatives were excreted in reduced

Table 2 Effect of ursodiol treatment on urinary bile acids in patients with primary biliary cirrhosis[a]

	Bile acids (μmol/g creatinine)				
		Uncommon		*Others[d]*	*Total*
	Endogenous[b]	*Hydroxylated[c]*	*Ursodiol*		
Patients					
Pretreatment[e]	37.3 ± 16.7	14.2 ± 10.2	2.9 ± 0.5	7.8 ± 2.8	62.2 ± 22.2
Placebo[f]	35.7 ± 14.7	12.4 ± 8.9	2.7 ± 0.6	8.1 ± 2.4	58.9 ± 18.6
Ursodiol[g] (6 months)	23.5 ± 8.7[h]	13.7 ± 5.4	77.9 ± 19.7[i]	23.9 ± 7.8	139.0 ± 28.9[i]
Ursodiol[g] (12 months)	24.9 ± 7.8[h]	15.0 ± 4.8	120.1 ± 33.6[i]	38.6 ± 12.7	198.6 ± 42.7[i]
Ursodiol[g] (24 months)	18.5 ± 4.5[h]	11.5 ± 4.7	96.9 ± 23.9[i]	35.0 ± 8.7	161.9 ± 34.7[i]
Controls[j]					
Pretreatment	1.7 ± 0.3	–	0.3 ± 0.1	0.5 ± 0.1	2.5 ± 0.4
Ursodiol (2 weeks)	2.5 ± 0.5	2.1 ± 0.3	33.0 ± 6.7	11.1 ± 2.2	48.7 ± 7.3

[a] Urinary bile acids were quantified by capillary gas–liquid chromatography.
[b] Chenodeoxycholic acid, cholic acid, deoxycholic acid, lithocholic acid.
[c] 1β,3α,12α-Trihydroxy-5β-cholanoic acid, 1β,3α,7β-trihydroxy-5β-cholanoic acid, 1β,3α,7α,12α-tetrahydroxy-5β-cholanoic acid.
[d] Iso-ursodeoxycholic acid, ursocholic acid, hyocholic acid, ω-muricholic acid.
[e] Early-morning urine was obtained immediately pretreatment. Values reported are mean ± SD ($n = 14$).
[f] Early-morning urine was obtained every month from patients receiving placebo. The average of the last two determinations for each patient was used to obtain mean ± SD ($n = 11$).
[g] Early-morning urine was obtained every month from patients receiving 900 mg/day ursodiol. The average of two determinations during months 5 and 6 (6-month effect, $n = 11$), 11 and 12 (12-month effect, $n = 8$), or 23 and 24 (24-month effect, $n = 8$) for each patient was used to obtain mean ± SD.
[h] p = n.s.
[i] $p<0.001$.
[j] Early-morning urine was obtained from four healthy subjects. Ursodiol (900 mg/day) was fed for 10 days, and serum was collected before and on the last day of bile acid fasting.

amounts. In addition, a small portion of ursodiol was excreted hydroxylated at 1-, 6-, and 21-positions.

Biliary bile acids

Before treatment the biliary bile acid pattern (Table 3) closely resembled that of serum bile acids (Table 1). Again, cholic acid was the major bile acid in all bile samples, and was approximately 1.9 times more abundant than chenodeoxycholic acid in bile, compared with 1.5 times in serum; secondary bile acids, lithocholic acid and deoxycholic acid, constituted only a small fraction of the total biliary bile acids. Unlike urine, in which up to 36% of 1β-hydroxycholic acid (1β-hydroxychenodeoxycholic acid) is present, only 1% or less of the extra hydroxylated primary bile acids were found in the bile of these patients (Table 4). The biliary bile acid pattern remained constant during the placebo period, but during treatment the proportion of ursodiol rose from 0.3% to 31%, and cholic acid declined from 62% to 33% (Table 3), whereas chenodeoxycholic acid dropped slightly from 33% to 29%.

Table 3 Effect of urdosiol on biliary bile acids in primary biliary cirrhosis[a]

Bile acids	*Patients*			*Controls[e]*	
	Pre[b]	*Placebo[c]*	*Ursodiol[d]*	*Pre*	*Ursodiol*
CDCA[f]	33 ± 8[g]	41 ± 2	29 ± 8	24 ± 5	18 ± 3
CA	62 ± 8	57 ± 2	33 ± 9[h]	49 ± 8	15 ± 2[i]
UDCA	0.3 ± 0.2	0.1 ± 0.1	31 ± 12[j]	1 ± 1	55 ± 7[j]
LCA	0.7 ± 0.3	0.5 ± 0.2	1 ± 1	1 ± 0.2	2 ± 0.4
DCA	3 ± 3	0.4 ± 0.2	5 ± 3	25 ± 6	9 ± 0.3
Others[k]	1 ± 0.2	1 ± 0.4	1 ± 1		1 ± 0.2

[a]Biliary bile acids were quantified by capillary gas–liquid chromatography.
[b]Values reported are mean ± SD for the pretreatment bile samples ($n = 6$).
[c]Duodenal bile was obtained from patients receiving placebo. Two measurements were averaged to obtain mean ± SD ($n = 3$).
[d]Duodenal bile was obtained from patients receiving 900 mg/day or ursodiol. Two values were averaged to obtain mean ± SD ($n = 3$).
[e]Bile was collected from four healthy subjects. Ursodiol (900 mg/day) was fed for 1 day, and bile was collected before and on the last day of bile acid feeding.
[f]CDCA, chenodeoxycholic acid; CA, cholic acid; UDCA, ursodiol; LCA, lithocholic acid; DCA, deoxycholic acid.
[g]The values represent total bile acids in the pretreatment, placebo or ursodiol-treated bile samples.
[h]$p<0.002$.
[i]$p<0.001$.
[j]$p<0.0001$
[k]Iso-ursodiol, ursocholic acid, hyocholic acid, 1β,3α,12α-trihydroxy-5β-cholanoic acid, 1β,3α,7α,12α-tetrahydroxy-5β-cholanoic acid, 1β,3α,7β-trihydroxy-5β-cholanoic acid, ω-muricholic acid.

The proportion of unconjugated bile acids in bile was determined by GLC analysis of the bile samples measured before deconjugation of bile salts (Table 4). Approximately 6% unconjugated bile acids were found in the bile samples, with cholic acid as the major component. In control subjects, 0.5% free bile acid was detected in bile. After ursodiol feeding there was a slight decline in the proportion of free bile acids, with ursodiol becoming the major bile acid, constituting 41% of total free bile acids.

DISCUSSION

In this study 14 symptomatic patients with primary biliary cirrhosis at various stages were treated with ursodiol for up to 24 months. We have demonstrated that clinical and biochemical improvements persisted in all patients for the duration of the study. Histological improvements, principally a reduction of inflammation, were documented by follow-up liver biopsy in three of four patients treated for 24 months.

Total serum endogenous bile acid concentration decreased with treatment. There was a statistically significant reduction in serum endogenous bile acids after 6 months, that persisted after 2 years of treatment. This may have resulted, at least in part, from improved hepatic clearance of endogenous bile acids, since the reduced serum bile acid concentration after ursodiol feeding was not attributable to increased urinary endogenous bile acid excretion alone. Urinary endogenous bile acid excretion was reduced during the last 12 months of therapy, whereas serum bile acids did not change appreciably. In addition to the bile acids measured at baseline, hydroxylated derivatives of ursodiol at C-1, C-6, and C-21 positions appeared in both the serum and urine.

Cholic acid was the major biliary bile acid in all patients with PBC, suggesting an active 12α-hydroxylation[6], and the bile acid pattern was similar to that found in the serum. Unusual extra hydroxylated bile acids such as 1β-hydroxycholic acid, 1β-hydroxydeoxycholic acid and hyocholic acid are preferentially excreted in the urine, and their biliary concentration was only 1%. Biliary bile acid patterns did not change during placebo administration but treatment with ursodiol caused a significant decline in the proportion of cholic acid with only a small decrease in chenodeoxycholic acid, whereas ursodiol constituted approximately 30% of the biliary bile acids (Table 4). This degree of enrichment is about 25% less than usually obtained when similar doses of urso-

Table 4 Unconjugated bile acid as percentage of total biliary bile acid in patient with primary cirrhosis[a]

Patients	*Treatment*	*Free bile acids as percentage of total bile acids*				
		CDCA[b]	*CA*	*DCA*	*UDCA*	*Total*
E.Z.	Pretreatment[c]	0.4[d]	5.1	0.5	–	6.0
	Placebo[e]	1.8	2.4	1.8	–	6.0
R.G.	Pretreatment	0.2	0.4	–	–	0.6
	Placebo	0.1	0.1	–	–	0.2
D.D.	Pretreatment	7.4	9.5	0.4	–	17.3
	Placebo	4.1	12.5	0.3	–	16.9
S.D.	Pretreatment	1.3	2.4	0.4	–	4.1
	UDCA[f]	0.2	0.7	0.6	4.9	6.4
M.E.	Pretreatment	0.1	1.2	–	–	1.3
	UDCA	0.3	0.4	0.1	0.5	1.3
E.A.	Pretreatment	2.6	5.4	0.5	–	8.5
	UDC	2.2	2.6	0.9	2.7	8.4
Control[g]	Pretreatment	–	0.5	–	–	0.5
	UDCA	–	–	–	0.6	0.6

[a]Biliary bile acids were quantified by capillary gas–liquid chromatography.
[b]CDCA, chenodeoxycholic acid; CA, cholic acid; UDCA, ursodiol; DCA, deoxycholic acid.
[c]Values reported are mean for the pretreatment bile samples (n = 6).
[d]The values represent percentage of total bile acids in the pretreatment, placebo or ursodiol-treated bile samples.
[e]Duodenal bile was obtained from patients receiving placebo. Two measurements were averaged to obtain mean (n = 3).
[f]Duodenal bile was obtained from patients receiving ursodiol. Two values were averaged to obtain mean (n = 3),
[g]Bile was collected from four healthy subjects. Ursodiol (900 mg/day) was fed for 10 days, and bile was collected before and on the last day of bile acid feeding.

diol are given to gallstone patients with normal hepatic function, and may reflect increased urinary excretion or inability of the abnormal liver to take up the fed bile acid efficiently in PBC. The changes in biliary bile acid composition were similar to those found in the serum, where 6 months of ursodiol feeding caused a significant decline in the concentration of cholic acid but not chenodeoxycholic acid, and accounted for almost 40% of the total serum bile acids (Table 2). In untreated patients only small amounts of lithocholic acid, the 7-dehydroxylated derivative of chenodeoxycholic acid and ursodiol, were secreted in the bile, which strongly argues against a pathogenic role of lithocholic acid in PBC. After ursodiol treatment the proportion of lithocholic acid rose slightly, and liver function tests improved.

It is important to emphasize that significant amounts of unconjugated bile acids were secreted in the bile of all patients. In both pretreatment and placebo bile samples, cholic acid was the major free bile acid, accounting for 4% of the total biliary bile acids. After administration of ursodiol the proportion of free bile acids was slightly reduced, with ursodiol becoming the most abundant biliary free bile acid. The secretion of free bile acids in the bile may result from the bypassing of the intrahepatic conjugating mechanism or, alternatively, from reduced cholehepatic shunting. The latter mechanism, whereby a free bile acid molecule is exchanged for HCO_3^- in the upper bile ductules, has been postulated to be responsible for alkalinization and the virtual absence of free bile acids in the bile.

Due to the destruction of intrahepatic bile ductules, hepatic uptake and secretion of bile acids are impaired, and bile acids accumulate in the liver tissue. As a result, increased amounts of bile acids overflow back into the serum and are excreted in the urine. Bile acid synthesis is also reduced in this disease, apparently due to feedback inhibition of the rate-determining enzyme, cholesterol-7α-hydroxylase, by the large retained hepatocyte bile acid pool. Since hepatic enzymes preferentially conjugate bile acids with taurine, the larger portion of taurine-conjugated bile acids secreted into the bile probably reflects very low synthesis. The situation is different when bile acid synthesis is normal (between 300 and 500 mg/day), and the need for conjugation is greater. Because the amount of hepatic taurine is limited, whereas the supply of glycine is almost unlimited, a larger portion of bile acids ends up glycine conjugated in healthy humans. Feeding free bile acid also greatly increases conjugation, and rapidly depletes the hepatic taurine pool, so that the fed bile acid is principally (90%) glycine conjugated. As expected, in patients with PBC, ursodiol was conjugated mainly with glycine. Endogenous bile acids were still substantially conjugated with taurine, reflecting slow clearance coupled with a reduced incorporation of ursodiol in bile.

In summary we have demonstrated that continued treatment with ursodiol improved symptoms and lowered the levels of endogenous serum bile acids in patients with PBC. Some histological improvement is seen after 24 months of therapy, although the histological stage is not changed. In addition, we found that the bile acid conjugation pattern is abnormal in these patients. A greater proportion of biliary bile acids is conjugated with taurine, consistent with a low synthetic rate of endogenous bile acids. In some patients a sizeable fraction of biliary bile acids was also secreted unconjugated. Ursodiol conjugated principally with glycine and also free in the bile constituted about 30% of the total biliary bile acids.

Acknowledgement

This work was supported by VA Research Service and USPHS Grant HL 17818.

References

1. James SP, Hoofnagle JH, Strober W *et al.* Primary biliary cirrhosis: a model autoimmune disease. Ann Intern Med. 1983;99:500–12.
2. Goldmann MA, Schwartz CC, Swell L *et al.* Bile acid metabolism in health and disease. Prog Liver Dis. 1979;6:225–41.
3. Summerfield JA, Cullen J, Barens S *et al.* Evidence for renal control of urinary excretion of bile acids and bile acid sulfates in the cholestatic syndrome. Clin Sci Mol Med. 1977;52:51–65.
4. Vlahcevic ZR, Prugh MF, Gregory DH *et al.* Disturbances of bile acid metabolism in parenchymal liver cell disease. Clin Gastroenterol. 1977;6:25–43.
5. Akashi Y, Mayazaki H, Yanagisawa J *et al.* Bile acid metabolism in cirrhotic liver tissue: altered synthesis and impaired hepatic secretion. Clin Chim. 1987;168:199–206.
6. Batta AK, Salen G, Michondoni R, *et al.* Effect of long-term treatment with ursodiol on clinical and biochemical features and biliary bile acid metabolism in patients with primary biliary cirrhosis. Am J Gastroenterol. 1993;88:691–700.

27
The influence of ursodeoxycholic acid on immune markers in primary biliary liver diseases

G. R. PAPE

Although direct proof is lacking, many immunological abnormalities in patients with primary biliary cirrhosis (PBC) give us indirect proof and circumstantial evidence that PBC is an autoimmune disease or at least that immune mechanisms may play a significant role in its pathogenesis[1–5]. This is less clear for primary sclerosing cholangitis (PSC)[6] and for the so-called autoimmune cholangitis[7].

Surprisingly, immunosuppressive treatment is not very efficient in PBC. Carefully done randomized controlled trials of treatment of this disease with immunosuppressive drugs, like methotrexate, azathioprine and cyclosporin A[8,9], have revealed statistically significant beneficial effects on several clinical and laboratory parameters, which were the objectives of the respective trial, yet the biological effect of these treatment forms was not impressive. In contrast, treatment with ursodeoxycholic acid (UDCA), which is not considered an immunosuppressive drug, improves not only clinical, biochemical and histological parameters but seems to have a significant favourable effect on survival of patients with PBC[8,10]. Thus one is inclined to attribute at least some of these effects on the capability of UDCA to interfere with immune mechanisms, which may be crucial for the pathogenesis of the disease.

UDCA has been proposed to work by several mechanisms:

1. It inhibits absorption of toxic, endogenous bile salts.
2. It inhibits secretion of toxic bile salts.
3. It dilutes toxic bile salts via a choleretic action.
4. It prevents increase in cytosolic ionized calcium.
5. It stabilizes hepatocyte membranes against toxic bile salts.
6. When incorporated in membranes, it alters antigen expression and free surface radicals.

During the past few years, the influence of UDCA on a relatively small number of immunological parameters in vivo and in vitro was analysed[9–23].

Lacaille and Paradis[11] studied human mononuclear cell proliferation as an in-vitro model of cell-mediated immunity in the presence of UDCA, its glycoconjugate and tauroconjugate and chenodeoxycholic acid at concentrations of 5, 25 and 50 μmol/L. Proliferation was inhibited in a dose-dependent manner compared with control values (15–54% depending on the type and the concentration of the bile acid as well as on the mitogen, PHA vs PMA, used for stimulation). Furthermore, they studied cell-surface receptors or antigens, respectively, CD3 (part of the T cell receptor), CD4 and CD8 (differentiating T cell subpopulations), interleukin-2 receptor (IL-2R), and the human leukocyte Class II antigen-DR (HLA-DR) as well as IL-2 production. The number of these cell-surface receptors (antigens) was not modified by bile acids. However, there seemed to be a functional interference with the IL-2 receptor, since the murine CTLL-2 cell line, which is IL-2 dependent, shows an inhibition of proliferation by bile acids in the presence of abundant IL-2. IL-2 production was decreased in a dose-dependent manner in the presence of UDCA (35–60% less IL-2 secreted than in the control cultures). The mechanisms of the demonstrated partially immunosuppressive effect of UDCA are unknown. However, the authors discuss that although the inhibition of an intracellular function cannot be excluded, UDCA act by incorporation into the cell membrane and could thus interact with many effectors of lymphocyte proliferation.

Yoshikawa *et al.*[12] measured the effects of UDCA on cytokine and immunoglobulin production in vitro. UDCA suppressed IL-2 and IL-4 production stimulated by ConA and IFN-γ production induced by poly I-C, whereas it affected neither IL-1 nor IL-6 production. The suppressive effects of UDCA on Ig production were Ig-class non-specific because IgM, IgG and IgA production were suppressed. UDCA reduced Ig production in human B lymphoma cell lines, suggesting that it could act directly on B cells. In addition, it is conceivable that UDCA suppresses Ig production via modifying lymphokine production by T cells. The authors speculated that UDCA reduces immune-mediated injuries against hepatocytes and bile duct epithelium through the suppression of IFN-γ production in the liver.

Kürktschiev *et al.*[13] demonstrated that the pokeweed-mitogen-induced IL-2 production, which is minimal in PBC patients before UDCA treatment, increases to normal levels compared with controls after 16–20 weeks of UDCA therapy.

The modulation of HLA Class II expression on hepatocytes and bile duct epithelial cells by UDCA in vitro and in vivo was more extensively studied by several groups. Töx and colleagues[14] have investigated the effect of bile acids on expression of HLA molecules on primary human hepatocytes in vitro. Addition of UDCA (optimal concentration at least 100 mmol/L) led to a marked reduction of IFN-γ-induced HLA Class I and, to a lesser extent, HLA Class II expression. Furthermore, the expression of the adhesion molecule, ICAM-1, on human primary hepatocytes *in vitro* was also reduced under UDCA. In 1990, Leuschner and colleages[15] demonstrated a marked reduction in HLA Class I and Class II molecule expression on the epithelia of small and medium-sized bile ducts and on hepatocytes in the majority (5/9) of patients with PBC undergoing UDCA treatment. A similar change was seen in HLA expression on hepatocytes.

Slightly different results were reported by Calmus and coworkers[16]. They have studied the effects of long-term administration of UDCA (at least one year) on hepatic HLA expression in patients with PBC. Aberrant biliary HLA Class II expression was not modified by chronic administration of UDCA. In contrast, hepatocyte HLA Class I expression was markedly reduced.

We have also studied the expression of HLA Class II molecules on bile-duct epithelial cells of PBC patients treated with UDCA[17]. There was no significant change in the expression of HLA DR, DP or DQ after therapy with UDCA (10 mg/kg, n = 10 patients) for one year (Figure 1). In contrast, treatment with Cyclosporin A (CicA) (3 mg/kg) for one and two years markedly reduced the expression of HLA-DR and -DQ on bile ducts (n = 9 patients). Furthermore, the production of tumour necrosis factor α and β (TNFα, TNFβ) of peripheral blood T cells and T cell lines and of liver-derived T cell lines were investigated in patients with PBC treated with UDCA or CicA[5,17]. As can be seen in Figure 2, TNFβ production of peripheral blood T cells increased after treatment with both substances compared with untreated PBC patients. This increase reached statistical significance only for CicA-treated patients.

Terasaki *et al.*[18] investigated immunohistochemically hepatocellular expression of HLA Class I antigens on hepatocytes before and after UDCA therapy in four patients with PBC and reported on the reduced expression of these molecules on hepatocytes following UDCA treatment.

The effects of bile acids on monocyte function of healthy individuals in vitro was investigated by Calmus *et al.*[19]. They report on the production of IL-1, IL-6 and TNFα by monocytes. In contrast to chenodeoxycholic acid (CDCA), UDCA only marginally reduced IL-1-, Il-6- and LPS-stimulated TNFα production.

Several authors report on the reduction in antimitochondrial antibody titres in patients with PBC on UDCA treatment[20] and on reduction of IgM (for review see Reference 21).

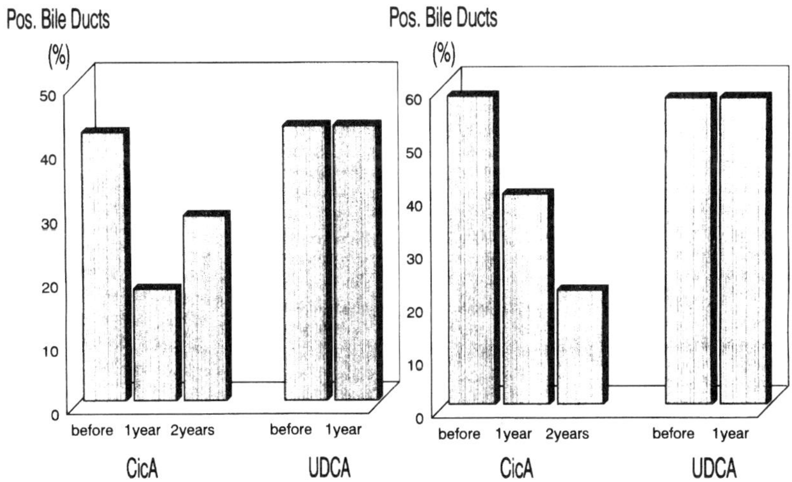

Fig. 1 Influence of UDCA and CicA treatment on expression of HLA-DQ (left) and HLA-DR (right) molecules on bile duct cells in patients with PBC. UDCA treatment: n = 10 patients; CicA treatment: n = 9 patients. HLA-DR and -DQ molecules were demonstrated immunohistologically by staining with monoclonal antibodies

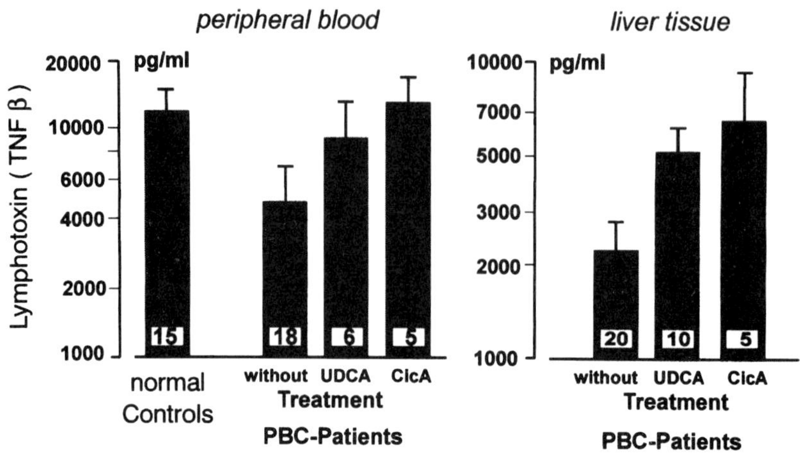

Fig. 2 Influence of UDCA and CicA treatment on TNFβ (lymphotoxin) production of peripheral-blood-derived and liver-tissue-derived T cells from patients with PBC[17]. For details of the method, see Reference 5

Taken together, the undoubtedly beneficial effect of UDCA treatment on laboratory parameters in patients with primary biliary liver diseases, which are believed to be at least in part immunologically mediated, as well as on the clinical outcome of patients with PBC, which is thought to be an autoimmune disease, suggests that this substance acts via immunomodulating effects. We have discussed the results of several carefully done studies on the effects of UDCA on immune parameters *in vitro* and *in vivo* in healthy individuals and in patients with PBC. The results show that UDCA exerts an immunosuppressive effect on several immune parameters. The majority of investigators unequivocally discuss their data as an indication that UDCA possibly exerts its favourable effect via modulating pathological immune mechanisms, which contribute to the pathogenesis of PBC.
However, one has to be very cautious with the interpretation of the results so far published.

1. The number of published relevant studies is small.
2. These studies cover only a limited scope of immunological parameters.
3. One has to be cautious when comparing data obtained *in vitro*, particularly from healthy individuals, with data from PBC patients under UDCA treatment.
4. The significance of the investigated parameters for the pathogenesis of primary biliary cirrhosis or primary sclerosing cholangitis is totally unknown.
5. The published data on reduction of HLA Class I and Class II expression by UDCA must not necessarily be interpreted as immunosuppressive, since:

a. T cells can only be activated by two signals. Signal one is delivered by the trimolecular interaction between the T cell receptor with the peptide presented by the appropriate HLA molecule on the surface of the antigen presenting cell (APC) and signal two is the costimulatory signal from the APC. Lack of the second signal, i.e. when non-professional APC-like biliary epithelial cells present antigen via their HLA Class II, does not result in activation but in anergy of the respective T cells; that is, the T cell can no longer respond to its specific antigen.

b. Recently, it was shown that downregulation of certain HLA Class I antigens (HLA-C) can also have a harmful effect, since HLA-C expression protects target cells from damage by a subpopulation of killer cells, preventing them from exerting their lytic capacity (D. Schendel, personal communication).

The scenario of tissue destruction in the liver in primary biliary liver disease is not understood. However, one can speculate that antigen-specific cells recruit many antigen-non-specific cells into their immediate vicinity. This process results in the formation of necroinflammatory foci, in which biliary epithelial cells and hepatocytes are damaged or destroyed. It is this specifically induced but non-specifically perpetuated smouldering and damaging process which may be positively influenced by UDCA.

Taken together, on the basis of our limited knowledge about the contribution of immunological mechanisms to the pathogenesis of PBC in general and the available experimental data of the influence of UDCA on these mechanisms in detail, it is at present very difficult if not impossible to explain the favourable effect of UDCA treatment in patients by its action via immune mechanisms.

References

1. Pape GR, Spengler U, Hoffmann RM, Jung MC. Pathogenesis of primary biliary cirrhosis. New aspects of the role of T lymphocytes. In: Krawitt EL, Wiesner RH, eds. Autoimmune liver diseases. Raven Press 1991:43.
2. Hoffmann RM, Pape GR, Spengler U *et al.* Clonal analysis of liver derived T cells of patients with primary biliary cirrhosis. Clin Exp Immunol. 1989;76:210–15.
3. Björkland A, Tötterman TH. Is primary biliary cirrhosis an autoimmune disease? Scand J Gastroenterol. 1994;29S204:32–9.
4. Spengler U, Pape GR, Hoffmann RM *et al.* Differential expression of MHC class II subregion products on bile duct epithelial cells and hepatocytes in patients with primary biliary cirrhosis. Hepatology. 1988;8:459.
5. Spengler U, Möller A, Jung MC *et al.* T lymphocytes from patients with primary biliary cirrhosis produce reduced amounts of lymphotoxin, tumor necrosis factor and interferon gamma upon mitogen stimulation. J Hepatol. 1992;15:129.
6. Boberg KM, Lundin KE, Schrumpf E. Etiology and pathogenesis in primary sclerosing cholangitis. Scand J Gastroenterol. 1994;29S204:47–58.
7. Ben-Ari Z, Dhillon AP, Sherlock S. Autoimmune cholangiopathy: Part of the spectrum of autoimmune chronic active hepatitis. Hepatology. 1993;18:10–15.
8. Poupon RE, Poupon R, Balkau B, UDCA–PBC Study Group. Ursodiol for the long-term treatment of primary biliary cirrhosis. N Engl J Med. 1994;330:1342–7.
9. Lombard M, Portmann B, Neuberger J *et al.* Cyclosporin A treatment in primary biliary cirrhosis. Results of a long-term placebo controlled trial. Gastroenterology. 1993;104:519.
10. Kaplan MM. Primary biliary cirrhosis–A first step in prolonging survival. N Engl J Med. 1994;330:1386–7.

11. Lacaille F, Paradis K. The immunosuppressive effect of UDCA: A comparative in vitro study on human peripheral blood mononuclear cells. Hepatology. 1993;18:165–71.
12. Yoshikawa M, Tsujii T, Matsumura K *et al.* Immunomodulatory effects of UDCA on immune responses. Hepatology. 1992;16:358–64.
13. Kürktschiev D, Subat S, Adler D, Schentke KU. Immunomodulating effect of UDCA therapy in patients with primary biliary cirrhosis. J Hepatol. 1993;18:373–7.
14. Töx U, Arnold JC, Theilmann L, Otto G, Stremmel W, Stiehl A. Effect of bile acids on expression of HLA on primary human hepatocytes. Proceedings of the Bile Acid Meeting, San Diego, 1994. Lancaster, UK: Klüwer Academic publishers; [In press].
15. Leuschner U, Dienes HP, Güldütuna S, Birkenfeld G, Leuschner M. UDCA influences immune parameters in patients with primary biliary cirrhosis. Hepatology. 1990;12:957(abstract).
16. Calmus Y, Gane P, Rouger P, Poupon R. Hepatic expression of class I and class II major histocompatibility complex molecules in primary biliary cirrhosis: Effect of UDCA. Hepatology. 1990;11:12–15.
17. Spengler U, Jung MC, Hoffmann RM *et al.* Influence of cyclosporin A and ursodeoxycholic acid on MHC class II expression and lymphokine production in primary biliary cirrhosis. German J Gastroenterol. 1991;12:725(abstract).
18. Terasaki S, Nakanuma Y, Ogino H, Unoura M, Kobayashi K. Hepatocellular and biliary expression of HLA antigens in primary biliary cirrhosis before and after UDCA therapy. Am J Gastroenterol. 1991;86:1194–9.
19. Calmus Y, Guechot J, Podevin P, Bonnefis M-T, Giboudeau J, Poupon R. Differential effects of chenodeoxycholic and ursodeoxycholic acids on interleukin 1, interleukin 6 and tumor necrosis factor-alpha production by monocytes. Hepatology. 1992;16:719–23.
20. Poupon RE, Balkau B, Eschwege E, Poupon R, UDCA–PBC Study Group. A multicenter, controlled trial of ursodiol for the treatment of primary biliary cirrhosis. N Engl J Med. 1991;324:1548–54.
21. Leuschner U. Ursodeoxycholic acid therapy in primary biliary cirrhosis. Scand J Gastroenterol. 1994;29S204:40–46.
22. Keane RM, Gadacz TR, Munster AM, Birmingham W, Winchurch RA. Impairment of human lymphocyte function by bile salts. Surgery. 1984;95:439–43.
23. Calmus Y, Weill B, Ozier Y, Chereau C, Houssin D, Poupon R. Immunosuppressive properties of chenodeoxycholic and ursodeoxycholic acids in the mouse. Gastroenterology. 1992;103:617–21.
24. Calmus Y, Podevin P, Robert A, Poupon R. Differential effects of CDCA and UDCA on expression of procoagulant activity by human monocytes. J Hepatol. 1994;20:466–72.

28 Putative mechanisms of hepatoprotective effects of ursodeoxycholate in chronic cholestatic liver diseases

S. GÜLDÜTUNA, G. ZIMMER and U. LEUSCHNER

INTRODUCTION

The beneficial effect of ursodeoxycholate (UDC) in different cholestatic liver diseases has been clearly shown in numerous studies[1–4]. Cholestatic liver diseases, independent of their pathogenesis, can result in accumulation of bile salts in the hepatocyte and regurgitate across the basolateral membrane into the space of Disse, causing an increase in plasma bile acids[5]. Chenodeoxycholate (CDC), an α-dihydroxy bile salt, frequently produces elevations of serum transaminases during treatment of patients for gallstone dissolution[6]. In cholestasis, a correlation between the feathery degeneration and the intrahepatic concentration of α-dihydroxy bile salts like CDC or deoxycholate (DC) has been demonstrated[7].

BILE SALT CYTOTOXICITY

Bile salt toxicity depends on the hydrophobicity of the individual bile salt, which can be defined using high performance liquid chromatography[8]. Hydrophilicity decreases in the following order:

$$UDC > C > CDC > DC > LC$$

The α-dihydroxy bile salts, CDC and DC, induce necrosis and cholestasis of the liver[9–13]. The mean bile salt concentration in the human hepatocyte is estimated[13] to be 50 μmol/L; higher local concentrations exist, especially in cholestasis. CDC concentrations of 50 μmol/L were shown to induce alterations in the membrane permeability of large unilamellar vesicles[14,15]. The changes in membrane permeability depend on membrane binding and the increase in the energy potential between the inner and the outer leaflet. This induces the redistribution of the bound bile salt from the outer to the inner leaflet of the bilayer, leading to transient pore formation[15,16]. This non-detergent mechanism of bile salts permits cations, such as Ca^{2+} and Mg^{2+} to enter the cell via the plasma membrane[17]. Increased concentrations of Ca^{2+} and Mg^{2+} could induce apoptosis in hepatocytes by stimulation of Mg^{2+}-dependent endonucleasis following cell death[18]. Alterations in the lipid structure of the membrane by low concentrations of bile salts could also induced inhibition of the Na-K-ATPase accompanied by cholestasis[19], an enzyme which is located at the basolateral liver plasma membrane. Increasing the bile salt concentration to the critical micellar concentration causes solubilization of the membranes[14,15] *in vitro*. In liver perfusion studies, disruption of the canalicular domain of liver plasma membrane occurred in perfusion concentrations as low as 0.3 mmol/L CDC, indicating that the bile salts are enriched in the hepatocyte, especially in this domain. When the CDC concentration was increased to 0.5 mmol/L, damage of cell organelles, like mitochondria, could be detected by electron microscopy (unpublished data).

MODE OF ACTION OF UDC

UDC and its conjugates could prevent the liver damage caused by apolar bile salts *in vivo* and *in vitro*[21–24]. The mechanisms by which UDC protects the liver against injury remain obscure. However, the fact that UDC therapy is of such uniform benefit in a broad variety of liver diseases argues for a more general hepatoprotective action. UDC could reduce the toxicity of apolar bile salts in a number of ways:

1. Changes in the bile acid pool composition during UDC therapy,
2. Hypercholoresis,
3. Activation of intracellular metabolic pathways,
4. Interaction of UDC with plasma membranes.

Changes in the bile acid pool composition during UDC therapy

Inhibition of intestinal uptake of more hydrophobic bile salts[25] and an increased fractional turnover rate in the enterohepatic circulation during UDC therapy[26] have been suggested to be responsible for the hepatoprotective effect of UDC. During UDC therapy, UDC becomes the dominant bile acid in serum and bile, comprising about 30–50% of the total bile acid pool[2,26]. The concentrations of the endogenous bile acids drop accordingly, although this does not occur to the same extent in all studies[2,26–28]. However, altered bile salt metabolism is not crucial for the hepatoprotective effect of UDC, since bile acid binding resins, such as cholestyramine (which also replaces apolar bile salts), do not lead to improvement in cholestatic liver diseases[29]. In addition, one clinical study showed that the drop in GLDH (an enzyme localized exclusively in liver mitochondria) during UDC therapy occurs prior to the decrease in apolar bile acids[30]. Furthermore, intravenous administration of UDC can also protect liver cells against damage induced by toxic bile salts[23]. This effect indicates that the mode of action of UDC is at the hepatocellular level.

Hypercholoresis

The role of choloresis in the hepatoprotective action of UDC appears to be minor. Unconjugated UDC does induce hypercholoresis, but this effect is abolished by conjugation[31]. In studies with the conjugated form, similar clinical results were obtained with cholestatic liver diseases. Furthermore, the choloretic potency of UDC is similar to that of other common bile salts, such as taurohydrocholate, which lacks its protective properties.

Activation of intracellular metabolic pathways

The effects of bile salts on metabolic activity and their compartmentation within the hepatocyte are currently a subject of active research. One interesting study of Beuers and collegues[32] has shown that TUDC leads to a sustained stimulation of biliary exocytosis following mobilization of extracellular Ca^{2+}. Thus, TUDC stimulates hepatocellular secretion by activating a Ca^{2+}- and PKC-dependent signal pathway. The relevance of this effect to the therapy of cholestatic liver diseases is still to be evaluated. UDC protects isolated hepatocytes, gastric cell cultures, and erythrocytes against the damaging effect of toxic bile salts[24,33]. These studies indicate that the protective effect of UDC is not dependent on liver metabolism, but seems to be of a more general nature.

Interaction of UDC with plasma membranes

Since the initial effects of bile salt toxicity were observed on hepatocyte plasma membranes, we focused our investigations on alterations of the plasma membrane. Hydrophobic bile salts increased the membrane permeability below the critical micellar concentration without causing solubilization of membrane lipids[14–15]. The increase in membrane permeability depended on the cholesterol content. Membranes without cholesterol and membranes with extremely high concentrations of cholesterol (cholesterol:phospholipid ratio above 0.7) were very sensitive to permeability changes induced by bile salts[14,15]. UDC was able to prevent the increased membrane permeability induced by hydrophobic bile salts[34]. In studies with electron paramagnetic resonance spectroscopy (EPR), we demonstrated that toxic bile salts create polar compartments in the apolar domain of the membrane bilayer, indicating the presence of membrane pores[35]. The increase in membrane polarity by bile salts also depends on the membrane cholesterol concentration[35]. Parallel to the experiments on measuring the membrane permeability, UDC and its conjugates also prevents the membrane polarity changes induced by toxic bile salts when measured using EPR[35]. This is important, since increased membrane permeability and polarity could cause an increase in intracellular Ca^{2+} and Mg^{2+} stores and thus induce hepatocellular apoptosis followed by cell death[17,18].

Membrane stabilization by UDC is due to membrane binding. The pKa of UDC is higher than that of CDC[36] and, in membranes, pH increases by several units[37,38]. Under physiological conditions, UDC is probably protonated and membrane bound. In NMR experiments, Saito *et al.* reported that α-dihydroxy bile salts are inserted into the membrane as dimers[39], whereas cholic acid molecules lie flat on the membrane surface[40]. In EPR experiments using different lipid spin labels, we found that the steroid nucleus of UDC is located in the apolar domain, whereas the conjugates bind at the interphase[35]. The binding site of UDC is similar to cholesterol.

Experiments with the differential scanning calorimetry (DSC) have shown that UDC influences the thermal behaviour of lipids[41]. As with cholesterol, UDC reduced the enthalpy and this was accompanied by a broadening of the transition peak[41,42]. These studies show that the protective effect of UDC is due to the decreased freedom of movement of the hydrocarbon chains. The stabilization and rigidization of the membrane by UDC could also impede the insertion of apolar bile salts and probably also of cholesterol. UDC stabilize model membranes, not only against the damaging effect of toxic bile salts, but also against gravitational and centrifugal forces in a similar fashion to cholesterol[42–44].

Since cholesterol is increased in hepatocyte plasma membranes, long-term administration of UDC could downregulate the membrane cholesterol content. Data on the membrane diffusion time of UDC are not available; however, this may be similar to that of cholic acid where $t_{1/2}$ is about 10–30 s[37,38], depending on the cholesterol concentration of the membrane[15,16].

Insertion of UDC into the membrane could preserve membrane function, e.g. HLA antigen expression or alterations in the activity of membrane-bound enzyme[45–47]. In *in-vitro* studies, HLA expression of hepatocytes and human gallbladder epithelial cells could be reduced by UDC and all the other bile salts[48,49]. This phenomenon could be induced by alterations in membrane structure or by a direct effect on RNA synthesis. However, data on quantitation of mRNA failed. Similar results on LDL-receptor expression were obtained by incubation of hamster hepatocytes at 4°C with UDC for 60 and 20 min. UDC led to increased receptor-dependent low density lipoprotein binding up to 3.5-fold[50].

CONCLUSIONS

UDC seems to have several different modes of action, both extra- and intracellularly. The similarities between cholesterol and UDC concerning their interaction with plasma membranes may be of relevance for the therapeutic effect of UDC. However, the next decade may well bring new insights into the role of UDC and other bile salts in pathophysiology and therapy of chronic liver diseases.

References

1. Leuschner U, Leuschner M, Sieratzki J *et al.* Gallstone dissolution with ursodeoxycholic acid in patients with chronic active hepatitis and two years follow-up. A pilot study. Dig Dis Sci. 1985;40:642–9.
2. Leuschner U, Fischer H, Kurtz W *et al.* Ursodeoxycholic acid in primary biliary cirrhosis: Results of a controlled double blind trial. Gastroenterology. 1989;87:1268–74.
3. Colombo C, Setchell KD, Podda M *et al.* Effects of ursodeoxycholic acid therapy for liver disease associated with cystic fibrosis. J Pediatr. 1990;117:482–9.
4. Chazouillères O, Poupon R, Capron J-P *et al.* Ursodeoxycholic acid for primary sclerosing cholangitis. J Hepatol. 1990;11:120–3.
5. Festi D, Labate AMM, Roda A *et al.* Diagnostic effectiveness of serum bile acids in liver diseases as evaluated by multivariate statistical methods. Hepatology. 1983;3:707–13.

6. Fromm H, Holtz-Slomczy KM, Zobi H. Studies of liver function and structure in patients with gallstones before and during treatment with chenodeoxycholic acid. Acta Hepatogastroenterol. 1975;22:359–69.
7. Greim H, Trülzsch D, Czygan P *et al.* Mechanism of cholestasis. 6. Bile acids in human livers with or without biliary obstruction. Gastroenterology. 1972;63:846–50.
8. Attili AF, Angelico M, Cantafora A, Alvaro D, Capocaccia L. Bile acid induced liver toxicity: relation to the hydrophobic balance of bile acids. Med Hypoth. 1986;19:57–69.
9. Drew R, Priestly BG. Choloretic and cholestatic effects of infused bile salts in the rat. Experientia. 1978;35:809.
10. Dryska H, Chen T, Salen G, Mosbach EH. Toxicity of chenodeoxycholic acid in the rhesus monkey. Gastroenterology. 1975;69:333–7.
11. Miyai K, Price VM, Fisher MM. Bile acid metabolism in mammals. Ultrastructural studies on intrahepatic cholestasis induced by lithocholic and chenodeoxycholic acids in the rat. Lab Invest. 1971;24:292–302.
12. Miyazaki K, Nakayama F, Koga A. Effect of chenodeoxycholic and ursodeoxycholic acid on isolated adult human hepatocytes. Dig Dis Sci. 1984;29:1123–30.
13. Hofman AF. Bile acid secretion, bile flow and biliary lipid secretion in humans. Hepatology. 1990;12:17S–25S.
14. Güldütuna S, Weiß A, Deisinger B *et al.* The effect of chenodeoxycholate (CDC) on large unilamellar vesicles (LUV) with variable cholesterol concentration. Gastroenterology. 1994;106:A902.
15. Schubert R, Schmidt KH. Structural changes in vesicle membranes and mixed micelles of various lipid compositions after binding of different bile salts. Biochemistry. 1988;27:8787–94.
16. Schubert R, Beyer K, Wolburg H, Schmidt KH. Structural changes in membranes of large unilamellar vesicles after binding of sodium cholate. Biochemistry. 1986;25:5263–9.
17. Anwer MS, Engelking LR, Nolan K *et al.* Hepatotoxic bile acids increase cytosolic calcium activity of isolated rat hepatocytes. Hepatology. 1991;8:887–91.
18. Patel T, Bronk SF, Gores GJ. Increases of intracellular magnesium promote glycodeoxycholate-induced apoptosis in rat hepatocytes. J Clin Invest. 1994;94:2183–92.
19. Keeffe EB, Scharschmidt BF, Blankenship NB, Ockner RK. Studies on relationship among bile flow, liver plasma membrane NaK-ATPase and membrane viscosity in the rat. J Clin Invest. 1979;64:1590–8.
20. Kanai S, Kitani K. Glycoursodeoxycholate (GU) is as effective as tauroursodeoxycholate (TU) in preventing the taurocholate induced cholestasis in the rat. (Abstract). Hepatology. 1983;3:810.
21. Kitani K, Ohta M, Kanai S. Tauroursodeoxycholate prevents biliary protein excretion induced by other bile salts in the rat. Am J Physiol. 1985;248:G407–17.
22. Kitani K, Kanai S. Effect of ursodeoxycholate on the bile flow in the rat. Life Sci. 1982;31:1973–85.
23. Kitani K, Kanai S. Tauroursodeoxycholate prevents taurocholate induced cholestasis in the rat. Life Sci. 1982;30:515–23.
24. Heuman DM, Pandak WM, Hylemon PB, Vlahcevic ZR. Conjugates of ursodeoxycholate protect against cytotoxicity of more hydrophobic bile salts: In vitro studies in rat hepatocytes and human erythrocytes. Hepatology. 1991;14:920–6.
25. Eusufzai S, Ericson S, Cederlund T *et al.* Effect of ursodeoxycholic acid treatment on ileal absorption of bile acids in man as determined by the SeHCAT test. Gut. 1991;32:1044–8.
26. Mazzella G, Parini P, Bazzoli F *et al.* Ursodeoxycholic acid administration on bile acid metabolism in patients with early stages of primary biliary cirrhosis. Dig Dis Sci. 1993;38:896–902.
27. Stiehl A, Rudolph G, Raedsch R *et al.* Ursodeoxycholic acid-induced changes of plasma and urinary bile acids in patients with primary biliary cirrhosis. Hepatology. 1990;3:482–7.
28. Crosignani A, Podda M, Battezzati PM *et al.* Changes in the acid composition in patients with primary biliary cirrhosis induced by ursodeoxycholic acid administration. Hepatology. 1991;14:1000–7.
29. Carey JBJ, Williams G. Relief in the pruritus of jaundice with a bile acid sequestering resin. JAMA. 1961;176:432–5.
30. Güldütuna S, Leuschner M, Wunderlich N. Cholic acid and ursodeoxycholic acid therapy in primary biliary cirrhosis. Changes in bile acid pattern and their correlation with liver function. Eur J Clin Pharmacol. 1993;45:221–5.
31. Erlinger S. Hypercholoretic bile acids: a clue to the mechanism. Hepatology. 1990;11:888–90.

32. Beuers U, Nathanson MH, Boyer JL. Effects of tauroursodeoxycholic acid on cytosolic Ca^{++} signals in isolated rat hepatocytes. Gastroenterology. 1993;104:604–12.
33. Ota S, Tsukahara H, Terano A *et al.* Protective effect of tauroursodeoxycholate against chenodeoxycholate-induced damage to cultured rabbit gastric cells. Dig Dis Sci. 1991;36:409–16.
34. Güldütuna S, Weiß A, Deisinger B *et al.* Ursodeoxycholate (UDC) mimics the membrane stabilizing effect of cholesterol on large unilamellar vesicles (LUV). Gastroenterology. 1994;106:A902.
35. Güldütuna S, Zimmer G, Imhof M, Bhatti S, You T, Leuschner U. Molecular aspects of membrane stabilization by ursodeoxycholate. Gastroenterology. 1993;104:1736–44.
36. Igimi H, Carey MC. Ph-solubility relations of chenodeoxycholic and ursodeoxycholic acids: physical–chemical basis for dissimilar solution and membrane phenomena. 1980;21:72–90.
37. Kamp F, Hamilton JA. Movement of fatty acid analogues, and bile acids across phospholipid bilayers. Biochemistry. 1993;32:11074–86.
38. Cabral DJ, Small DM, Lilly HS, Hamilton JA. Transbilayer movement of bile acids in model membranes. Biochemistry. 1987;26:1801–4.
39. Saito H, Sugimoto Y, Tabeta R *et al.* Incorporation of bile acids of low concentration into model and biological membranes studied by ^{2}H and ^{31}P NMR. J Biochem (Tokyo). 1983;94:1877–87.
40. Ulmius J, Lindblom G, Wennerström H *et al.* Molecular organization in the liquid-crystalline phases of lecithin–sodium cholate–water systems studied by nuclear magnetic resonance. Biochemistry. 1982;21:1553–60.
41. Güldütuna S, Deisinger B, Weiß A, Sippos P, Freisleben HJ, Leuschner U. Ursodeoxycholate (UDC) mimics the effect of cholesterol on the phase transition of egg yolk lecithin (EYL). Hepatology. 1994;20:A1029.
42. Yeagle PL. Cholesterol and the cell membrane. Biochim Biophys Acta. 1985;822:267–87.
43. Güldütuna S, Deisinger B, Weiß A, Sippos P, Freisleben HJ, Leuschner U. Cholesterol like effects of ursodeoxycholate (UDC) on large unilamellar vesicles (LUV). Hepatology. 1994;20:A262.
44. El-Sayed MY, Guion TA, Fayer MD. Effect of cholesterol on visoelastic properties of dipalmitoylphosphatidylcholine multibilayers as measured by laser-induced ultrasonic probe. Biochemistry. 1986;25:4825–30.
45. Leuschner U, Güldütuna S, Dienes HP *et al.* Bile acids during treatment of primary biliary cirrhosis: Ursodeoxycholic acid improves membrane stability and influences immune reactions in liver tissue. In: Paumgartner G, Stiehl A, Gerok W, eds. Bile acids as therapeutic agents. Lancaster, UK: Kluwer Academic Publ.; 1991:297–9.
46. Schachter D. Fluidity and function of hepatocyte plasma membranes. Hepatology. 1984;4:140–51.
47. Smith DJ, Gordon ER. Membrane fluidity and cholestasis. J Hepatol. 1987;5:362–5.
48. Töx U, Arnold JC, Otto G, Theilmann L, Kommerell B, Stiehl A. Differences in the effect of ursodeoxycholic acid and chenodeoxycholic acid on the expression of HLA-molecules of human primary hepatocytes. XIII International Bile Acid Meeting, San Diego, Poster Abstracts. 1994:51.
49. Gökce Y, Güldütuna S, Hottenrott C, Leuschner U. The effect of bile acids on HLA-antigens of human gallbladder epithelial cells (GBECs) in vitro. Gastroenterology. [In press].
50. Bouscarel B, Fromm H, Ceryak S, Cassidy MM. Ursodeoxycholic acid increases low density lipoprotein binding, uptake and degradation in isolated hamster hepatocytes. Biochem J. 1991;280:589.

29
Treatment of primary biliary cirrhosis with ursodeoxycholic acid: adjuvant therapeutic strategies are required

U. LEUSCHNER, S. GÜLDÜTUNA, S. BHATTI and M. LEUSCHNER

INTRODUCTION

In 1981 we introduced ursodeoxycholic acid (UDCA) therapy into the treatment of chronic active hepatitis[1] and in 1985 into the treatment of primary biliary cirrhosis (PBC), primary sclerosing cholangitis and Caroli's syndrome[2]. In the first prospective, placebo-controlled trial[3] we were able to show significantly lowered transaminases, cholestasis enzymes and IgM, but UDCA had no influence on antimitochondrial antibodies and no significant effect on liver histology. The therapeutic dose used was 10 mg/kg body weight daily[1–3], which is still considered to be an optimal therapeutic dosage. Nine controlled studies[4–12] revealed no significant new aspects, except that in some patients serum bilirubin also decreased (Table 1). In a long-term trial covering a maximum of 12 years[13] we demonstrated that withdrawal of UDCA induced a marked rebound effect, and that in the late stages of PBC complications typical of cirrhosis would develop, although laboratory values remained low. Thus UDCA obviously did not cure the disease; however, it had no side-effects even after 12 years of treatment.

If we summarize the positive results of these trials then we can conclude that UDCA lowers serum levels of liver enzymes, bilirubin (in our trials this was elevated only in a few patients) and IgM, and causes no side-effects.

Problems and open questions regarding UDCA therapy

The therapeutic goals of UDCA treatment are usually quoted under the following five headings:

1. improvement of symptoms,
2. improvement of liver histology,
3. prolongation of the time span up to liver transplantation,
4. prolongation of life expectancy,
5. complete cure.

Table 1 UDC treatment in primary biliary cirrhosis: controlled trials

First author, date	*No. of patients*	*PBC stage*	*Dose per (mg/kg per day)*	*Duration of treatment (months)*	*Laboratory tests*	*Histology*	*Time until transplantation*
Leuschner, 1989	20	I–III	10	9	+	(n.s.+)	0
Hadziyannis, 1989	45	II–IV	12–15	12	+/–	(+)/–	(n.s.+)
Oka, 1990	45	I–IV	8–12	6	+	0	0
Combes, 1993	153	I–IV	Bili <2 mg%	24	+	+	0
			Bili >2 mg%	24	(+)	–	0
Battezzati, 1993	88	I–III	8.7	12	+	0	0
Hwang, 1993	12	I–IV	10	3	+	0	0
Turner, 1993	64	I–IV	10	24	+	(n.s.+)	0
Poupon, 1994	145	I–IV	13–15	24/24 open	+[a]	+	+
Heathcote, 1994	222	I–IV	14	24	+	(n.s.+)	(n.s.+)
Lindor, 1994	180	I–IV	13–15	48	+	–	(n.s.+)

(n.s.+), not significant, but positive trend;
+, significant improvement;
–, no therapeutic effect;
0, not investigated.
[a] Previous evaluation (1991).

At present none of these therapeutic goals has been attained, although UDCA has now been prescribed for the treatment of PBC for more than 10 years.

Symptoms

The influence of UDCA on symptoms is assessed unequally in the individual trials (Table 2). The symptoms listed include not only pruritus, but also uncharacteristic abdominal complaints and fatigue, which are not well defined and are therefore difficult to assess. One study from 1991 reported a positive effect on symptoms; however, in the final evaluation in 1994 this effect is no longer quoted.

Histology

A significant improvement in histological findings has been found in only one out of 10 controlled trials with approximately 1000 patients (Table 1[10]). In three further studies there was a trend towards improvement[3,9,11] and in one study[6] improvement was found in patients with serum bilirubin levels below 2 mg%. We conclude from these results that it is not justified to assume that UDCA has a positive influence on histology. This is basically for two reasons: in the majority of studies no morphometric investigations were performed; instead the results were assessed according to a simple score system. However, since different PBC stages can occur simultaneously in one organ one would in fact need to take nine liver biopsies simultaneously in order to get a sustained verdict[14], and this is obviously not possible. Therefore, in order to state that UDCA has a positive influence on histology, this needs to be confirmed by highly significant results of several well-documented studies.

Time span until liver transplantation and life expectancy

The prolongation of the time up to liver transplantation has also hitherto been positively assessed in only one out of four studies covering this aspect[10]. In three further studies there was a positive trend[4,11,12]. A recently presented summary of these three studies[10–12,15] has shown a significant prolongation of the time up to liver transplantation under UDCA; however, the result needs to be critically assessed, for three reasons: (a) it is not known whether in all three studies the time span of the disease up to transplantation was of the same duration; (b) it is not certain whether the criteria for transplantation were the same in all three centres, and (c) although the results were statistically significant ($p = 0.014$), UDCA led to an absolute prolongation of life of only 2–3 months (3.66 vs. 3.45 years). It seems doubtful whether this result is of clinical relevance in a disease that has a natural course of up to 20 years. Likewise, a prolongation of life expectancy has not yet been described under UDCA therapy. However, since the natural course of the disease is not well documented, and all future patients will undergo liver transplantation before a drastic deterioration of the disease takes place, the effect of UDCA therapy on life expectancy can no longer be investigated. Nevertheless, in one study[13] it was shown that UDCA might prevent the development of oesophageal varices, splenomegaly and ascites in stages I and II. The results of this study could be compared only to results from the literature, as no untreated control group was available.

Table 2 Influence of UDC on symptoms in primary biliary cirrhosis: results of controlled trials

First author, date	*No. of patients*	*Dose (mg/kg per day)*	*Months*	*Symptoms*	*Improved*	*Worsened*	*Result*
Leuschner, 1989	20	10	9	Pruritus	2/3 UDC, 1/2 placebo	–	Positive
				Well-being	8/10 UDC, 4/7 placebo		
Hadziyannis, 1989	45	12–15	12	Pruritus	83% UDC, 26% no therapy		Positive
Oka, 1990	45	8–12	6	Pruritus	4/9 UDC, 2/7 placebo		Negative
Combes, 1993	153	10–12	24	Pruritus	UDC, Bili <2 mg%	placebo	Positive
Battezzati, 1993	88	8, 7	12	Pruritus	11/25 UDC 5/19 placebo	2/25 UDC 1/19 placebo	Negative
Hwang, 1993	12	10	3	Pruritus	90% UDC	100% placebo	Positive
Turner, 1993	64	10	24	Pruritus	No effect		Negative
				Well-being	No effect		
Poupon, 1994	145	13–15	24	Not given	But positive effects in the study from 1991		
Heathcote, 1994	222	14	24	Pruritus Fatigue	No differences between UDC and placebo group		Negative
Lindor, 1994	180	13–15	48	Pruritus	18/71	15/71	Negative
				Fatigue	23/71	10/71	

To the present date there has been no report of a cure. The rebound effect which occurred even after $5\frac{1}{2}$ years of continuous UDCA therapy when treatment was discontinued[13] indicates that UDCA has no influence on the pathogenic mechanisms underlying PBC or the influence of UDCA was too weak due to an insufficient therapeutic dosage. However, there are no controlled long-term trials with higher dosages of UDCA.

After 10 years administration of UDCA we can safely say that at present UDCA is the preferable treatment for the therapy of PBC. It can be given for many years without any side-effects; however, UDCA alone will not solve the problem of treatment of primary biliary liver diseases, and it is therefore essential to look for other therapy concepts. In future we should consider treatment with UDCA conjugates or the combination of UDCA with immunosuppressive and antifibrotic substances.

NEW PERSPECTIVES FOR THE TREATMENT OF PBC WITH UDCA

There are no clinical studies available with tauro- or glycoursodeoxycholate. Four studies have been performed with UDCA and colchicine[16–19]. The results were unequal, the histology did not improve[16]. Similarly, treatment with UDCA and methotrexate produced no real improvement compared to the results of UDCA monotherapy[20–22]. Combination of UDCA with prednisolone has been examined in only one study in six patients retrospectively[23] and another study using a triple combination of UDCA, azathioprine and prednisolone has not yet been completed[24] In our own trial (submitted for publication) with UDCA and prednisolone we found a highly significant improvement in liver histology compared to monotherapy with UDCA and placebo (Table 3), a result not found in any of our previous three trials with monotherapy[2,3,13]. The histological results of this prospective double-blind trial correspond to the results of an earlier trial with prednisolone monotherapy[25], which suggests that combination of UDCA with immunosuppressive and/or antifibrotic substances could improve the effect of UDCA. Thus we appear to be faced with a new therapeutic concept that might be further enhanced by the above-mentioned triple therapy[24].

SUMMARY

Today ursodeoxycholic acid is the preferable treatment for the therapy of primary biliary cirrhosis, despite the fact that several goals, such as improvement of histology, prolongation of time up to liver transplantation, prolongation of life expectancy, and a cure for the disease, cannot yet be reached. It is possible that combination of UDCA with immunosuppressive and antifibrotic substances could be helpful, as suggested by the preliminary results of recent studies.

Table 3 Treatment of primary biliary cirrhosis with combination therapy

First author, date	*Therapy*	*Design*	*No. of patients*	*Histology*	*Laboratory data*
Schaffner, 1991	UDCA, colch vs. colch	O	45	n.i.	+
Shibata, 1992	UDCA, colch vs. UDCA	O	12	n.i.	–
Raedsch, 1993	UDCA, colch vs. UDCA	RCT	22	–	–
Podda, 1993	UDCA, colch vs. UDCA	RCT	88	–	–
Kaplan, 1992	UDCA, MTX vs. MTX	O	14	n.i.	+
Buscher, 1993	UDCA, MTX vs. UDCA	O	8	n.i.	+
van Steenbergen, 1994	UDCA, MTX vs. no therapy	O	14	–	+
Wolfhagen, 1994	UDCA, pred	r	7	n.i.	+
Leuschner, 1995	UDCA, pred vs. UDCA	RCT	30	+	+
Dutch Multicentre Study	UDCA, pred, aza vs. UDCA	RCT	41	on-going study	on-going study

Aza, azathioprine; colch, colchicine; MTX, methotrexate; pred, prednisolone, UDCA, ursodeoxycholic acid; O, open; RCT, randomized controlled trials; r, retrospective evaluation; n.i., not investigated; –, no difference; +, improved.

References

1. Leuschner U, Leuschner M, Hübner K. Gallstone dissolution in patients with chronic active hepatitis. Gastroenterology 1981;80:1208 (abstract).
2. David R, Kurtz W, Strohm WD, Leuschner U. Die Wirkung von Ursodesoxycholsäure bei chronischen Leberkrankheiten. Z Gastroenterol. 1985;23:420 (abstract).
3. Leuschner U, Fischer H, Kurtz W *et al.* Ursodeoxycholic acid in primary biliary cirrhosis: results of a controlled double blind trial. Gastroenterology. 1989;97:1268–74.
4. Hadziyannis SJ, Hadziyannis ES, Lianidou E, Markis A. Long-term treatment of primary biliary cirrhosis with ursodeoxycholic acid: the third year of a controlled trial. In: Paumgartner G, Stiehl A, Gerok W, editors.: Bile acids as therapeutic agents. Dordrecht: Kluwer; 1991:287–96.
5. Oka H, Toda G. Ikeda Y *et al.* A multi-center double-blind controlled trial of ursodeoxycholic acid for primary biliary cirrhosis. Gastroenterol Jpn. 1990;25:774–80.
6. Combes B, Carithers RL, Maddrey WC *et al.* A randomized, double-blind, placebo-controlled trial of ursodeoxycholic acid in primary biliary cirrhosis. In: Paumgartner G, Stiehl A, Gerok W, editors.: Bile acids and the hepatobiliary system. Dordrecht: Kluwer; 1993:289–91.
7. Battezzati PM, Podda M, Bianchi FB *et al.* Ursodeoxycholic acid for symptomatic primary biliary cirrhosis. Preliminary analysis of a double-blind multicenter trial. J Hepatol. 1993;17:332–8.
8. Hwang S-J, Chan C-Y, Lee S-D, Wu J-C, Tsay S-H, Lo K-J. Ursodeoxycholic acid in the treatment of primary biliary cirrhosis: a short-term, randomized, double blind controlled, cross-over study with long-term follow up. J Gastroenterol Hepatol. 1993;8:217–23.
9. Turner IB, Myszor M, Mitchison HC, Bennet MK, Burt AD, James OFW. A two year controlled trial examining the effectiveness of ursodeoxycholic acid in primary biliary cirrhosis. J Gastroenterol Hepatol. 1994;4:162–8.
10. Poupon RE, Poupon R, Balkau B, and the UDC–PBC Study Group. Ursodiol for the long-term treatment of primary biliary cirrhosis. N Engl J Med. 1994;300:1342–7.
11. Heathcote EJ, Cauch-Dudek K, Walker V *et al.* The Canadian multicenter double-blind randomized controlled trial of ursodeoxycholic acid in primary biliary cirrhosis. Hepatology. 1994;19:1149–56.

12. Lindor KD, Dickson ER, Baldus WP *et al.* Ursodeoxycholic acid in the treatment of primary biliary cirrhosis. Gastroenterology. 1994;106:1284–90.
13. Leuschner U, Güldütuna S, Imhof M, Hübner K, Benjaminov A, Leuschner M. Effects of ursodeoxycholic acid after 4 to 12 years therapy in early and late stages of primary biliary cirrhosis. J Hepatol. 1994;21:624–33.
14. Leuschner U. Ursodeoxycholic acid therapy in primary biliary cirrhosis. Scand J Gastroenterol. 1994;29(Suppl. 204):40–6.
15. Heathcote EJ, Lindor KD, Poupon ER *et al.* Combined analysis of French, American and Canadian randomized controlled trials of ursodeoxycholic acid therapy in primary biliary cirrhosis. AGA, 14–17 May 1995 (abstract).
16. Raedsch R, Stiehl A, Walker S *et al.* Controlled study on the effects of a combined ursodeoxycholic acid plus colchicine treatment in primary biliary cirrhosis. In: Paumgartner G, Stiehl A, Gerok W, editors. Bile acids and the hepatobiliary system. Dordrecht: Kluwer; 1993:303–9.
17. Podda M, Almasio P, Battezzati PM, Crosignani A and the Italian multicentre group for the study of UDC in PBC. Long-term effect of the administration of ursodeoxycholic acid alone or with colchicine in patients with primary biliary cirrhosis. A double-blind multicenter study. In: Paumgartner G, Stiehl A, Gerok W, editors. Bile acids and the hepatobiliary system. Dordrecht: Kluwer; 1993:310–15.
18. Shibata J, Fujiyama S, Honda Y, Sato T. Combination therapy with ursodeoxycholic acid and colchicine for primary biliary cirrhosis. J Gastroenterol Hepatol. 1992;7:277–82.
19. Schaffner F. Ursodeoxycholic acid (U) + colchicine (C) for treatment of primary biliary cirrhosis (PBC). Hepatology. 1991;14:62A (abstract).
20. Kaplan MM. The therapeutic effects of ursodiol and methotrexate are additive and well tolerated in primary biliary cirrhosis. Hepatology. 1992;16:92A (abstract).
21. Buscher H-P, Zietzschmann Y, Gerok W. Positive responses to methotrexate and ursodeoxycholic acid in patients with primary biliary cirrhosis responding insufficiently to ursodeoxycholic acid alone. J Hepatol. 1993;18:9–14.
22. Van Steenbergen W, Sciot R, van Eyken P, Desmet V, Fevery J. Methotrexate alone or in combination with ursodeoxycholic acid as possible treatment in primary biliary cirrhosis. In: Van Berge Henegouwen GP, van Hoek B, de Groote J, Matern S, editors. Cholestatic liver diseases. New strategies for prevention and treatment of hepatobiliary and cholestatic liver diseases. Dordrecht: Kluwer; 1994:246–54.
23. Wolfhagen FHJ, van Buuren HR, Schalm SW. Combined treatment with ursodeoxycholic acid and prednisolone in primary biliary cirrhosis. Neth J Med. 1994;44:84–90.
24. Van Buuren HR, Wolfhagen FHJ, Schalm SW. Treatment with ursodeoxycholic acid, as monotherapy and in combination with other agents, in primary biliary cirrhosis. In: Van Berge Henegouwen GP, van Hoek B, de Groote J, Matern S, editors. Cholestatic liver diseases. New strategies for prevention and treatment of hepatobiliary and cholestatic liver diseases. Dordrecht: Kluwer; 1994:236–45.
25. Mitchison HC, Palmer JM, Bassendine MF, Watson AJ, Record CO, James OFW. A controlled trial of prednisolone treatment in primary biliary cirrhosis. Three-year results. J Hepatol. 1992;15:336–44.

30
The Netherlands Multicentre Trial on ursodeoxycholic acid in primary biliary cirrhosis

F. H. J. WOLFHAGEN and G. P. VAN BERGE-HENEGOUWEN for the DUTCH MULTICENTRE PBC STUDY GROUP

INTRODUCTION

Primary biliary cirrhosis (PBC) is usually a slowly progressive disease of unknown cause with many features of an autoimmune disorder. Initially there is mainly involvement of the small intrahepatic bile ducts; in the later stages progressive fibrosis and ultimately cirrhosis with secondary copper overload may develop[1].

Ursodeoxycholic acid (UDCA) is nowadays considered as the first-line treatment option for PBC. Several controlled trials have shown clear beneficial effects of UDCA on biochemical and immunological parameters in PBC[2–7]. Uncontrolled studies suggested impressive amelioration of symptoms, but this effect was less convincing in controlled studies[2,7]. Some studies have also indicated improvement in liver histology[2,3]. Reports of up to 4 years of placebo-controlled follow-up showed no improvements in survival[8–10], although in one study significantly less liver transplants were performed in patients receiving UDCA during 4 years compared to patients with 2 years of UDCA[10]. Current data suggest that UDCA slows down the progression of the disease, but does not seem capable of inducing a complete inactivation of the disease in most patients.

Due to the protracted course and relative rarity of the disease, trials evaluating survival are hardly feasible, and alternative parameters to assess treatment efficacy are needed. It seems likely that any drug which could potentially alter the natural course of the disease should exert marked effects on clinical, biochemical and histological parameters. In analogy with other autoimmune diseases, e.g. chronic active autoimmune hepatitis, disease remission has therefore been proposed as the first and main treatment goal in PBC[11,12]. Surprisingly, no studies have been published evaluating the potential of UDCA to induce disease remission. This prospective study was initiated to assess how many patients with

PBC achieve a complete (symptomatic, biochemical and histological) remission during UDCA treatment.

PATIENTS AND METHODS

In October 1990 a prospective multicentre study was initiated in The Netherlands to evaluate new treatments in PBC. The design of this project aims to reflect the general therapeutic approach to diseases for which no established effective treatment is available: patients are first treated with the current best monotherapy, and when this is not sufficiently effective are offered an alternative (or additional) treatment. Patients who do not satisfactorily respond to the standard therapy, *in casu* UDCA, are candidates, for subsequent enrolment in controlled evaluations of additional new treatment options. To date 180 patients in 38 centres (four university and 34 non-university clinics) are participating in this project.

The first 110 patients completing the first phase of the project, i.e. an open 1-year study with UDCA, are the subjects of this report. Before the start of the study it was determined that the first evaluation would be performed as soon as the complete follow-up data of at least 100 patients became available.

Patient selection

Newly diagnosed patients, as well as patients with a longer-standing diagnosis of PBC, were included. Patients who were already being treated with UDCA were withdrawn from this treatment for at least 3 months before entry.

PBC was diagnosed when two major and two minor diagnostic criteria, or one major and four minor criteria, according to Taal *et al.*[13], were present. Major criteria are: level of antimitochondrial antibodies ≥1/20 and liver biopsy showing duct lesions. Minor criteria are: pruritus, jaundice with normal clotting factors, alkaline phosphatase ≥2 × upper limit of normal, serum IgM above normal, Schirmer test showing <10 mm tear secretion in 5 min. Exclusion criteria were: age >75 years, presence of another life-expectancy-limiting disease, evidence of extrahepatic bile duct disease on ultrasound, pregnancy or risk of pregnancy due to lack of suitable contraception, absence of manifest disease (= fulfilment of criteria for complete response – see below) and the use of UDCA within 3 months prior to entry. Furthermore patients with advanced disease (Child–Pugh class B or C) were excluded, as these patients are likely candidates for liver transplantation in the near future and in general seem unlikely to benefit from medical treatment[12].

Study design

Patients received UDCA (Ursochol® 300 mg tablets; Zambon BV, Amersfoort, The Netherlands) as one bedtime dose. The dose was adjusted according to body weight: 450 mg if <50 kg, 600 mg if 50–70 kg and 750 mg if >70 kg, thus corresponding to ± 10 mg/kg daily.

At entry, and at 3-monthly follow-up visits, a clinical examination was performed, including assessment of pruritus and fatigue as either being absent or present, and laboratory investigations (bilirubin, alkaline phosphatase (APh), aspartate aminotransferases (AST) and IgM). Furthermore creatinine, albumin, Hb, WBC, platelets, prothrombin time, and antithrombin-III were measured at entry.

For all patients admitted to the study liver biopsies were available for diagnostic review. Considering the non-controlled design of the study it was decided not to insist on performing a new liver biopsy at entry. For this study evaluation of repeat biopsies was demanded only in patients who had attained both symptomatic and biochemical remission after 1 year of UDCA, as it is unlikely that patients with clinical disease activity will have a histological remission. All biopsies were reviewed by one pathologist, who was not aware of the clinical results.

Definitions for remission as proposed by Beukers and Schalm were used[12]. These include disappearance of PBC-related complaints, especially pruritus and fatigue, (*symptomatic remission*); normal values for bilirubin, AST and IgM, with APh not exceeding 1.5 × the upper limit of normal (*biochemical remission*), and inflammatory infiltrate absent or restricted to the portal tracts without bile duct destruction and absence of granulomas (*histological remission*). *Complete remission* was defined as symptomatic, biochemical ànd histological remission.

A steering committee was established to address scientific, methodological and ethical problems arising during the study. Informed consent was obtained from each patient and the study was approved by all local ethical committees.

Statistical analysis

Quantitative data are expressed as multiples of the upper limit of normal (ULN) of each centre. Differences between the levels at entry and after 1 year were analysed using the Wilcoxon signed-rank test. Differences in the number of patients with abnormal parameters and complaints between entry and 1 year were compared by McNemar's-test. A p-value ≤ 0.05 was considered significant.

RESULTS

At the time of evaluation 104 of the 110 included patients had completed one year of treatment with UDCA (Fig. 1).

Six patients stopped treatment and were excluded from analysis; four of them stopped UDCA treatment because of supposed adverse effects: three patients experienced abdominal discomfort (nausea, vomiting) and one had increased itching, fatigue and malaise not responding to dose reduction; two asymptomatic patients were no longer motivated to continue the medication. In five of the six patients, biochemical abnormalities clearly improved during UDCA, and deteriorated after withdrawal. None of them attained a spontaneous clinical remission.

Deterioration of disease (defined as doubling of bilirubin, decrease of albumin >6 g/l, variceal bleeding, ascites, death or liver transplantation according to Mitchison *et al.*[14] was noted in one non-cirrhotic patient who showed a decrease of albumin of 10 g/l. Main entry characteristics of the 110 included, as well as the 104 evaluated patients, are given in Table 1.

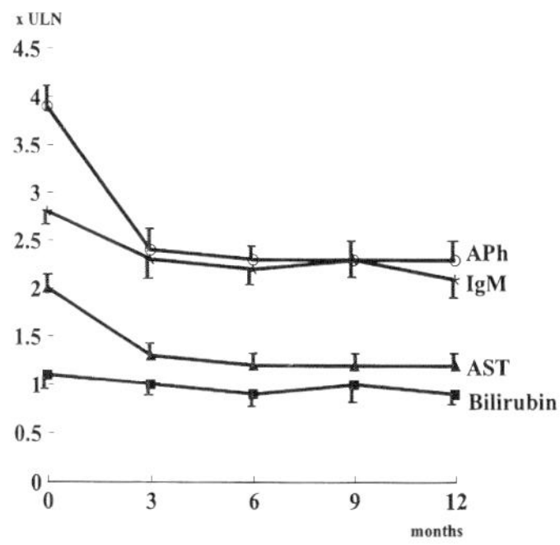

Fig. 1 Changes (means ± SE) in bilirubin, APh, AST and IgM in 104 patients completing 1 year of UDCA treatment. All parameters improved significantly (bilirubin $p = 0.02$, others all $p<0.001$)

Table 1 Patient characteristics at entry

	Patients included	*Patients evaluated*
No. of patients	110	104
Median range age (years)	58 [33–75]	58 [33–75]
Median [range] disease duration (years)	5 [0–19]	5 [0–17]
No. of males	14 (13%)	14 (14%)
Histology		
Cirrhosis[a]	20 (18%)	20 (19%)
No cirrhosis[b]	39 (36%)	39 (38%)
No recent data	51 (46%)	45 (43%)

[a]As histologically documented previously.
[b]Liver biopsy performed <1 year before entry.

Symptomatic remission

Numbers and percentages of patients with pruritus and fatigue at entry and after 1 year are shown in Table 2. At entry 63% (65/104) of the patients complained of fatigue and 42% (44/104) of itching. After 1 year these figures were 49% (51/104) and 29% (30/104), respectively. This decrease was significant for both fatigue ($p<0.03$) and pruritus ($p<0.01$). The percentage of symptomatic patients significantly decreased from 68% (71/104) to 51% (53/104) ($p<0.01$).

Biochemical remission

Bilirubin ($p = 0.02$), APh, AST and IgM (all $p<0.001$) improved significantly during the year of treatment (Fig. 1). There were no differences in changes between cirrhotic and non-cirrhotic patients.

The number and percentage of patients with abnormal biochemical parameters at entry and after 1 year are shown in Table 2. After 12 months of treatment 29 patients had only one abnormal parameter: IgM was still elevated in 19, APh was more than 1.5 times the upper normal value in eight and AST was still above normal in two patients.

Table 2 Presence of symptoms and abnormal biochemical parameters at entry and 1 year

	Entry	*1 year*	p-*Value*[a]
Symptoms			
Pruritus	42% (44/104)	29% (30/104)	<0.03
Fatigue	63% (65/104)	49% (51/104)	<0.01
Biochemical parameters			
Bilirubin	32% (33/104)	26% (27/104)	>0.1
APh	96% (100/104)	60% (62/104)	<0.001
AST	86% (89/104)	42% (44/104)	<0.001
IgM	93% (97/104)	75% (78/104)	<0.001

[a]*p* Value with respect to the difference between entry and 1 year of treatment within each group (McNemar's test).

Twelve of the 104 (12%) patients achieved a biochemical remission on UDCA. The majority of these patients had mild liver function abnormalities at entry, and all had normal bilirubin levels. Characteristics at entry of these patients are given in Table 3.

At 12 months 10 of the 12 patients with a biochemical remission were without pruritus and seven did not have fatigue at 12 months. One patient had developed

Table 3 Characteristics at entry of patients attaining biochemical, symptomatic and/or histological remission

No.	*Age (years)*	*Sex*	*Histological stage*	*Disease duration (years)*	*Bili*	*APh* (× ULN)	*AST* (× ULN)	*IgM*	*Pruritus (yes/no)*	*Fatigue (yes/no)*
Biochemical remission										
1.	56	f	III	<0.5	0.8	4.1	2.8	1.9	Yes	Yes
2.	73	f	III	10	0.7	2.0	1.0	0.7	Yes	Yes
3.	51	f	II	<0.5	0.4	2.0	0.9	4.0	Yes	Yes
4.	71	f	–[a]	15	0.8	2.2	0.9	1.3	No	No
5.	57	f	II	1	0.3	4.1	0.9	0.6	No	No
Biochemical and symptomatic remission										
6.	56	f	I	5	0.2	1.8	0.6	1.4	No	No
7.	75	f	II	<0.5	0.5	1.7	1.1	1.4	No	Yes
8.[b]	61	f	–[a]	9	0.7	2.1	0.9	1.2	No	No
9.	53	f	I	8	0.5	1.8	0.7	1.5	No	Yes
Biochemical, symptomatic and histological remission										
10.	66	f	–[a]	10	0.7	1.7	1.3	2.0	No	Yes
11.	46	m	IV	<0.5	0.7	1.0	1.4	1.0	No	Yes
12.	69	f	I	<0.5	0.5	2.8	1.3	0.6	No	No

[a]No liver biopsy within 1 year before entry available and no cirrhosis established in previous biopsies.
[b]No liver biopsy after UDCA treatment available.

persistent fatigue after 3 months of treatment, which seemed to be (at least partly) attributable to an intercurrent vital depression; therefore 7/104 (7%) patients achieved a symptomatic and biochemical remission.

Histological remission

One patient died of cardiac arrest shortly after her 1-year visit; a liver biopsy was performed in the remaining six patients with a symptomatic and biochemical remission. One patient displayed no histological signs of active PBC and presented only aspecific reactive changes (slight portal and periportal fibrosis). In the other five patients a predominantly lymphocellular portal infiltrate was found. In three of them the infiltrate affected the biliary epithelium, without evidence of actual bile duct destruction; in one of these three patients granulomas were found, and in another patient granulomas and a periportal infiltrate with piecemeal necrosis. In the remaining two patients the biliary epithelium was not affected by the portal infiltrate; in one of them a periportal infiltrate with piecemeal necrosis was found. Thus the criteria for histological remission were fulfilled in three of the six biopsied patients.

Complete (biochemical, symptomatic and histological) remission

Seven of the 110 initial patients (6%; 95% confidence interval 2–10%) achieved biochemical and symptomatic remission, and three patients also attained histological remission. The patient in whom no biopsy could be performed might also have attained a histological remission; thus the maximal number of patients attaining a complete remission according to our criteria was four (4%; 95% CI 0–8%) (Fig. 2).

DISCUSSION

The results of this study confirm the already well-established effects of UDCA on biochemical and immunological parameters of the disease in a homogeneous group of patients with non-advanced PBC. However, despite these marked overall improvements in laboratory parameters, an assessment of the effect of UDCA on an individual basis shows that a biochemical, symptomatic and histological inactivation of the disease is rarely achieved. Our results further suggest that a remission may occur only in patients with mild disease activity. It is also clear that, although the number of symptomatic patients decreased, a large number of patients remain symptomatic on UDCA treatment.

To define remission we used recently proposed, strict criteria[12]. These criteria are based on the definitions which have been extensively used in chronic autoimmune hepatitis[15]. Since PBC is a cholestatic disorder with primarily involvement of the bile ducts, the criteria were slightly modified, especially with regard to alkaline phosphatase.

To the best of our knowledge this is the first study in PBC in which the main outcome variable was remission of disease. This might be due to the absence of generally accepted criteria for remission. Obviously the validity of these

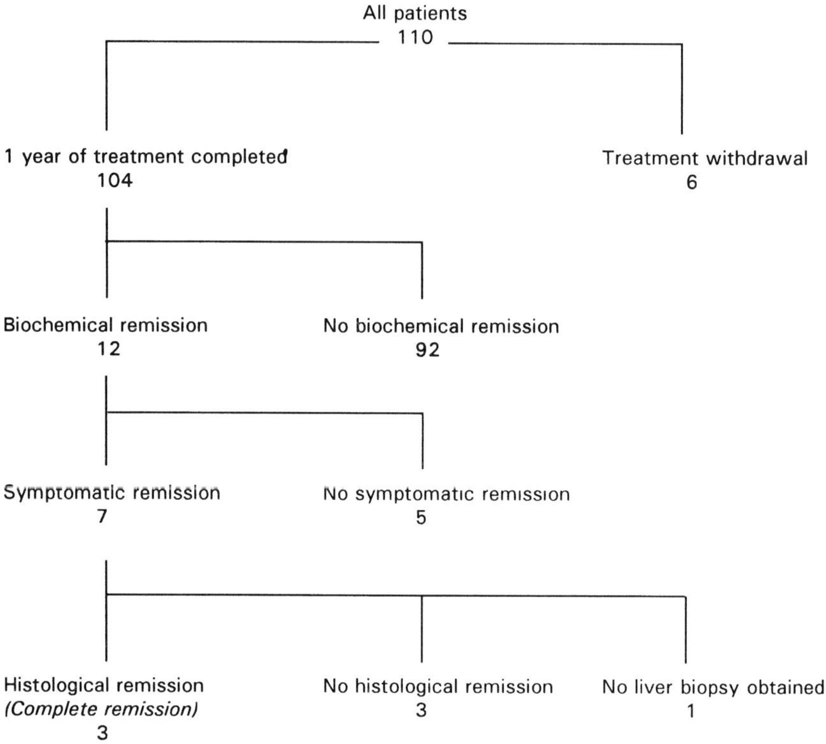

Fig. 2 Flowchart of the 110 patients entering the study, indicating the number of patients stopping treatment and of patients attaining biochemical, clinical (biochemical + symptomatic) and complete (biochemical, symptomatic and histological) remissions

criteria, and the relation between clinical and histological remission, must be further explored in future studies.

With regard to establishing histological remission possible sample errors constitute a problem, and may lead to underestimation of disease activity. Therefore, in our study the absence of clear histological activity in three of the liver biopsies after UDCA treatment can only be considered as suggestive for complete remission.

We administered a dose of about 10 mg/kg UDCA in this study, in agreement with several other authors[3,7]. It could be argued that a higher dose might lead to a higher remission frequency. However, this seems unlikely, since the quantitative changes in our study population are comparable with those reported in studies using higher doses[2,8,9]. Furthermore, the only dose–response study with UDCA performed in chronic liver diseases indicated no extra benefit of a 750 mg dose over a 500 mg dose[16].

In the present study we found no differences between cirrhotic and noncirrhotic patients with respect to their response to UDCA, as suggested by others[17–19]. No cirrhotic patient deteriorated during this 1-year treatment period.

This finding contrasts with the results of some uncontrolled studies[20–22]. However, in these studies patients with Child–Pugh Class B/C cirrhosis were not explicitly excluded. The majority of patients deteriorating on UDCA had evidence of advanced disease, indicated by the presence of Child–Pugh Class B cirrhosis, jaundice or bilirubin levels over twice the upper limit of normal. Furthermore, Battezzati *et al.*[7] found UDCA to be well tolerated and to improve liver biochemistry in a placebo-controlled study in 88 patients with advanced PBC (bilirubin >34 umol/l and/or pruritus) of which 50% had cirrhosis. Whether UDCA really alters the eventual outcome in patients with cirrhosis remains to be established but, based on the currently available data, UDCA treatment should not be withheld from patients with compensated (Child–Pugh Class A) cirrhosis.

In conclusion, our findings confirm that UDCA improves biochemical parameters and complaints in PBC. However, in spite of overall improvement, complete remission of disease activity in individual patients is rare.

EPILOGUE

It may not be surprising that UDCA monotherapy is not sufficient to induce disease inactivation in PBC. UDCA seems to interfere mainly with the consequences of cholestasis and not, or only to a minor extent, with the underlying immunological disorder[23]. Combined therapy of PBC with bile acids and other treatment modalities is proposed as a logical next step[24–27], and has already been tried by several workers[28–35]. Additional treatment with colchicine does not seem to be of major benefit[28–32]. Methotrexate treatment has also been tried in addition to UDCA, and seems to induce further improvements of liver tests[33,34], but bears a high risk of complications, particularly interstitial pneumonitis[36].

We initiated a 1-year, double-blind, placebo-controlled trial with combined low-dose prednisone and azathioprine. Both drugs have been shown to be of some benefit in PBC[14,37], and form a well-known and effective combination in the treatment of chronic autoimmune hepatitis[15]. Moreover, we had noted synergistic effects of UDCA with prednisone (with or without azathioprine) in seven patients treated with this combination[27].

Fifty patients, without disease remission in the first study phase, have now entered this trial. An interim analysis, concerning the first 36 patients completing the study, showed clear additional improvement of pruritus ($p<0.01$), AST (mean difference in percentage change [Δ]: 44%, $p<0.001$), alkaline phosphatase (Δ: 36%, $p<0.001$) and IgM (Δ 20%, $p<0.001$). In 24 patients procollagen-III-propeptide, a marker of active fibrogenesis[38] with prognostic significance in PBC[39,40], was monitored. It normalized in four of eight patients in the treatment group compared to none of five in the placebo group (Δ 26%, $p<0.001$). Bilirubin stabilized in the treatment group, but tended to increase in the placebo group. Moreover, although no effect could be established on histological stage of disease in this small, short-term trial, a decrease in inflammatory features was noted in the treatment group ($p<0.05$) but not in the placebo group. The main side-effect was weight gain, which was considered cosmetically hindering by three patients, but did not necessitate treatment withdrawal in any of them. Three other patients in the prednisone/azathioprine group withdrew from treatment within 1 month (two general malaise, one after a period of spontaneous bacterial peritonitis). In the placebo group two patients needed a liver transplantation, and were withdrawn from treatment after 6 and 9 months, respectively.

The main potential drawback of corticosteroid treatment in PBC is the enhancement of bone loss[41]. In a simultaneously performed controlled study in 12 patients, comparing biphosphonate treatment, in the form of cyclical etidronate + calcium (Didrokit®, Procter & Gamble, Rotterdam, The Netherlands) to calcium alone, we have shown that etidronate may obviate this problem. In the prednisone-treated patients receiving etidronate, mean loss in lumbar bone mineral content, as measured by dual energy X-ray absorptiometry, was 0.8% compared to 3.5% in the untreated group ($p<0.03$). For comparison, in the overall PBC population at the University Hospital Rotterdam, the mean annual bone loss had been found to be 1.3% (unpublished data).

These preliminary data show increased beneficial effects of the addition of immunosuppressives in the form of a combination of low-dose prednisone and azathioprine to UDCA. The short term benefit/risk ratio of the triple (UDCA/prednisone/azathioprine) treatment, under biphosphonate protection, appears to be positive, and justifies the long-term evaluation of this regimen.

Acknowledgements

We thank the members of the Dutch Multicentre PBC Study Group, who have contributed to this study: P. L. Batenburg, Zuiderziekenhuis, Rotterdam; J. G. S. Breed, St Jans Ziekenhuis, Weert; H. R. van Buuren, Academisch Ziekenhuis, Rotterdam; L. G. J. B. Engels, Maasland Ziekenhuis, Sittard; F. A. L. M. Eskens, Canisius Ziekenhuis, Nijmegen; J. Ferwerda, Elisabeth Ziekenhuis, Haarlem; J. van Hattum, Academisch Ziekenhuis Utrecht; K. J. Heering, Bleuland Ziekenhuis, Gouda; E. W. van der Hoek, Carolus Ziekenhuis, Den Bosch; J. W. Kappelle, Medisch Centrum Leeuwarden; M. J. Kerbert-Dreteler, Medisch Spectrum Twente, Enschede; I. J. Klompmaker, Academisch Ziekenhuis, Groningen; J. H. van Lijf, Medisch Spectrum Twente, Enschede; B. J. Looij, Maasland Ziekenhuis, Geleen; J. W. den Ouden-Muller, St Franciscus Gasthuis, Rotterdam; A. M. Smit, Carolus Ziekenhuis, Den Bosch; H. J. Metselaar, Academisch Ziekenhuis Dijkzigt, Rotterdam; D. Overbosch, Rode Kruis Ziekenhuis, Den Haag; J. Scherpenisse, Reinier de Graaf Ziekenhuis, Delft; S. W. Schalm, Academisch Ziekenhuis Rotterdam; J. E. Thies, Rijnstate Ziekenhuis, Arnhem; J. C. Thijs, Bethesda Ziekenhuis, Hoogeveen; V. M. C. Verstappen, St Maartens Ziekenhuis, Venlo; R. A. de Vries, Rijnstate Ziekenhuis, Arnhem; R. M. Valentijn, Rode Kruis Ziekenhuis, Den Haag; M. M. Vidakovic-Vukic, St. Lucas Ziekenhuis, Amsterdam. *Pathologist*: F. J. W. ten Kate, Academisch Medisch Centrum, Amsterdam; *Members of Steering Committee*: R. Beukers, Drechtsteden Ziekenhuis, Dordrecht; J. H. P. Wilson, Academisch Ziekenhuis Dijkzigt, Rotterdam. This project is supported by Zambon Nederland BV, The Wellcome Foundation, Procter & Gamble and the Dutch Digestive Disease Foundation.

References

1. Kaplan MM. Primary biliary cirrhosis. N Engl J Med. 1987;316:521–8.
2. Poupon RE, Balkau B, Eschwège E, Poupon R and the UDCA–PBC Study Group. A multicenter controlled trial of ursodiol for the treatment of primary biliary cirrhosis. N Engl J Med. 1991;324:1548–54.
3. Leuschner U, Fischer H, Kurtz *et al.* Ursodeoxycholic acid in primary biliary cirrhosis; results of a controlled double-blind study. Gastroenterology. 1989;97:1268–74.
4. Oka H, Toda G, Ikeda Y *et al.* A multi-center double-blind controlled trial of ursodeoxycholic acid for primary biliary cirrhosis. Gastroenterol Jpn. 1990;25:774–80.
5. Combes B, Carithers RL Jr, Maddrey WC *et al.* A randomized double-blind, placebo-controlled trial of ursodeoxycholic acid therapy in primary biliary cirrhosis. Hepatology. 1993;18:A175 (abstract).
6. O'Brien CB, Senior JR, Sternlieb JM *et al.* Ursodiol treatment of primary biliary cirrhosis. Gastroenterology. 1989;98:A617 (abstract).
7. Battezzati PM, Podda M, Bianchi R and the Italian Multicentre Group for the Study of UDCA in PBC. Ursodeoxycholic acid for symptomatic primary biliary cirrhosis: preliminary analysis of a double-blind controlled multicentre trial. J Hepatol. 1993;17:332–8.
8. Lindor KD, Dickson ER, Baldus WB *et al.* Ursodeoxycholic acid in the treatment of primary biliary cirrhosis. Gastroenterology. 1994;106:1284–90.
9. Heathcote EJL, Cauch-Dudek K, Walker V *et al.* The Canadian multicenter double-blind randomized controlled trial of ursodeoxycholic acid in primary biliary cirrhosis. Hepatology. 1994;19:1149–56.
10. Poupon RE, Poupon R, Balkau B and the UDCA–PBC Study Group. Ursodiol for the long term treatment of primary biliary cirrhosis. N Engl J Med. 1994;330:1342–7.
11. Wiesner RH. Is continued enthusiasm for ursodeoxycholic acid therapy for the treatment of primary biliary cirrhosis warranted? Hepatology. 1992;15:971–3.
12. Beukers R, Schalm SW. Immunosuppressive therapy for primary biliary cirrhosis. J Hepatol. 1992;14:1–6.
13. Taal BG, Schalm SW, Kate ten FWJ, Hermans J, Geertzen GM, Feltkamp BEW. Clinical diagnosis of primary biliary cirrhosis: a classification based on major and minor criteria. Hepatogastroenterology. 1983;30:178–82.
14. Mitchison HC, Palmer JM, Bassendine MF, Watson AJ, Record CO, James OFW. A controlled trial of prednisolone treatment in primary biliary cirrhosis: three year results. J Hepatol. 1992;15:336–44.
15. Davis GL, Czaja AJ. Immediate and long-term results of corticosteroid therapy for severe idiopathic chronic active hepatitis. In: Czaja AJ, Dickson ER, editors. Chronic active hepatitis: the Mayo Clinic experience. New York: Marcel Dekker; 1986:269–83.
16. Podda M, Ghezzi C, Battezzati PM *et al.* Effect of different doses of ursodeoxycholic acid in chronic liver disease. Dig Dis Sci. 1989;34:59S–65S.
17. Floreani A, Zappalà F, Mazzetto M, Naccarato R, Plebani M, Chiaramonte M. Different response to ursodeoxycholic acid in primary biliary cirrhosis according to severity of disease. Dig Dis Sci. 1994;39:9–14.
18. Raedsch R, Stiehl A, Theilman L, Galle P, Möller B, Hopf U. Influence of ursodeoxycholic acid on primary biliary cirrhosis depending on stage of the disease. Gastroenterology. 1989;96:A647 (abstract).
19. Hadzyannis SJ, Hadzyannis ES, Lianidou E, Makris L. Long term treatment of primary biliary cirrhosis with ursodeoxycholic acid: the third year of a controlled trial. In: Paumgartner G, Stiehl A, Gerok W, editors. Bile acids as therapeutic agents. Dordrecht: Kluwer; 1991:287–96.
20. Kneppelhout JC, Mulder CJJ, Van Berge Henegouwen GP, De Vries RA, Brandt KH. Ursodeoxycholic acid treatment in primary biliary cirrhosis with the emphasis on late stage disease. Neth J Med. 1992;41:11–16.
21. Vogel W, Kathrein H, Judmaier G, Braunsteiner H. Deterioration of primary biliary cirrhosis during treatment with ursodeoxycholic acid. Lancet. 1988;1:1163.
22. Lotterer E, Stiehl A, Raedsch R, Foelsch UR, Bircher J. Ursodeoxycholic acid in primary biliary cirrhosis: no evidence for toxicity in stage I to III. J Hepatol. 1990;10:284–90.
23. Van Erpecum KJ, Van de Meeberg PC, Van Berge Henegouwen GP. Rationale for therapy with ursodeoxycholic acid in patients with cholestatic liver disease. Neth J Med. 1993;43:233–8.

24. Caestecker JS de, Jazrawi RP, Petroni ML, Northfield TC. Ursodeoxycholic acid in chronic liver disease. Gut. 1991;32:1061–5.
25. Jansen PLM. Antifibrotic therapy of liver cirrhosis, with special reference to primary biliary cirrhosis. Neth J Med. 1992;40:209–14.
26. Kaplan MM. New strategies needed for treatment of primary biliary cirrhosis? Gastroenterology. 1993;104:651–3.
27. Wolfhagen FHJ, Van Buuren HR, Schalm SW. Combined treatment with ursodeoxycholic acid and prednisone in primary biliary cirrhosis. Neth J Med. 1994;44:84–90.
28. Shibata J, Fujiyama S, Honda Y, Sato T. Combination therapy with ursodeoxycholic acid and colchicine for primary biliary cirrhosis. J Gastroenterol Hepatol. 1992;7:277–82.
29. Raedsch R, Stiehl A, Walker S, Shermann JM, Kommerel B. Kombinierte Ursodeoxycholsäure plus Colchizinbehandlung bei primär biliärer Zirrhose: Ergebnisse einer Placebo-kontrollierten Doppelblindstudie. Z Gastroenterologie. 1992;30(Suppl. 1):55–7.
30. Podda M and the Italian multicentre group for the study of UDCA in PBC. Long-term effects of the administration of ursodeoxycholic acid (UDCA) alone or with colchicine in patients with primary biliary cirrhosis (PBC). A double-blind multicenter study. Proceedings of the XII international Falk bile acid meeting. Basel, 1992:50–1.
31. Poupon RE, Niard AM, Huet PM *et al.* A randomized trial comparing the combination ursodeoxycholic acid (UDCA) and colchicine to UDCA alone in primary biliary cirrhosis. Hepatology. 1994;20:151A (abstract).
32. Goddard CJR, Hunt L, Smith A, Fallowfield G, Rowan B, Warnes TW. A trial of ursodeoxycholic acid and colchicine in primary biliary cirrhosis. Hepatology. 1994;20:151A (abstract).
33. Kaplan MM. The therapeutic effects of ursodiol and methotrexate are additive and well tolerated in primary biliary cirrhosis. Hepatology. 1992;16:92A (abstract).
34. Buscher HP, Zietschmann Y, Gerok W. Positive responses to methotrexate and ursodeoxycholic acid in patients with primary biliary cirrhosis responding insufficiently to ursodeoxycholic acid alone. J Hepatol. 1993;18:9–14.
35. Van Buuren HR, Wolfhagen FHJ, Schalm SW. Treatment with ursodeoxycholic acid, as monotherapy and in combination with other agents, in primary biliary cirrhosis. In: Van Berge Henegouwen GP, Van Hoek B, De Groote J, Matern S, Stockbrügger RW, editors. Cholestatic liver diseases: new strategies for prevention and treatment of hepatobiliary and cholestatic liver diseases. Dordrecht: Kluwer; 1994:236–45.
36. Sharma A, Provenzale D, McKusick A, Kaplan MM. Interstitial pneumonitis after low-dose methotrexate therapy in primary biliary cirrhosis. Gastroenterology. 1994:107:266–70.
37. Christensen E, Neuberger J, Crowe J *et al.* Beneficial effect of azathioprine and prediction of prognosis in primary biliary cirrhosis. Gastroenterology. 1985;89:1084–91.
38. Plebani M, Burlina A. Biochemical markers of hepatic fibrosis. Clin Biochem. 1991;24:219–39.
39. Babbs C, Hunt LP, Haroubi NY, Smith A, Rowas BP, Warnes TW. Type III procollagen peptide: a marker of disease activity and prognosis in primary biliary cirrhosis. Lancet. 1988;1:1021–4.
40. Poupon RE, Balkau B, Guéchot J, Heintzmann F. Predictive factors in ursodeoxycholic acid-treated patients with primary biliary cirrhosis: role of serum markers of connective tissue. Hepatology. 1994;19:635–40.
41. Sherlock S, Dooley J. Diseases of the liver and biliary system, 9th edn. London: Blackwell Scientific Publications; 1993:237–48.

31 Ursodeoxycholic acid as therapy for primary sclerosing cholangitis

U. SPENGLER

INTRODUCTION

Primary sclerosing cholangitis (PSC) is a disease of unknown aetiology characterized by chronic inflammation, fibrosis and scarring of intra- and extrahepatic bile ducts. It may eventually lead to cirrhosis and liver failure, and is an important risk factor for developing cholangiocellular carcinoma. The frequent association with ulcerative colitis, an inflammatory bowel disease attributed to autoimmune processes, and the association with certain histocompatibility antigens suggest that immunological mechanisms may also be involved in PSC. However, the precise role of autoimmunity has not yet been defined in this disease. Interestingly, in more than 80% of patients with PSC antibodies to an unidentified autoantigen in the cytoplasm of neutrophils (ANCA) have been detected, and may help to establish the diagnosis of PSC more easily.

Treatment of PSC patients was not very successful with most immunosuppressive, anti-inflammatory or antifibrotic agents[1]. Initial reports on beneficial effects with oral methotrexate[2] and tacrolimus[3] could not be confirmed in controlled trials[4] or, as in the case of tacrolimus, still await confirmation.

The success of ursodeoxycholic acid therapy in primary biliary cirrhosis with virtually no adverse effects has also prompted several pilot trials[5–7] and two controlled studies[8,9] on therapy with this bile acid in PSC patients. Chazouillères and co-workers[6] presented data on 15 patients with PSC treated by ursodeoxycholic acid in an uncontrolled manner; O'Brien and his group[7] analysed periodic treatment with ursodeoxycholic acid in an open-label pilot trial; Beuers *et al.*[8] studied 14 PSC patients in a placebo-controlled pilot trial; and Stiehl and his co-workers, after pretreating patients for 1 year with open-label ursodeoxycholic acid, randomized their patients to either continued ursodeoxycholic acid or placebo[5,9]. After 3 months the placebo group had to be discontinued in Stiehl's study according to ethical guidelines. Thereafter, in this study all patients were continued on ursodeoxycholic acid for up to 4 years. This chapter attempts to summarize the experience with ursodeoxycholic acid therapy in PSC, in order to define its potential role in the treatment of this disease.

EFFECTS OF URSODEOXYCHOLIC ACID ON MARKERS OF CHOLESTASIS

All authors agree that ursodeoxycholic acid leads to marked reductions of serum alkaline phosphatase (range 36–67%), γ-glutamyl transpeptidase (range 53–64%), and aminotransferases (range 36–48%), which occur within 3 months of therapy. Some controversy still exists as to whether ursodeoxycholic acid can also lower serum bilirubin, as Stiehl's group failed to detect significant reductions of serum bilirubin levels. Ursodeoxycholic acid therapy also improves parameters which are elevated as a consequence of cholestasis. Thus, O'Brien *et al.* noted significant reductions of serum cholesterol[7]. Furthermore, reductions of increased serum copper levels[8] and a hepatic sulphur-rich copperthionein[10] were observed. Usually laboratory results become abnormal again when ursodeoxycholic acid therapy is discontinued[7,9]. However, in some patients with early intrahepatic PSC, continued amelioration of cholestatic parameters was observed after prolonged ursodeoxycholic acid therapy, which persisted even after discontinuation of this bile acid therapy[11] (own unpublished observation). Taken together, to date there is little doubt that in PSC ursodeoxycholic acid also improves laboratory parameters of cholestasis.

EFFECTS OF URSODEOXYCHOLIC ACID ON IMMUNE PARAMETERS IN PSC

In the mouse and human, various effects of ursodeoxycholic acid have been observed on functions of the immune system, resulting either in immunosuppression or the opposite effect, namely the decrease of immunosuppression induced by other bile acids. Ursodeoxycholic acid itself induces suppression of lymphocyte proliferative responses[12,13], reduces secretion of cytokines such as interleukin-2 and interleukin-4, and suppresses *in-vitro* production of immunoglobulins G, M and A[14]. However, its suppressive effects on interleukin-1, interleukin-6 and tumour necrosis factor alpha production are weaker than those of the more hydrophobic bile acids[15]. Moreover, we were able to demonstrate recovery of blunted lymphotoxin and tumour necrosis factor responses to mitogens in ursodeoxycholic-acid-treated patients with primary biliary cirrhosis[16]. Most importantly ursodeoxycholic acid can modulate HLA class I expression on hepatocytes, thus affecting immune recognition by cytotoxic lymphocytes[17].

Despite this bulk of *in-vitro* data, little has been reported on immune parameters in patients with PSC during ursodeoxycholic acid therapy. Similar to primary biliary cirrhosis, HLA class I antigens decreased on hepatocytes during ursodeoxycholic acid therapy[8]. However, in this pilot study no effect was noted on the aberrant biliary expression of HLA class II antigens and the adhesion molecule ICAM-1. In contrast, Lo and co-workers[18] could detect aberrant HLA-

DR expression on bile duct epithelial cells in only four of seven ursodeoxy-cholic-acid-treated patients with PSC, but in all of six patients from the placebo-treated control group. Thus, biliary HLA class II expression might also be reduced by ursodeoxycholic acid. Although ursodeoxycholic acid can reduce imunoglobulin secretion *in vitro*, none of the studies in PSC could demonstrate any effect of ursodeoxycholic acid therapy on serum levels of immunoglobulins G, M and A[6,8,9]. In particular, titres of the antineutrophil cytoplasmic antibodies (ANCA) associated with PSC were not affected by ursodeoxycholic acid[19]. Unfortunately no data are available on cytokine profiles in patients with PSC, either untreated or under ursodeoxycholic acid therapy. Thus, the immunomodulatory effects of ursodeoxycholic acid in PSC – if any exist – are presently only poorly understood.

EFFECTS OF URSODEOXYCHOLIC ACID ON BILE ACID METABOLISM IN PSC

In patients with primary sclerosing cholangitis total serum bile acids can increase up to five-fold, and cholic acid constitutes the major serum bile acid as compared to chenodeoxycholic acid in healthy controls[7]. At pharmacological doses ursodeoxycholic acid can increase up to 50% of total serum bile acids in treated patients with PSC. Whether the total bile acid level remains the same or increases during ursodeoxycholic acid therapy is controversial[7,8]. With ursodeoxycholic acid therapy serum levels of cholic acid[7–9,20] and 1-OH-deoxy-cholic acid[9] tend to decline, with no significant changes in the other bile acid serum levels. However, changes in plasma bile acids during ursodeoxycholic acid treatment are not due to changes in bile acid pool sizes. Pool sizes were considerably smaller in untreated PSC patients for cholic, chenodeoxycholic and deoxycholic acids, and remained essentially the same during ursodeoxycholic acid therapy[20,21]. However, fractional turnover increased significantly for cholic and chenodeoxycholic acids, while synthesis was higher only for cholic acid. Decreasing serum levels of endogenous bile acids during ursodeoxycholic acid therapy despite unchanged pool sizes indicates redistribution of these bile acids into the enterohepatic circulation, probably because ursodeoxycholic acid improves bile acid hepatic transit time and excretory rates[22].

EFFECTS OF URSODEOXYCHOLIC ACID ON LIVER HISTOLOGY IN PSC

Histological results during ursodeoxycholic acid therapy have been reported only on a limited number of patients. As inflammation and fibrosis around bile ducts occur focally throughout the liver in PSC, results based on the histology of liver biopsies from only a few patients have only limited value, due to the large selection bias in this disease. Two studies evaluated changes in liver biopsies. Beuers and co-workers compared five biopsies on ursodeoxycholic acid to six on placebo by means of a histological score[8]. This score was significantly better in patients treated with ursodeoxycholic acid, mainly due to a reduction of cellular infiltrates in the portal fields. Stiehl and his group analysed 14 biopsies of 10 patients taken after 1 and 2 years of ursodeoxycholic acid therapy with respect to the corresponding pretreatment histology, and confirmed loss of cellular infiltrates, while all other parameters were not changed significantly[9].

EFFECTS OF URSODEOXYCHOLIC ACID ON SYMPTOMS AND SIDE-EFFECTS IN PSC

The effects of ursodeoxycholic acid on symptoms of PSC are much more heterogeneous than its effects on biochemical parameters. While Chazouillères *et al.* did not note any symptomatic improvements[6], O'Brien *et al.* reported a reduction of fatigue from 60% to 20% of treated patients, and a reduction of pruritus from 33% to 20% of treated patients. In the Stiehl *et al.* study fatigue improved during uncontrolled ursodeoxycholic acid therapy in seven of 11 patients; during the controlled study phase it became worse in two of 10 patients randomized to the placebo group and in one of 10 patients randomized to continued ursodeoxycholic acid therapy. Similarly, pruritus improved in two of five patients during open-label ursodeoxycholic acid therapy; in the controlled study period pruritus deteriorated in two of 10 patients on placebo and one of 10 patients on continued ursodeoxycholic acid. The changes in fatigue and pruritus were not statistically significant. In the placebo-controlled pilot study two patients in each group had a new onset of pruritus and one patient had remarkable recovery of his liver function with loss of ascites on ursodeoxycholic acid therapy[8]. Although considerable improvements can be observed in some individuals, ursodeoxycholic acid therapy has not been proven beneficial with regard to symptoms on a statistical basis. Otherwise, therapy with ursodeoxycholic acid is well tolerated in PSC. As the only major complication of ursodeoxycholic acid diarrhoea has been noted in a small number (<10%) of patients with PSC and ulcerative colitis which could be controlled by dose reductions in most patients.

EFFECTS OF URSODEOXYCHOLIC ACID ON BILE LUCT LESIONS

Since bile duct alterations on cholangiography are the hallmark of PSC, endoscopic retrograde cholangiography appears to be the most appropriate tool for assessing disease progression. However, information on the progress of bile duct lesions is only scanty. Most remarkably, Lebovics and his collaborators reported on a PSC patient with extensive intrahepatic biliary as well as pancreatic duct strictures that radiologically resolved to normal on ursodeoxycholic acid therapy[23]. A further case report suggests that ursodeoxycholic acid therapy may be particularly useful as combination therapy with endoscopic stenting[11]. In Stiehl *et al.*'s controlled study, endoscopic cholangiography was performed at yearly intervals over more than 3 years in 20 patients; and he noted progression of bile duct disease in only one patient treated with ursodeoxycholic acid. In this patient a major bile duct stenosis could be treated successfully by endoscopic dilatation[9]. In a follow-up study with 43 PSC patients on open-label ursodeoxycholic acid therapy Stiehl observed major bile duct stenosis developing in only seven patients[24]. Furthermore, combination therapy with ursodeoxycholic acid and endoscopic dilatation led to significant improvement of cholestatic markers in all these patients except those with end-stage liver cirrhosis.

EFFECTS OF URSODEOXYCHOLIC ACID ON PROGNOSIS OF PSC

Death from liver failure, cholangiocarcinoma and nowadays liver transplantation are the end-points of liver disease in PSC. However, thus far, no study in PSC has sufficient power to assess the effects of ursodeoxycholic acid therapy on survival. The evaluation of surrogate markers of prognosis, such as the aminopyrine breath test (a sensitive index of microsomal metabolism) or the Mayo risk score, has not demonstrated any short- or long-term improvement on ursodeoxycholic acid therapy[8,9]. Nevertheless, when comparing survival in 43 patients on continued ursodeoxycholic acid therapy to 14 drop-outs of this therapy, Stiehl's group found that two patients succumbed due to cholangiocellular carcinoma in the treatment group, while three drop-outs needed orthotopic liver transplantation and one more drop-out died from myocardial infarction[24,25]. Thus, survival appeared to be significantly better ($p<0.05$) in ursodeoxycholic-acid-treated patients. Nevertheless, this study cannot replace a prospectively randomized placebo-controlled clinical trial with survival as the predefined end-point for statistical analysis. However, given the many beneficial effects of ursodeoxycholic acid such a trial is already considered unethical by some experts in the field of chronic cholestatic liver diseases[24].

CONCLUSION

Ursodeoxycholic acid has an overall beneficial effect in PSC. Patients should be treated as early as possible, to prevent or delay progression to the advanced stages of this disease. Similar to primary biliary cirrhosis ursodeoxycholic acid appears not to be effective in patients with advanced PSC. Although generally ursodeoxycholic acid leads to improvement but not cure of PSC, there may be some patients with very early disease who have permanent benefit from ursodeoxycholic acid even after discontinuation of therapy. Nevertheless, prolonged or permanent therapy must be recommended. This should be possible for the majority of patients with PSC, as virtually no major side-effects have been noted. A problem in the treatment of PSC is the development of cholangiocarcinoma, which can be detected unexpectedly in up to 20% of explanted livers[26]. At present it is not clear whether ursodeoxycholic acid has any effect on this grave complication of PSC.

References

1. Kaplan MM. Medical approaches to primary sclerosing cholangitis. Sem Liver Dis. 1991;11:56–63.
2. Kaplan MM, Arora S, Pincus SH. Primary sclerosing cholangitis and low-dose oral pulse methotrexate therapy: clinical and histologic response. Ann Intern Med. 1987;106:231–5.

3. Van Thiel DH, Carrol P, Abu-Elmagd K *et al.* Tacrolimus (FK506), a treatment for primary sclerosing cholangitis: results of an open-label preliminary trial. Am J Gastroenterol. 1995;90:455–9.
4. Knox TA, Kaplan MM. A double-blind controlled trial of oral-pulse methotrexate therapy in the treatment of primary sclerosing cholangitis. Gastroenterology. 1994;106:494–9.
5. Stiehl A, Raedsch R, Kommerell B. The effect of ursodeoxycholic acid (URSO) in primary sclerosing cholangitis. A comparison to primary biliary cirrhosis. Gastroenterology. 1988;94:A595 (abstract).
6. Chazouillères O, Poupon R, Capron J-P *et al.* Ursodeoxycholic acid for primary sclerosing cholangitis. J Hepatol. 1990;11:120–3.
7. O'Brien CB, Senior JR, Arora-Mirchandani R, Batta AK, Salen G. Ursodeoxycholic acid for the treatment of primary sclerosing cholangitis: a 30-month pilot study. Hepatology. 1991;14:838–47.
8. Beuers U, Spengler U, Kruis W *et al.* Ursodeoxycholic acid for the treatment of primary sclerosing cholangitis: a placebo-controlled trial. Hepatology. 1992;16:707–14.
9. Stiehl A, Walker S, Stiehl L, Rudolph G, Hofmann WJ, Theilmann L. Effect of ursodeoxycholic acid on liver and bile duct disease in primary sclerosing cholangitis. A 3-year pilot study with a placebo-controlled study period. J Hepatol. 1994;20:57–64.
10. Hayashi H, Higuchi T, Ichimiya H, Hishida N, Sakamot N. Asymptomatic primary sclerosing cholangitis treated with ursodeoxycholic acid. Gastroenterology. 1990;99:533–5.
11. Springer DJ, Gaing AA, Slegel JH. Radiologic regression of primary sclerosing cholangitis following combination therapy with an endoprosthesis and ursodeoxycholic acid. Am J Gastroenterol. 1993;88:1957–9.
12. Calmus Y, Weill B, Ozier Y, Chèreau C, Houssin D, Poupon R. Immunosuppressive properties of chenodoxycholic and ursodeoxycholic acids in the mouse. Gastroenterology. 1992;103:617–21.
13. Lagaille F, Paradis K. The immunosuppressive effect of ursodeoxycholic acid: a comparative *in vitro* study on human peripheral blood mononuclear cells. Hepatology. 1993;18:165–72.
14. Yoshikawa M, Tsujii T, Matsumura K *et al.* Immunomodulatory effects of ursodeoxycholic acid on immune responses. Hepatology. 1992;16:358–64.
15. Calmus Y, Guechot J, Podevin P, Bonnefis M-T, Giboudeau J, Poupon R. Differential effects of chenodeoxycholic and ursodeoxycholic acids on interleukin 1, interleukin 6 and tumor necrosis factor alpha production by monocytes. Hepatology. 1992;16:719–23.
16. Spengler U, Jung MC, Hoffmann RM *et al.* Effects of ciclosporin A (CiA) and ursodeoxycholic acid (UDCA) on MHC class II expression and lymphokine expression in primary biliary cirrhosis. Hepatology. 1990;12:A842 (abstract).
17. Hillaire S, Boucher E, Calmus Y *et al.* Effects of bile acids and cholestasis on major histocompatibility complex class I in human and rat hepatocytes. Gastroenterology. 1994;107:781–8.
18. Lo SK, Chapman RW, Dooley JS, Fleming KA. Aberrant HLA-DR antigen expression by bile duct epithelium in primary sclerosing cholangitis is down-regulated by ursodeoxycholic acid. Gastroenterology. 1993;105:A943 (abstract).
19. Lo SK, Fleming KA, Chapman RW. A 2-year follow-up study of anti-neutrophil antibody in primary sclerosing cholangitis: relationship to clinical activity, liver biochemistry, and ursodeoxycholic acid treatment. J Hepatol. 1994;21:974–8.
20. Rudolph G, Endele R, Senn M, Stiehl A. Effect of ursodeoxycholic acid on the kinetics of cholic and chenodeoxycholic acid in patients with primary sclerosing cholangitis. Hepatology. 1993;17:1028–32.
21. Beuers U, Spengler U, Zwiebel FM, Pauletzki J, Fischer S, Paumgartner G. Effect of ursodeoxycholic acid on the kinetics of the major hydrophobic bile acids in health and in chronic cholestatic liver disease. Hepatology. 1992;15:603–8.
22. Jazrawi RP, De Caestecker JS, Goggin PM *et al.* Kinetics of hepatic bile acid handling in cholestatic liver disease: effect of ursodeoxycholic acid. Gastroenterology. 1994;106:134–42.
23. Lebovics E, Salame M, Elhosseiny A, Rosenthal WS. Resolution of radiographic abnormalities with ursodeoxycholic acid therapy of primary sclerosing cholangitis. Gastroenterology. 1992;102:2143–7.
24. Stiehl A. Ursodeoxycholic acid therapy in treatment of primary sclerosing cholangitis. Scand J Gastroenterol. 1994;29 (Suppl. 204):59–61.

25. Stiehl A, Walker S, Rudolph G, Sauer P, Theilmann L. Survival in patients with PSC treated with ursodeoxycholic acid (UDCA) and by endoscopic dilatations of common duct stenosis: a controlled study. Hepatology. 1993;18:219A (abstract).
26. Strasser S, Sheil AGR, Gallagher ND, Waugh R, McCaughan GW. Liver transplantation for primary sclerosing cholangitis versus primary biliary cirrhosis: a comparison of complications and outcome. J Gastroenterol Hepatol. 1993;8:238–43.

32
Ursodeoxycholic acid therapy after liver transplantation

C. SAMA, A. M. MORSELLI-LABATE, G. DANESI, A. MASTROIANNI, F. BAGNATO and L. BARBARA

The development of liver transplantation can now offer an effective therapeutic option for many patients with end-stage and untreatable liver disease. The management of transplanted patients includes the prevention and treatment of rejection, infection and other medical and surgical complications. Many drugs are currently under investigation for the purpose of improving mangement of the transplant recipient.

Ursodeoxycholic acid (UDCA), the 7β-epimer of chenodeoxycholic acid, is a hydrophilic non-hepatotoxic bile acid which exhibits beneficial effects in patients with cholestatic disorders. Four basic mechanisms might account for the beneficial effects of UDCA:

1. Enrichment of the bile acid pool with UDCA and decrease in endogenous bile acids;
2. A cytoprotective effect toward hepatocytes;
3. An effect on the immune system;
4. Induction of a bicarbonate-rich hypercholeresis.

Based on these mechanisms, UDCA has been administered to liver transplant recipients in order to evaluate its effect on:

1. Bile flow and bile acid secretion;
2. Drug-induced cholestasis;
3. Prevention of acute rejection;
4. Bioavailability of cyclosporin.

Let us examine the available data on these topics.

BILE FLOW AND BILE ACID SECRETION

Normal bile secretion is critical for maintenance of liver function. Secretion of bile is the most important sign which demonstrates the recovery of hepatic func-

tion after liver transplantation (OLT). Bile secretion after OLT is dependent on the ability of the liver to secrete bile acids[1]. An unexplained cholestasis is observed in some patients after OLT in the absence of rejection, extrahepatic biliary obstruction and other known causes. A possible explanation could be impaired bile acid secretion. We decided to evaluate the possible therapeutic effects of UDCA on bile flow and bile acid secretion in a group of transplanted patients[2]. UDCA (600 mg/day) was administered to 15 randomly selected OLT recipients starting 7 days after surgery. Fifteen patients matched for age, sex and OLT indications were chosen as controls. Bile flow and bile acid secretion were measured in the two groups, starting from OLT, until the T tube was clamped (12 days). Bile samples were collected on days 1, 6, 8 and 12 after OLT for evaluation of bile acids (BA), phospholipids (PL) and cholesterol (XOL) by enzymatic methods. Patients who presented episodes of rejection, cholestasis or other major problems were excluded from the study which refers to six UDCA-treated patients and five controls. Bile flow and BA secretion increased in controls from day 1 to 12 after OLT (ANOVA trend: $p<0.05$ and $p<0.01$, respectively; Figure 1). UDCA administration induced a significant increase ($p<0.05$) both in bile flow and biliary BA secretion (Figure 2). XOL/BA and PL/BA ratios were not significantly different between controls and UDCA-treated patients and did not show time-related variations.
In conclusion, we found that:

1. Following OLT, the liver shows a time-related recovery of its ability to secrete bile acids;
2. UDCA administration induces a dramatic increase in bile flow and bile acid secretion.

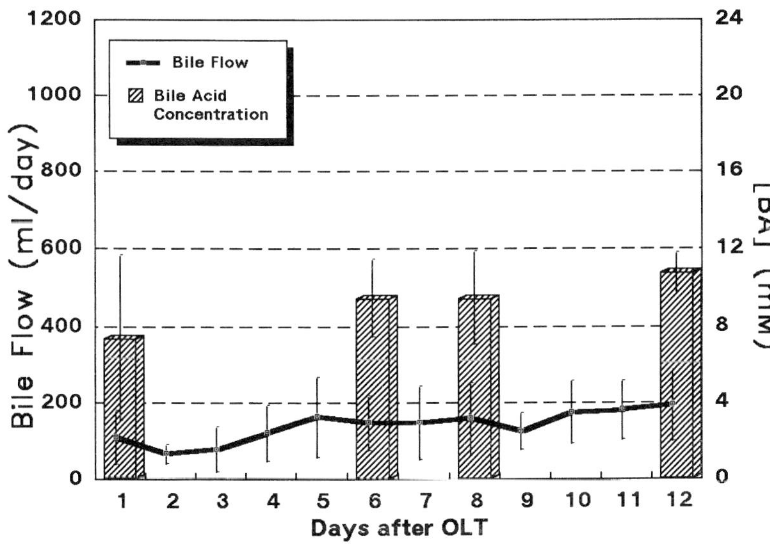

Fig. 1 Bile flow and bile acid concentration in five patients after liver transplantation (mean ± SD)

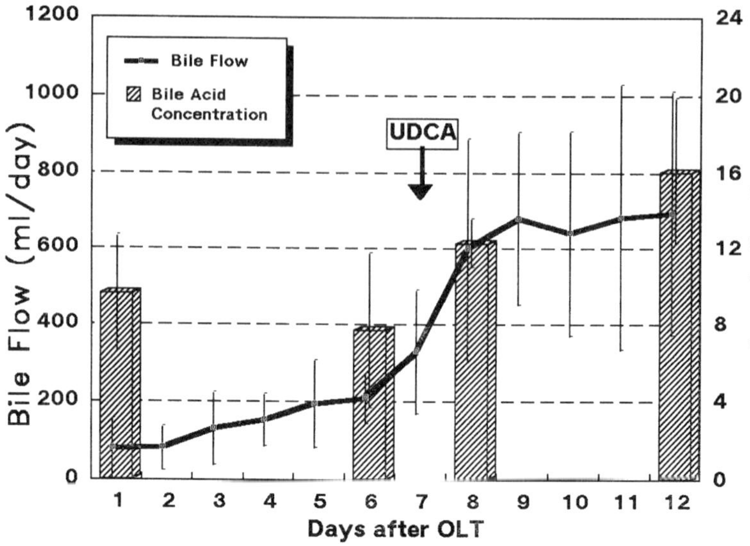

Fig. 2 Bile flow and bile acid concentration in six transplanted patients before and after UDCA administration (mean ± SD)

We concluded that, if unexplained cholestasis after OLT is related to insufficient bile acid secretion, UDCA could be the treatment of choice.

DRUG-INDUCED CHOLESTASIS

Cholestasis is a frequently observed feature of transplanted patients. In addition to rejection, biliary obstruction, hepatitis and poor arterial vascularization, cholestasis may be related to drug toxicity. Cyclosporin, the principal immunosuppressive drug used by the liver transplant recipient, can also induce cholestasis. The mechanisms are not fully understood but one possible explanation is the inhibition of the acidic pathway of bile acid synthesis. The process of bile acid synthesis from cholesterol takes place via two pathways, i.e. the 'neutral' and 'acidic' pathways. Recent data suggest that the contribution of the 'acidic' pathway may be larger than previously expected. Mitochondrial 27-hydrolase catalyses the initial step in the 'acidic' pathway, the conversion of cholesterol to 27-hydrocholesterol, and the final end product of the pathway is chenodeoxycholic acid. Studies in cultured rat hepatocytes showed that inhibition of sterol 27-hydrolase by cyclosporin may result in a 50% inhibition of bile acid synthesis[3].

Cholestasis induced by cyclosporin may be improved by UDCA administration, as suggested by the results of the Heidelberg group[4].

In this study, five heart-transplant recipients who developed cholestasis during immunosuppressive therapy involving cyclosporin, were treated with UDCA. Alkaline phosphatase, GGT, ALT and bilirubin levels were markedly reduced during therapy; when UDCA was discontinued, all five patients developed cholestasis again; this was again resolved with UDCA.

PREVENTION OF ACUTE REJECTION

One of the most frequent complications observed after liver transplantation is acute rejection. In fact, as many as 60–80% of transplant recipients suffer from at least one episode of acute rejection. The majority of rejection episodes occur early in the postoperative period, between the 7th and the 30th day after OLT. Rejection of the transplanted liver is a process characterized by multiple cell interactions, involving a variety of cell-associated and soluble mediators. Although the cellular mechanisms of liver allograft rejection are not completely understood, infiltrating host lymphocytes, which appear in the portal tract and central vein endothelia, are generally presumed to play a major role in allograft rejection.

There are some similarities between primary biliary cirrhosis (PBC) and liver rejection:

1. Similar histological lesions,
2. In both cases, there is abnormal expression of Class I and Class II HLA molecules in the liver, and
3. Both conditions are associated with cholestasis and the destruction of interlobular bile ducts.

In PBC, UDCA reduces HLA Class I expression in the liver[5], prevents direct destruction and improves cholestasis. Based on these facts, it has been postulated that UDCA could be effective against rejection. The results of a Swedish study are in favour of a preventive effect of UDCA on early acute rejection[6]. UDCA, at a dose of 10 mg kg^{-1} day^{-1} was administered to 33 consecutive OLT recipients, starting within the first 5 days after the transplant. All patients had primary graft function and were undergoing quadruple immunosuppression treatment (cyclosporin, steroids, azathioprine, ATG). Patients were monitored clinically, biochemically and histologically. Five episodes of acute rejection were observed during the first month after OLT (5/33, 15%). These results were compared with a group of 8 patients transplanted previously in the same Institution, which served as historical controls. In this group of patients, rejection had occurred in 6 of them (75%) during the first month after OLT.

We also decided to investigate the efficacy of UDCA in preventing acute liver rejection[7]. Forty consecutive adult liver transplant recipients, with primary graft function and no major intra-operative problems, were selected for the study.

UDCA (300 mg bid) was randomly administered to 20 patients starting on the 5th–7th postoperative day for 6 months. The remaining 20 patients served as controls. All patients were on a standard immunosuppressive regimen (steroids–cyclosporin). During the 6 months of the study, the occurrence of rejection episodes was assessed clinically and histologically.

Five patients in the UDCA-treated group, and six in the control group, were subsequently excluded from calculation because of death, retransplantation or the occurrence of major postoperative problems.

The results of the study were as follows:

- Twelve rejection episodes were observed in 8 out of 15 patients treated with UDCA (53%);
- Ten episodes of rejection were observed in 7 out of 14 untreated patients (50%);
- The majority of rejection episodes were observed during the first month after OLT, 67% and 90% in the treated and non-treated groups respectively (Figure 3).

All rejection episodes were treated with bolus corticosteroids or OKT3 (3 cases). No irreversible rejection occurred in this group of patients.

We concluded that, in our experience, UDCA administration does not prevent early rejection after liver transplantation.

No data are available so far on the possible preventive effect of UDCA on late or chronic rejection.

BIOAVAILABILITY OF CYCLOSPORIN

UDCA has been proposed for ameliorating bioavailability of cyclosporin after oral administration.

Cyclosporin is a lipophilic drug which is absorbed in the ileum. As with most lipid-soluble drugs, the absorption of cyclosporin from the intestine depends upon the availability of bile and bile acids.

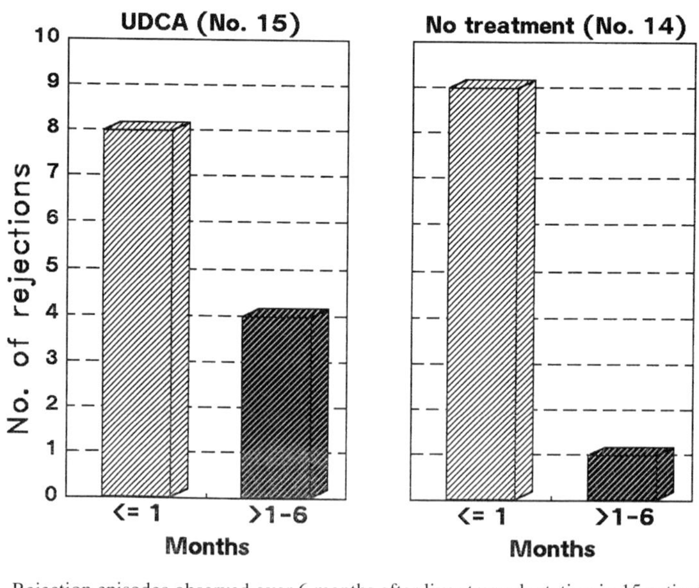

Fig. 3 Rejection episodes observed over 6 months after liver transplantation in 15 patients treated with UDCA and in 14 controls

Cyclosporin bioavailability after oral administration is low and highly variable, mainly in the early post-transplant period and is reduced in cholestatic conditions. Bile refeeding[8] and chenodeoxycholic acid administration[9] have been shown to increase cyclosporin absorption in animals and man; however, the first method necessitates an open T-tube and a nasoduodenal tube, while chenodeoxycholic acid administration can worsen a cholestatic condition. Therefore, UDCA was investigated in order to evaluate its efficacy in promoting cyclosporin intestinal absorption.

The Heidelberg group[10] has recently demonstrated that UDCA can favourably improve bioavailability of cyclosporin. Cyclosporin kinetics were measured in 4 patients who had undergone heart or liver transplantation before and during UDCA administration (250 mg qid); one patient had a short bowel and, in one, the T-tube was open. Despite the fact that UDCA has only a weak micelle-forming capacity, the data from this study showed that concomitant oral UDCA administration significantly increases the biovailability of cyclosporin in patients with both normal and impaired enterohepatic circulation (Table 1).

A recent paper from King's College[11] arrived at different conclusions. They studied the acute effect of a single dose of UDCA (10 mg/kg) on cyclosporin pharmacokinetics, during paired studies, in 12 liver transplant recipients, six of whom were cholestatic. UDCA resulted in a more rapid absorption of cyclosporin in 8 of 12 cases (67%), but had no effect in 4 patients (two with cholestasis). Median T_{max} did not change significantly after UDCA, and only 7 patients showed a rise in the amount of cyclosporin absorbed over 24 hours, with the AUC not having changed significantly. However, they showed an increased clearance of cyclosporin metabolites by choleresis in cholestatic subjects. They concluded that, although their study failed to demonstrate a consistent improvement in cyclosporin pharmacokinetics, benefit from UDCA may be greater at higher doses or after prolonged administration.

Table 1 Effect of UDCA on CyA AUC

No.	*Organ*	*CyA AUC (ng/ml × h)*		*Difference*
		Control	*UDCA*	
1	Heart	8850	11 200	+27%
2	Liver	4820	6 260	+30%
3a	Liver	2100	2 910	+39%[a]
3b	Liver	6430	7 170	+12%[b]
4a	Heart	1010	2 360	+134%[c]
4b	Heart	1010	2 250	+123%[c]

[a] Open T-tube; [b] clamped T-tube; [c] short bowel. From Gutzler *et al.* 1992[10]

References

1. Shiffman ML, Carithers RL Jr, Posner MP, Moore EW. Recovery of bile secretion following orthotopic liver transplantation. J Hepatol. 1991;12:351–61.
2. Sama C, Morselli Labate AM, Roda A *et al.* UDCA after liver transplantation. J Hepatol. 1990;11(suppl 2):S54.

3. Princen HMG, Meijer P, Wolthers B *et al.* Cyclosporin A blocks bile acid synthesis in cultured hepatocytes by specific inhibition of chenodeoxycholic acid synthesis. Biochem J. 1991;275:501–5.
4. Kallinowski B, Theilmann L, Zimmerman R, Gams E, Kommerell B, Stiehl A. Effective treatment of cyclosporin-induced cholestasis in heart-transplanted patients treated with ursodeoxycholic acid. Transplantation. 1991;51:1128–9.
5. Calmus Y, Gane P, Rouger P, Poupon R. Hepatic expression of class I and class II major histocompatibility complex molecules in primary biliary cirrhosis. Effect of ursodeoxycholic acid. Hepatology. 1990;11:12–13.
6. Friman S, Persson H, Scherstén T, Svanvik J, Karlberg I. Adjuvant treatment with ursodeoxycholic acid reduces acute rejection after liver transplantation. Transplant Proc. 1992;24:389–90.
7. Sama C, Mazziotti A, Grigioni W *et al.* Ursodeoxycholic acid administration does not prevent rejection after OLT. J Hepatol. 1991;13(suppl 2):S68.
8. Merion RM, Gorski GH, Burtch GD, Turcotte JG, Colletti LM, Campbell DA. Bile refeeding after liver transplantation and avoidance of intravenous cyclosporin. Surgery. 1989;106:604–10.
9. Ericzon BG, Todo S, Lynch S *et al.* Role of bile and bile salts on cyclosporin absorption in dogs. Transplant Proc. 1987;19:1248–9.
10. Gutzler F, Fischer G, Sauer P *et al.* Improved bioavailability of cyclosporin by coadministration of ursodeoxycholic acid. Gastroenterology. 1992;102:816.
11. Al-Quaiz MN, O'Grady JG, Tredger JM, Williams R. Variable effects of ursodeoxycholic acid on cyclosporin absorption after orthotopic liver transplantation. Transplant Int. 1994;7:190–4.

33
Ursodeoxycholic acid in the treatment of paediatric liver disease

W. F. BALISTRERI

INTRODUCTION

There are several forms of chronic cholestasis unique to the paediatric population which present vexing problems for the patient and the clinician (Table 1). These disease entities are poorly understood, their aetiopathogenesis is unknown, their clinical course is associated with a high morbidity and often a high mortality rate, and there are no specific therapeutic strategies available. Several medical and surgical approaches have been tried in an effort to forestall the complications, ameliorate the manifestations or retard the progression of these disorders. For many patients the only effective modality is liver transplantation.

Ursodeoxycholic acid (UDCA) has been frequently utilized in the strategic management of these unique chronic cholestatic diseases in children. In order to place the experience in perspective, in this chapter we will discuss these disorders, indicate the major clinical concerns, review the preliminary results from therapeutic trials of UDCA in the condition, and offer our recommendations for therapy.

Table 1 Chronic cholestatic diseases in the paediatric patient

A. Chronic intrahepatic cholestasis
   1. Syndromic paucity of the interlobular bile ducts (Alagille syndrome)
   2. Non-syndromic paucity of the interlobular bile ducts
   3. Progressive familial intrahepatic cholestasis (Byler's)

B. Biliary atresia

C. Inborn errors of bile acid biosynthesis
   1. Δ^4-3-Oxosteroid-5β reductase deficiency
   2. 3β-Hydroxy C_{27} steroid dehydrogenase/isomerase deficiency

D. Liver disease associated with systemic disease
   1. CF-associated liver disease
   2. TPN-associated liver disease

CHRONIC INTRAHEPATIC CHOLESTASIS

An intriguing group of cholestatic diseases which beg clear definition are the heterogeneous subset characterized by intrahepatic cholestasis, with or without bile duct alterations, i.e. hypoplasia or paucity[1–4]. The latter term (paucity) is preferable, since it is descriptive and does not imply a specific pathogenesis[1]. 'Paucity' indicates that within the portal triad there is either an absence or marked reduction in the number of interlobular bile ducts (<0.5 interlobular bile ducts per triad) in the presence of the normal-sized branches of the portal venule and hepatic arteriole.

Syndromic paucity of the intrahepatic bile ducts (Alagille syndrome)

This disease is characterized by chronic cholestasis, a decreased number of interlobular bile ducts and various congenital malformations (Table 2)[1,5–9]. In view of the characteristic extrahepatic anomalies, which are of variable expression, the disease is readily recognized.

Major clinical manifestations

Intense pruritus is almost universally present; this is often noted by the fourth to sixth months of life. The pruritus may be intractable, and of such severity as to interfere with sleep and daily activities[10]. There is also a progressive increase in serum cholesterol levels, often reaching levels greater than 1000 mg/dl; hypercholesterolaemia is often associated with cutaneous xanthoma formation. These patients are also at risk of developing fat-soluble vitamin deficiency due to intraluminal bile acid deficiency, manifest by complications such as a degenerative neurological disease characterized by ataxia and ophthalmoplegia due to vitamin E deficiency[11]. While there is a high degree of

Table 2 Alagille's syndrome (arteriohepatic dysplasia)[(5,6)]

Criteria and Features	*Incidence (%)*
Major features	
Bile duct paucity (decreased number of interlobular ducts and chronic cholestasis)	91
Extrahepatic anomalies (variable expression)	
Unusual facies (broad forehead; deeply set, widely spaced eyes; long straight nose)	95
Vertebral arch defects (butterfly vertebrae; hemivertebrae)	87
Cardiovascular abnormalities (peripheral pulmonic stenosis)	70
Posterior embryotoxon	89
*Associated features**	
Renal abnormalities	68
Growth retardation	50
Mental retardation	16
Hypogonadism	<10
Bone disease	<10
High-pitched voice	<10

*Many of the associated features may be secondary to chronic cholestasis, for example, vitamin E deficiency with attendant neuromuscular disease

morbidity in view of the cholestasis, it is uncommon for the disorder to be associated with cirrhosis; therefore there is a low mortality rate. There have been rare reports of hepatocellular carcinoma occurring in patients with Alagille syndrome[12]. The relatively good prognosis emphasizes the need for a precise diagnosis, avoidance of surgical procedures that alter the narrow, but patent biliary tract (e.g. hepatoportoenterostomy)[13], as well as attempts to manage the complications aggressively.

Pathogenesis

The genesis of paucity is undefined, but possibly due to a failure to form (a defect in remodelling), atrophy related to decreased bile flow, or progressive injury mediated by an unknown insult, analogous to the disappearing bile duct syndrome[1–3].

Role of UDCA in Alagille syndrome

The administration of UDCA to patients with Alagille syndrome has been associated with improvement of clinical and biochemical parameters, including: (1) an alleviation of pruritus in many of the patients; (2) a decrease in serum levels of bilirubin, aminotransferase, and alkaline phosphatase; and (3) a decrease in the markedly elevated serum cholesterol levels[10,14].

In our pilot study of 31 patients with Alagille syndrome, 15 had a beneficial clinical response after 1 month of UDCA therapy, as documented by a decrease in the degree of pruritus[10,14]. For the 16 non-responsive patients the UDCA dose was increased, and pruritus was ameliorated in an additional 11. Five patients were non-responsive to doses as high as 45 mg/kg per day: in three of these non-responsive patients partial external biliary diversion was carried out. Diversion combined with UDCA therapy was effective in relieving the pruritus. In general, the responsive patients in each group were older (mean age 10.1 years) than the non-responsive patients (mean age 3.5 years). During the 6 months of UDCA administration the mean serum aminotransferase levels decreased, the total serum bilirubin decreased, and the conjugated fraction decreased (all $p<0.05$ compared to values at entry). UDCA was effective in significantly decreasing the serum cholesterol level, from a baseline mean of >620 mg/day to <390 mg/day after 3 months of therapy ($p<0.05$)[10,14]. There are no data regarding the correlation of the successful achievement of these end-points and the degree of enrichment of bile with UDCA.

Levy *et al.* also noted a beneficial effect of UDCA in a patient with Alagille syndrome[15]. They reported a decrease in serum cholesterol, triglyceride and phospholipid levels. In this patient liver synthetic function did not improve, therefore the authors ascribed the changes to the choleretic effect of UDCA.

Krawinkel *et al.* reported a decrease in pruritus, serum bilirubin, alkaline phosphatase, aminotransferase and serum cholesterol levels in a patient with Alagille syndrome during UDCA administration (15 mg/kg per day); this was associated with a complete disappearance of cutaneous xanthomas[16]. UDCA did not forestall the progression of the liver disease in this patient.

Conclusion

Controlled trials are needed to truly define the role of UDCA in Alagille syndrome. In view of the beneficial effect noted in preliminary studies of many patients, pending definitive studies, it appears that UDCA should be the drug of choice for pruritus and hypercholesterolaemia in patients with this syndrome[1,10,17,18]. A beneficial response is not universal[19]; in order to achieve desired end-points it may be necessary to administer high doses of UDCA (up to 45 mg/kg per day in divided doses). In addition, *persistence* with UDCA therapy is required, since early in the course of therapy many patients will experience an exacerbation of the pruritus. There are no data as to whether UDCA will halt any potential progression of the disease, or affect other complications, such as poor growth.

Progressive familial intrahepatic cholestasis (PFIC; also known as Byler's disease)

A severe form of intrahepatic cholestasis with progressive hepatocellular damage has been noted to occur sporadically or on a familial basis[20–26]. The clinical features and natural history of progression have been noted to be variable among this group of patients. These patients may overlap with the group of patients with inborn errors of bile acid biosynthesis.

Clinical manifestations

PFIC (or Byler's disease) is usually manifest in the first 6 months of life; the major clinical manifestations are jaundice and hepatomegaly, often accompanied by diarrhoea and poor growth[1,22–26]. Of note, despite the significant cholestasis (as manifested by elevated serum bile acid levels), the serum cholesterol levels and γ-glutamyl transpeptidase (GGTP) levels may be normal to low[20,23–26]. The latter feature, which has been associated with a poor prognosis, may be a relatively specific feature of Byler's disease or PFIC[1,20,25,26]. Inheritance is autosomal recessive. There is a high rate of progression to cirrhosis and end-stage liver disease; liver transplantation has been utilized in the management of these patients[27]. In view of the progression, therapeutic efforts have been aimed at relieving symptoms and retarding the rate of decompensation.

Pathogenesis

Recent data have suggested the existence of a defect in canalicular transport of bile acids in patients with PFIC[28]. This hypothesis is based on the observation of a distinct compartmentalization of individual bile acids in affected subjects; biliary bile acid concentrations are low (cholic acid predominates); however, chenodeoxycholic acid predominates in serum, suggesting altered canalicular excretion[28,29].

Role of UDCA in progressive familial intrahepatic cholestasis

UDCA has been administered to a large number of patients with PFIC, often in combination with partial external biliary diversion[10,14,30]. In these patients there has been a relief of pruritus, improvement in biochemical parameters and, in selected patients, an apparent retardation of the rate of progression.

In our pilot study of 27 patients with idiopathic intrahepatic cholestasis (predominantly PFIC)[10], 23 noted an improvement in the degree of pruritus following adminstration of UDCA at the initial dose of 15 mg/kg per day. For the four non-responsive patients the dose was increased or combined with partial external biliary diversion; this was effective in reducing the degree of pruritus in two of the refractory patients. There was a decline in biochemical indices of liver injury during UDCA therapy.

Conclusion

Controlled trials are needed to define the safety and efficacy of bile acid therapy; however, at present it appears that UDCA therapy is of short-term benefit to patients with PFIC, often leading to an amelioration in the severity of their pruritus.

INBORN ERRORS OF BILE ACID BIOSYNTHESIS

In recent years primary enzyme deficiencies or disorders of bile acid biosynthesis or metabolism arising secondary to specific organelle dysfunction have been recognized[1,31–41]. Defective bile acid biosynthesis or metabolism appears to be an initiating or perpetuating factor in neonatal cholestasis[3,31,34–36]; however, the true incidence is unknown. Delineation of this new category of metabolic liver disease is an important development; recognition of these disorders not only provides insight into normal hepatobiliary physiology but also offers the clinician a treatable form of liver injury. There is a dramatic clinical response to bile acid replacement therapy in the disorders recognized to date[31]. Precise and widespread screening of patients with cholestatic diseases, as well as further investigation into their pathophysiology, is needed. *Defective* bile acid biosynthesis may occur in the presence of a primary enzyme deficiency or may arise secondary to specific organelle dysfunction (Table 3)[1,31,34].

Primary defects

Our *hypothesis* was that primary inborn errors in bile acid biosynthesis, resulting from an inherent enzyme deficiency, will lead to the underproduction of the normal trophic and choleretic primary bile acids, as well as over-production of potentially hepatotoxic primitive bile acid metabolites[1,31,34].

Patients affected by these disorders have previously been considered to have idiopathic disease, such as ‘idiopathic’ neonatal hepatitis or intrahepatic cholestasis. Recognition has allowed the sub-segmentation of those broader categories[31,37–39]. At present two distinct disorders related to defective transformation of the steroid nucleus have been described: (1) Δ^4-3-oxosteroid 5β-reductase deficiency, and (2) 3β-hydroxy-C_{27}-steroid dehydrogenase/isomerase deficiency. It is possible that these defects account for up to 5% of the patients with idiopathic intrahepatic cholestatic disorders; however, the true incidence is not known. These disorders are recognized by screening with fast atom bombardment–mass spectrometry (FAB-MS) and confirmed by gas chromato-

Table 3 Inborn errors of bile acid biosynthesis and metabolism(1)

- *Primary enzymopathies*
  - Defective degradation of cholesterol side chain
    - Cerebrotendinous xanthomatosis
  - Defective transformation of steroid nucleus
    - 3β-Hydroxy-Δ^5-C_{27} steroid dehydrogenase/isomerase deficiency
    - Δ^4-3-Oxosteroid 5β-reductase deficiency
- *Secondary Defects*
  - Peroxisomal disorders
    - Disorders of peroxisome biogenesis with *general* loss of peroxisomal function
      - Zellweger's (cerebrohepatorenal) syndrome
      - Neonatal adrenoleukodystrophy
      - Infantile Refsum's disease
      - Hyperpipecolic acidaemia
      - Leber's congenital amaurosis
    - Disorders with loss of *limited* number of peroxisomal functions (structure intact)
      - Rhizomelic chondrodysplasia punctata
      - Zellweger-like syndrome
    - Disorders with loss of a *single* peroxisomal function (structure intact)
      - Adrenoleukodystrophy (X-linked)
      - Thiolase deficiency (pseudo-Zellweger's syndrome)
      - Bifunctional protein deficiency
      - Acyl-CoA oxidase deficiency (pseudo-neonatal adrenoleukodystrophy)
      - Hyperoxaluria type I
      - Acatalasaemia
  - Hepatic synthetic dysfunction
    - Tyrosinaemia
    - Fulminant hepatic failure

graphy–mass spectrometry (GC-MS). The limitation to greater recognition is the lack of widespread availability of sensitive and specific screening methodology such as FAB-MS[31,37,38,42,43].

Δ^4-3-Oxosteroid 5β-reductase deficiency

Clinical features

Patients with 5β-reductase deficiency described to date have presented with *severe neonatal cholestasis* accompanied by a coagulopathy[31,34,40,44]. This phenotype resembles other forms of severe neonatal metabolic liver disease, including tyrosinaemia and neonatal iron storage disease[31]. The histology is that of 'giant cell' neonatal hepatitis. Patients with 5β-reductase deficiency can be distinguished morphologically from patients with other forms of neonatal cholestasis by the presence of a uniform mosaic of altered and unaltered canaliculi, the relative lack of large bile plugs and the generalized complex membrane contours and canalicular diverticula[44].

Pathophysiology

The mechanism of liver injury is unclear; hepatocellular and bile ductular injury may be directly attributable to the accumulation of hepatotoxic Δ^4-3-oxo bile acids, or due to inadequate synthesis of the primary bile acids needed to generate bile acid dependent bile flow.

Role of UDCA in Δ^4-3-oxosteroid 5β-reductase deficiency

UDCA was administered to displace the hepatotoxic compounds and thereby aid in reversal of hepatic injury[45]. Oral cholic acid therapy was instituted to specifically replace the absent primary bile acids and down-regulate endogenous bile acid synthesis via feedback inhibition of cholesterol 7α-hydroxylase, and thereby prevent the further accumulation of potentially hepatotoxic Δ^4-3-oxo bile acids[31,40]. This drug combination, given orally to patients documented to have 5β-reductase deficiency, led to suppression of Δ^4-3-oxo-bile acid synthesis and normalization of liver function tests[31,44]. In these patients hepatocellular cholestasis and giant-cell transformation resolved in parallel with clinical and biochemical recovery during oral bile acid administration[31,44]

Conclusion

These patients represent a subset of familial 'idiopathic' neonatal hepatitis[1,3,31]; the proportion of such cases explained by 5β-reductase deficiency and the variability of presentation of the defect remain to be defined[31,44]. This favourable outcome indicates that treatment is lifesaving, and that early treatment prevents the development of liver failure[31].

3β-Hydroxy-C_{27}-steroid dehydrogenase/isomerase (3β-HSD) deficiency

Clinical features

Reported patients have presented at various ages with jaundice, hepatomegaly and elevated aminotransferase levels[39,46–52]. They may have malabsorption of fat and fat-soluble vitamins, and poor growth[49]; pruritus is surprisingly uncommon[52]. There appears to be bimodal presentation either as neonatal hepatitis or chronic hepatitis in older children. The GGTP and serum bile acid levels are normal despite elevated conjugated bilirubin levels, which is in contrast to most forms of neonatal cholestasis[31,48]. The serum cholesterol levels may also be low[52]. Liver biopsy specimens are heterogeneous, ranging from giant cell hepatitis to micronodular cirrhosis[49]. In many documented cases a similar clinical picture is present in siblings. There is an association with consanguinity. The disorder may be transmitted in an autosomal recessive fashion. This clinical phenotype overlaps with that noted in patients with PFIC, discussed above.

Pathophysiology

The liver injury may be related to the absent choleretic effect of the primary bile acids or the cholestatic effect of the atypical bile acids. 3β,7α-Dihydroxy-5-cholenoic acid is normally metabolized to chenodeoxycholic acid by 3β-hydroxy-C_{27}-steroid dehydrogenase/isomerase; this will not occur in patients with deficiency of this enzyme[31,37–39].

Role of UDCA in 3β-hydroxy-C_{27}-steroid dehydrogenase/isomerase (3β-HSD) deficiency

As in Δ^4-3-oxosteroid 5β-reductase deficiency, UDCA has been administered, often in conjunction with cholic acid, as replacement and displacement therapy in 3β-HSD deficiency in an attempt to reverse the hepatic injury. It appears that with combination therapy there is suppression of abnormal bile acid biosynthesis, normalization of liver function tests and bile canalicular morphology, as well as clinical recovery[31,38,44,48].

Jacquemin *et al.* successfully treated five patients with 3β-hydroxy-C_{27}-steroid dehydrogenase/isomerase deficiency with UDCA alone (600 mg/m^2 per day, by mouth)[52]. However, they suggested that replacement therapy, using primary bile acids, should be co-administered in order to suppress endogenous bile acid synthesis and prevent synthesis of atypical 3β-hydroxy-Δ^5 bile acids[52].

Conclusion

It appears that in patients with this potentially fatal disorder, characterized by a specific inborn error of bile acid biosynthesis (3β-hydroxy-C_{27}-steroid dehydrogenase/isomerase) deficiency, the use of bile acid therapy has been lifesaving. Therefore prompt recognition is imperative.

BILIARY ATRESIA

Biliary atresia is an idiopathic, localized, complete obliteration or discontinuity of the hepatic or common bile ducts at any point from the porta hepatis to the duodenum. Total obstruction of bile flow leads to cholestasis, progressive fibrosis and ultimately cirrhosis, which is usually fatal without surgical intervention[1].

Clinical manifestations

Affected patients present early in life (<1–2 months of age) with persistent cholestasis. The liver biopsy is fairly characteristic, showing ductular proliferation, canalicular and cellular bile stasis, and portal or perilobular oedema or fibrosis. The extrahepatic bile duct is obliterated.

Patients with biliary atresia are subject to progressive and rapid development of end-stage liver disease due to the persistent intrahepatic inflammatory process[1,53,54]. This occurs often, despite the attempt at drainage via hepatoportoenterostomy. Other postoperative complications include a high incidence of bacterial cholangitis and failure to thrive. Biliary atresia is the major indication for liver transplantation in the paediatric population; therefore, in view of the high morbidity and mortality, multiple therapeutic trials have been carried out[1,53]. These have been unsuccessful.

Pathophysiology

The aetiopathogesis is unknown. However, it appears that a progressive inflammatory process results in complete or partial obliteration of the extrahepatic and often the intrahepatic bile ducts[1,53,55–57].

Role of ursodeoxycholic acid in patients with biliary atresia

There have been two previous studies of the utility of UDCA therapy in patients with biliary atresia. Ullrich *et al.* administered UDCA to two children with biliary atresia in whom growth arrest had occurred despite maximization of calories with nasogastric feedings and supplementation with medium-chain triglycerides and fat-soluble vitamins; there had also been deterioration in hepatic function[58]. UDCA therapy (17 mg/kg per day orally at bedtime) was associated with an increase in body weight and in length; in one of the children there was a trend towards a decrease in the indices of hepatobiliary dysfunction. Nittono *et al.* administered UDCA (10–15 mg/kg per day) to six patients with biliary atresia, four had a decrease in serum bilirubin and bile acids while two did not respond[59].

In our preliminary studies of patients with biliary atresia, UDCA has been unsuccessful in halting the progression of the disease despite an apparent improvement in weight gain and a decrease in serum aminotransferase and bilirubin levels[10]. In selected patients, however, UDCA was associated with a reduction in the degree of pruritus. We also noted a decrease in pruritus in several patients following in transition from placebo to UDCA. At the 1- and 2-year follow-up points there were no observed differences in survival or the need for transplantation between the two groups. No side-effects were noted. UDCA in a dose range of 15–30 mg/kg per day, while possibly mediating an amelioration of clinical symptoms such as pruritus, does not appear to affect the outcome for patients with biliary atresia.

Conclusion

While preliminary trials have not indicated a role for UDCA in forestalling the progression of hepatic injury, UDCA therapy may be attempted in hopes of ameliorating pruritus.

CYSTIC FIBROSIS ASSOCIATED LIVER DISEASE

The life expectancy for patients with cystic fibrosis (CF) continues to be extended, initially through improved pulmonary and general medical care and perhaps in the future through gene therapy. Concomitant with the increased median survival the incidence of recognizable hepatobiliary complications has increased[60–66]. There is a wide spectrum of hepatobiliary disease reported in patients with cystic fibrosis (Table 4). Hepatobiliary disease, while often asymptomatic, can be severe; the major concern is focal biliary cirrhosis progressing to multilobular biliary cirrhosis.

Pathogenesis

The pathogenesis of these lesions, while not completely understood, has been ascribed to the accumulation or inspissation of eosinophilic material in the intrahepatic ducts; this material serves to occlude the duct, leading to chronic inflammatory infiltrate, bile duct proliferation and fibrosis with extension and coalescence, culminating in cirrhosis[1,61–65].

Table 4 Hepatobiliary diseases reported in patients with cystic fibrosis

Specific to cystic fibrosis
Hepatic
Focal biliary cirrhosis with inspissation
Multilobular cirrhosis with inspissation
Biliary
Microgallbladder
Mucous hyperplasia of gallbladder
Mucocoele
Secondary to extrahepatic disease
Lesions associated with cardiopulmonary disease
Centrilobular necrosis
Cirrhosis
Lesions associated with pancreatic disease
Pancreatic duct sludge (obstruction)
Pancreatic fibrosis (leading to bile duct compression or stricture)
Lesions that occur with higher frequency in patients with cystic fibrosis
Hepatic
Fatty liver
Neonatal cholestasis
Drug hepatotoxicity
Endotoxaemia
Viral hepatitis
Biliary
Biliary sludge
Cholelithiasis
Sclerosing cholangitis
Cholangiocarcinoma

Modified from Balistreri WF. Spectrum of liver disease in patients with cystic fibrosis. Pediatr Pulmonol. 1990;S5:71–3

Clinical manifestations

The major clinical manifestations of CF-associated liver disease are hepatomegaly, splenomegaly and variceal haemorrhage. Liver transplantation has been carried out in patients with end-stage liver disease.

The role of UDCA in cystic fibrosis

Since the presumed underlying pathogenesis of CF-associated liver disease is the accumulation of abnormal, hyperviscid secretions with bile stasis, a strong rationale for UDCA therapy can be presented. The goals are to attempt to decrease the viscosity of bile, and to replace or displace hepatotoxic bile acids. In patients with CF, UDCA therapy has been associated with an improvement in biochemical parameters[63,67–77]. There has also been scintigraphic documentation of an improvement in bile flow during UDCA therapy[73]. Colombo *et al.* reported a significant and sustained improvement ($p<0.01$) in indices of cytolysis and cholestasis in 19 patients with CF and liver disease treated with UDCA (20 mg/kg per day) for periods ranging from 33 to 66 months; these effects were maintained throughout treatment[71]. Over the follow-up period no deterioration occurred in indices reflecting hepatic synthesis or nutritional status. No significant change in the coefficient of fat absorption was observed; growth rates improved in seven patients. Hepatobiliary scintigraphy revealed a consistent reduction in the time of intestinal appearance of isotope, suggesting an improvement in bile flow. The degree of improvement of scintigraphic parameters was greater in patients without cirrhosis. During the follow-up, two patients with multilobular biliary cirrhosis developed portal hypertension, whereas no clinical and ultrasonographic signs of liver cirrhosis occurred in the seven patients without cirrhosis at entry. These data suggest UDCA treatment is safe and effective in CF patients with liver disease; however, it may not be able to prevent the development of portal hypertension once cirrhosis is present[71].

Conclusion

UDCA therapy should be instituted in all patients with CF-associated liver disease. Further trials are needed to document whether UDCA therapy is associated with a forestalling of the progression to cirrhosis in patients with CF. A long-term controlled trial to establish whether UDCA is of any value in *prevention* of CF-associated liver disease in patients at high risk would be of extreme benefit.

TPN-ASSOCIATED CHOLESTASIS

Advances in neonatal care have permitted the long-term survival of extremely low birth weight premature infants. However, many of these low birth weight infants are unable to ingest oral nutrients, therefore nutrient intake must be provided exclusively via the parenteral route. This leads to numerous adverse hepatobiliary consequences. The most frequent and predictable complication of total parenteral nutrition (TPN) is cholestasis; this is especially prominent in infants of extreme low birth weight (<1500 g) or in those with short gut syndrome[78–81].

Major clinical manifestations

The incidence of cholestasis is inversely related to gestational age, and directly to the duration of infusion. TPN-associated cholestasis is most frequently noted in small critically ill infants whose clinical picture is dominated by the features of sepsis or multi-organ failure[1,81]. In addition to low birth weight, most affected infants have confounding variables such as sepsis and necrotizing enterocolitis; they are often the recipient of blood transfusions and drugs[1,81]. The onset is insidious; cholestasis is most often noted during routine serial monitoring by a rise in serum bilirubin or bile acids. Serum aminotransferase levels might be midly elevated while hepatic synthetic function is typically normal[78,82]. Hepatomegaly may be present.

Pathophysiology

The pathogenesis of the hepatobiliary injury engendered by the exclusive infusion of nutrients is poorly defined and is most likely multifactorial[1,81]. Presumably there is an interaction of epidemiological features (low birth weight, bowel disease, sepsis and multi-organ failure), and the predisposing role of immaturity of hepatic function and physiological cholestasis[1,83–86]. In the immature liver, bile flow rates, both basal and bile acid-stimulated, are lower than in the adult. This physiological feature suggests a rationale for UDCA; the goal being to increase bile flow.

The role of ursodeoxycholic acid in TPN-associated cholestasis (TPN-AC)

UDCA might be of benefit to patients at risk for TPN-AC; this compound could theoretically improve bile flow[45,78], exert a cytoprotective effect[87], or modify gut-derived endotoxaemia[88]. There have been no controlled trials of UDCA in the treatment of TPN-associated cholestasis. In a case report Lindor, *et al.* noted an improvement in an adult with TPN-associated cholestasis[89]. Beau *et al.* carried out a prospective study to determine the effects of short-term administration of UDCA in nine patients, all adults treated with long-term TPN[90]. UDCA administration (approximately 11 mg/kg per day) induced a significant reduction in GGTP and AST from baseline values; there was no significant change in alkaline phosphatase or bilirubin levels. Preliminary studies from Kowalski *et al.* suggested that administration of UDCA significantly reduced biochemical markers of cholestasis in adult patients receiving long-term TPN[91]. Cocjin *et al.* have reported preliminary results regarding the use of UDCA in an attempt to alter the course of TPN-associated cholestasis in neonates[92]. A major limitation to the use of UDCA is the poor degree of biliary enrichment attained in these low-birth-weight infants who often have reduced intestinal length[78].

Conclusion

Whether UDCA therapy alters histology or the natural history of the disease remains unknown; however, trials, especially in low-birth-weight infants and in children with short gut syndrome, are required. These issues have recently been discussed by Hofmann *et al.*[93].

SUMMARY

The enigmatic cholestatic liver diseases of children present unique challenges. Until a specific therapy is available it appears that UDCA may be part of an effective targeted strategic regimen of bile acid replacement or displacement[10]. In all patients UDCA was well tolerated; there were no significant side-effects, therefore UDCA appears to be a safe and effective therapeutic agent for children with chronic cholestasis. Controlled trials of the long-term effects of this agent in these disorders are needed.

Acknowledgements

This work was funded by FD-R-000357-03; ursodeoxycholic acid was supplied by the Falk Foundation, Freiburg, Germany. The authors wish to thank Al Patterson, Pharm. D., and Dennis Eling, R. Ph. for drug formulation and distribution; Joseph Santangelo for technical assistance and Ms. Patti Gubser for her assistance in manuscript preparation.

References

1. Balistreri WF, Schubert WK. Liver disease in infancy and childhood. In: Schiff L, Schiff ER, editors. Diseases of the liver, 7th edn. Philadelphia: Saunders; 1993:1099–1203.
2. Balistreri WF. Neonatal cholestasis: medical progress. J Pediatr. 1985;106:171.
3. Balistreri WF. neonatal cholestasis: lessons from the past, issues for the future (Foreword). Semin Liver Dis. 1987;7:1–3.
4. Bruguera M, Llach J, Rodes J. Nonsyndromic paucity of intrahepatic bile ducts in infancy and idiopathic ductopenia in adulthood: the same syndrome? Hepatology. 1992;15:830–4.
5. Alagille D *et al.* Hepatic ductular hypoplasia associated with characteristic facies, vertebral malformations, retarded physical, mental, and sexual development, and cardiac murmur. J Pediatr. 1975;86:63.
6. Alagille D, Estrada A, Hadchouel M, Gautier M, Odievre M, Dommergues JP. Syndromic paucity of interlobular bile ducts (Alagille syndrome or arteriohepatic dysplasia): review of 80 cases. J Pediatr. 1987;110:195–200.
7. Greenwood RD *et al.* Syndrome of intrahepatic biliary dysgenesis and cardiovascular malformations. Pediatrics. 1976;58:243.
8. Watson GH, Miller V. Arteriohepatic dysplasia: familial pulmonary arterial stenosis with neonatal liver disease. Arch Dis Child. 1973;43:459.
9. Brodsky MC, Cunniff C. Ocular anomalies in the Alagille syndrome (arteriohepatic dysplasia). Ophthalmology. 1993;100:1767–74.
10. Balistreri WF, Setchell KDR, Ryckman FC, and the UDCA Study Group. Bile acid therapy in paediatric liver disease. In Paumgartner G, Stiehl A, Gerok W, editors. Bile acids and the hepatobiliary system. London: Kluwer; 1993:271–82.
11. Sokol RJ, Heubi JE, Iannaccone ST, Bove KE, Balistreri WF. Vitamin E deficiency with normal serum vitamin E concentrations in children with chronic cholestasis. N Engl J Med. 1984;310:1209–12.
12. Kaufman SS, Wood RP, Shaw BW, Jr *et al.* Hepatocarcinoma in a child with the Alagille syndrome. Am J Dis Child. 1987;141:698–700.
13. Markowitz J *et al.* Arteriohepatic dysplasia. I. Pitfalls in diagnosis and management. Hepatology. 1983;3:74.
14. Balistreri WF, A-Kader HH, Setchell KDR and the UDCA Study Group. Ursodeoxycholic acid therapy in pediatric patients with chronic cholestasis. In: Lentze, Reichem, editors. Pediatric cholestasis: approaches to treatment, London: Kluwer; 1991:333–44.
15. Levy E, Bendayan M, Thibault L, Lambert M, Paradis K. Lipoprotein abnormalities in two children with minimal biliary excretion. J Pediatr Gastroenterol Nutr. 1995;20:432–9.
16. Krawinkel MB, Santer R, Oldigs HD. Ursodeoxycholic acid: effect on xanthomas in Alagille–Watson syndrome. J Pediatr Gastroenterol Nutr. 1994;19:476–7.
17. Janas RM, Tretter J, Warnawin K, Pawlowska J, Rujner J, Socha J. Methionine enkephalin and aminopeptidase-M activity in blood in children with cholestasis before and after treatment with ursodeoxycholic acid. In: van Berge Henegouwen GP, De Groote J, van Hoek B, Matern S, Stockbrugger RW, editors. Cholestatic liver diseases: new strategies for prevention and treatment of hepatobiliary and cholestatic liver diseases. London: Kluwer; 1994:226–35.
18. Janas RM, Tretter J, Warnawin K, Pawlowska J, Rujner J, Socha J. Methionine enkephalin concentration and enkephalin-degrading activity are elevated in blood in children with cholestasis. Eur J Gastroenterol Hepatol. 1994;6:539–45.
19. Narkewicz MR, Sokol RJ, Smith D, Gregory C, Lear J. Ursodeoxycholic acid does not improve quantitative tests of hepatic function in children with intrahepatic cholestasis despite clinical improvement. Hepatology. 1992;16:258A (abstract).
20. Maggiore G, Bernard O, Riely CA, Hadchouel M, Lemonnier A, Alagille D. Normal serum β-glutamyl-transpeptidase activity identified groups of infants with idiopathic cholestasis with poor prognosis. J Pediatr. 1987;111:251–2.
21. Jones EA *et al.* Progressive intrahepatic cholestasis of infancy and childhood: a clinicopathological study of a patient surviving to the age of 18 years. Gastroenterology. 1976; 71:675.
22. Odievre M *et al.* Severe familial intrahepatic cholestasis. Arch Dis Child. 1973;48:806.

23. Whitington PF, Freese DK, Alonso EM, Schwarzenberg SJ, Sharp J. Clinical and biochemical findings in progressive familial intrahepatic cholestasis. J Pediatr Gastroenterol Nutr. 1994;18:134–41.
24. Alonso EM, Snover DC, Montag A, Freese DK, Whitington PF. Histologic pathology of the liver in progressive familial intrahepatic cholestasis. J Pediatr Gastroenterol Nutr. 1994;18:128–33.
25. Chobert MN, Bernard O, Bulle F, Lemonnier A, Guellaen G, Alagille D. High hepatic b-glutamyltransferase (b-GT) activity with normal serum b-GT in children with progressive idiopathic cholestasis. J Hepatol. 1989;8:22–5.
26. Maggiore G, Bernard O, Hadchouel M, Lemmonnier A, Alagille D. Diagnostic value of serum b-glutamyl transpeptidase activity in liver diseases in children. J Pediatr Gastoenterol Nutr. 1991;12:21–6.
27. Soubrane O, Gauthier F, DeVictor D *et al.* Orthotopic liver transplantation for Byler disease. Transplantation. 1994;50:804–6.
28. Jacquemin E, Dumont M, Bernard O, Erlinger S, Hadchouel M. Evidence for defective primary bile acid secretion in children with progressive familial intrahepatic cholestasis. Eur J Pediatr. 1993;153:424–8.
29. Tazawa Y, Yamada M, Nakagawa M, Konno T, Tada K. Bile acid profiles in siblings with progressive intrahepatic cholestasis: absence of biliary chenodeoxycholic acid. J Pediatr Gastroenterol Nutr. 1985;4:32–7.
30. Whitington PF, Whitington GL. Partial external diversion of bile for the treatment of intractable pruritus associated with intrahepatic cholestasis. Gastroenterology. 1988;95:130–6.
31. Balistreri WF. Inborn errors of bile acid metabolism: clinical and therapeutic aspects. In: Hofmann AF, Paumgartner G, Stiehl A, eds. Bile acids in gastroenterology: basic and clinical advances. Boston, Dordrecht, London: Kluwer Academic Publishers; 1995: 333–53.
32. Eyssen H *et al.* Trihydroxycoprostanic acid in the duodenal bile of two children with intrahepatic bile duct anomalies. Biochim Biophys Acta. 1972;273:212.
33. Hanson RF *et al.* The metabolism of 3 alpha, 7 alpha, 12 alpha, trihydroxy-5β-cholestan-26-oic acid in two siblings with cholestasis due to intrahepatic bile duct anomalies. J Clin Invest. 1975;56:577.
34. Balistreri WF. Fetal and neonatal bile acid synthesis and metabolism: clinical implications. J Inher Metab Dis. 1991;14:459–77.
35. Balistreri WF, Hofmann AF, A-Kader HH, Setchell KDR. Successful bile acid therapy in 3 siblings with neonatal hepatitis due to an inborn error of bile acid biosynthesis. Pediatr Res. 1991;29:99A.
36. Balistreri WF, Setchell KDR. Clinical implications of bile acid metabolism. In: Silverger M, Daum F, editors. Textbook of pediatric gastroenterology. Chicago: Year Book Medical; 1987:72–89.
37. Setchell KDR, Street JM. Inborn errors of bile acid synthesis. Semin Liver Dis. 1987;7:85–9.
38. Setchell KDR, O'Connell NC. Inborn errors of bile acid metabolism. In: Suchy FJ, editor. Liver disease in children. Boston, MA: Mosby; 1994:835–51.
39. Clayton PT, Leonard JV, Lawson AM *et al.* Familial giant cell hepatitis associated with synthesis of 3β,7α-dihydroxy and 3β,7α,12α-trihydroxy-5-cholenoic acids. J Clin Invest. 1987;79:1031–8.
40. Setchell KDR, Suchy FJ, Welsh MB, Zimmer-Nechemias L, Heubi J, Balistreri WF. Δ^4-3-Oxosteroid 5β-reductase deficiency described in identical twins with neonatal hepatitis: a new inborn error in bile acid synthesis. J Clin Invest. 1988;82:2148–57.
41. Bjorkhem I, Boberg KM. Inborn errors in bile acid biosynthesis and storage of sterols other than cholesterol. In: Scriver C, Beaudet A, Sly C, Valle D, editors. Metabolic basis of inherited disease. 1995:2073–93.
42. Evans JE, Ghosh A, Evans BA, Natowicz MB. Screening techniques for the detection of inborn errors of bile acid metabolism by direct injection and micro-high performance liquid chromatography continuous flow/fast atom bombardment mass spectrometry. Biol Mass Spectrom. 1993;22:331–7.
43. Libert R, Hermans D, Draye JP, Van Hoof F, Sokal E, de Hoffmann E. Bile acids and conjugates identified in metabolic disorders by fast atom bombardment and tandem mass spectrometry. Clin Chem. 1991,27:2101–10.
44. Daugherty CC, Setchell KDR, Heubi JE, Balistreri WF. Resolution of liver biopsy alterations in 3 siblings with bile acid treatment of an inborn error of bile acid metabolism (Δ_4-3-oxosteroid 5β-reductase deficiency). Hepatology. 1993;18:1096–101.

45. Hofmann AF. Pharmacology of ursodeoxycholic acid, an enterohepatic drug. Scand J Gastroenterol. 1994;204:1–15.
46. Clayton PT. Inborn errors of bile acid metabolism. J Inher Metab Dis. 1991;14:478–96.
47. Witzleben CL, Piccoli DA, Setchell KDR. Case 3: A new category of causes of intrahepatic cholestasis. Pediatr Pathol. 1992;12:269–74.
48. Setchell KDR, Balistreri WF, Piccoli DA, Clerici C. Oral bile acid therapy in the treatment of inborn errors in bile acid synthesis associated with liver disease. In: Paumgartner G, Stichl A, Gerok W, editors. Bile acids as therapeutic agents. 1990:367–73.
49. Ichimiya H, Nazer H, Gunaskeran T, Clayton P, Sjovall J. Treatment of chronic liver disease caused by 3β-hydroxy-Δ^5-C_{27}-steroid hydrogenase deficiency with chenodeoxycholic acid. Arch Dis Child. 1990;65:1121–4.
50. Ichimiya H, Egestad B, Nazer H, Baginski ES, Clayton PT, Sjovall J. Bile acids and bile alcohols in a child with hepatic 3β-hydroxy-Δ^5-C_{27}-steroid dehydrogenase deficiency: effects of chenodeoxycholic acid treatment. J Lipid Res. 1991;32:829–41.
51. Horslen SP, Lawson AM, Malone M, Clayton PT. 3β-Hydroxy-Δ^5-C_{27} steroid dehydrogenase deficiency; effect of chenodeoxycholic acid therapy on liver histology. J Inher Metab Dis. 1992;15:38 46.
52. Jacquemin E, Setchell KDR, O'Connell NC *et al.* A new cause of progressive intrahepatic cholestasis: 3β-hydroxy-C_{27}-steroid dehydrogenase/isomerase deficiency. J Pediatr. 1994;125:379–84.
53. Ryckman FC, Noseworthy J. Neonatal cholestatic conditions requiring surgical reconstruction. Semin Liver Dis. 1987;7:134–54.
54. Ryckman FC, Ziegler MM, Pedersen SH, Dittrich V, Balistreri WF. Liver transplantation in children. In: Suchy FJ, editor. Liver disease in children. Boston: Mosby; 1994:930–50.
55. Dahms BB. Biliary atresia: Extrahepatic? Intrahepatic? Both? Neither?: Transplant Pathol. 1994;18:142–5.
56. Davenport M, Savage M, Mowat AP, Howard ER. Biliary atresia splenic malformation syndrome: an etiologic and prognostic subgroup. Surgery. 1993;113:662–8.
57. Mieli-Vergani G, Howard ER, Portmann B, Mowat AP. Late referral for biliary atresia: missed opportunities for effective surgery. Lancet. 1989;1:421–3.
58. Ullrich D, Rating D, Schroter W. Treatment with ursodeoxycholic acid renders children with biliary atresia suitable for liver transplantation. Lancet. 1987;2:1234 (letter).
59. Nittono H, Tokita A, Hayashi M *et al.* Ursodeoxycholic acid therapy in the treatment of biliary atresia. Biomed Pharmacother. 1989;43:37–41.
60. Taylor WF, Quaquandah BY. Neonatal jaundice associated with cystic fibrosis. Am J Dis Child. 1972;123:161.
61. Oppenheimer EH, Esterly JR. Hepatic changes in young infants with cystic fibrosis: possible relation to focal biliary cirrhosis. J Pediatr. 1975;86:683–9.
62. Park RW, Grand RJ. Gastrointestinal manifestations of cystic fibrosis: a review. Gastroenterology. 1981;81:1143.
63. Psarcharopoulos HT *et al.* Hepatic complications of cystic fibrosis. Lancet. 1981;2:78.
64. Roy CC, Weber Am, Morin CL *et al.* Hepatobiliary disease in cystic fibrosis: a survey of current issues and concepts. J Pediatr Gastroenterol Nutr. 1982;1:469–78.
65. Valman HB *et al.* Prolonged neonatal jaundice in cystic fibrosis. Arch Dis Child. 1971;46:805.
66. Craig JM *et al.* The pathological changes in the liver in cystic fibrosis of the pancreas. Am J Dis Child. 1957;93:357.
67. Colombo C, Setchell KDR, Podda M *et al.* Effects of ursodeoxycholic acid therapy for liver disease associated with cystic fibrosis. J Pediatr. 1990;117:482–9.
68. Cotting J, Lentze MJ, Reichen J. Effects of ursodeoxycholic acid treatment on nutrition and liver function in patients with cystic fibrosis and longstanding cholestasis. Gut. 1990;31:918–21.
69. Strandvik B, Lindblad A. Cystic fibrosis: is treatment with ursodeoxycholic acid of value? Scand J Gastroenterol. 1994;204:65–7.
70. Merli M, Bertasi S, Servi R *et al.* Effect of a medium dose of ursodeoxycholic acid with or without taurine supplementation on the nutritional status of patients with cystic fibrosis: a randomized, placebo-controlled, crossover trial. J Pediatr Gastroenterol Nutr. 1994;19:198–203.
71. Colombo C, Apostolo MG, Comi S, Glunta A. Long-term treatment with ursodeoxycholic acid (UDCA) in liver disease associated with cystic fibrosis (CF). J Pediatr Gastroenterol Nutr. 1995;20:470.

72. Colombo C. Cholestatic liver diseases in children. In: van Berge Henegouwen GP, van Hoek B, de Groote J, Matern S, Stockbrugger RW, editors. Cholestatic liver disease: new strategies for prevention and treatment of hepatobiliary and cholestatic liver disease. London: Kluwer; 1994:154–63.
73. Colombo C, Castellani MR, Balistreri WF, Seregni E, Assaisso ML, Giunta A. Scintigraphic documentation of an improvement in hepatobiliary excretory function after treatment with ursodeoxycholic acid in patients with cystic fibrosis and associated liver disease. Hepatology. 1992;15:677–84.
74. Colombo C, Podda M, Battezzati PM *et al.* Ursodeoxycholic acid for cystic fibrosis-associated liver disease: final report of a multicenter trial. Hepatology. 1993;18:142A (abstract).
75. Galabert C, Montet JC, Lengrand D *et al.* Effects of ursodeoxycholic acid on liver function in patients with cystic fibrosis and chronic cholestasis. J Pediatr. 1992;121:138–41.
76. Bittner P, Posselt HG, Sailer T *et al.* The effect of treatment with ursodeoxycholic acid in cystic fibrosis and hepatopathy: results of a placebo-controlled study. In: Paumgartner G, Stiehl A, Gerok W, editors. Bile acids as therapeutic agents – from basic science to clinical practice. Dordrecht: Kluwer; 1991:345–8.
77. O'Brien S, Fitzgerald MX, Hegarty JE. A controlled trial of ursodeoxycholic acid treatment in cystic fibrosis-related liver disease. Eur J Gastroenterol Hepatol. 1992;4:857–63.
78. Balistreri WF, Bove K. Hepatobiliary consequences of parenteral nutrition. In: Boyer JL, ed. Progress in liver disease, vol. 9. 1989:567–601.
79. Postuma R, Trevenen CL. Liver disease in infants receiving total parenteral nutrition. Pediatrics. 1979;63:110.
80. Whitington PF. Cholestasis associated with total parenteral nutrition in infants. Hepatology. 1985;5:693.
81. Balistreri WF, Bucuvalas JC, Farrell MF, Bove KE. Total parenteral nutrition-associated cholestasis: Factors responsible for the decreasing incidence. In Lentze M, Reichem J, editors. Paediatric cholestasis; novel approaches to treatment. London: Kluwer; 1991:191–206.
82. Farell MK *et al.* Serum-sulfated lithocholate as an indicator of cholestasis during parenteral nutrition in infants and children. J Parent Enter Nutr. 1982;6:30.
83. Balistreri WF *et al.* Immaturity of the enterohepatic circulation in early life: factors predisposing to 'physiologic' maldigestion and cholestasis. J Pediatr Gastroenterol Nutr. 1983;2:346.
84. Balistreri WF *et al.* Immaturity of enterohepatic circulation of bile acids in early life: factors responsible for increased peripheral serum bile acid concentration. In: editors. Proceedings of Falk Symposium No. 42, Eighth International Bile Acid Meeting, Berne. Lancaster: MTP Press; 1985:87–93.
85. Sondheimer JM *et al.* Cholestatic tendencies in premature infants on and off parenteral nutrition. Pediatrics. 1978;62:984.
86. Suchy FJ *et al.* Physiologic cholestasis: elevations of the primary serum bile acid concentrations in normal infants. Gastroenterology. 1981;80:1037.
87. Leuschner U, Guldutuna S, Bhatti S, Sipos P, You T, Zimmer G. Cytoprotection by ursodeoxycholic acid. In: van Berge Henegouwen GP, van Hoek B, de Groote J, Matern S, Stockbrugger RW, editors. Cholestatic liver diseases (Falk Symposium no. 75), London: Kluwer; 1994:218–25.
88. Schwarzenberg SJ, Bundy M. Ursodeoxycholic acid modifies gut-derived endotoxemia in neonatal rats. Pediatr Res. 1994;35:214–17.
89. Lindor KD, Burnes J. Ursodeoxycholic acid for the treatment of home parenteral nutrition-associated cholestasis. Gastroenterology. 1991;101:250–3.
90. Beau P, Labat-Labourdette J, Ingrand P, Beauchant M. Is ursodeoxycholic acid an effective therapy for total parenteral nutrition related liver disease? J Hepatol. 1994;20:240–4.
91. Kowalski TE, Bosse M, Mullen J, Holt PR, Tint G, Malet PF. Randomized double-blind trial of ursodeoxycholic acid versus placebo for the treatment of parenteral nutrition-associated cholestasis. Gastroenterology. 1994;106:A615.
92. Cocjin J, Watanabe F, Sehgal S, Vanderhal A, Rosenthal P. Does ursodeoxycholic acid alter the course of total parenteral nutrition-associated cholestasis in the neonate? Pediatr Res. 1995;35:126A.
93. Hofmann AF. Defective biliary secretion during total parenteral nutrition: probable mechanisms and possible solutions. J Pediatr Gastroenterol Nutr. 1995;20:376–90.

34
Indications for ursodeoxycholic acid therapy in chronic active hepatitis

M. PODDA, A. CROSIGNANI, A. LARGHI and M. ZUIN

INTRODUCTION

Ursodeoxycholic acid (UDCA) was shown to improve serum liver biochemistry[1–5], liver histology[4] and, more recently, survival[6,7] in primary biliary cirrhosis. The mechanism of action has been attributed to dilution and/or displacement of endogenous detergent hepatotoxic bile acids[8–10].

Endogenous bile acids may play a role also in chronic active hepatitis (CAH) by aggravating and perpetuating liver cell injury. Impaired bile acid secretion, with retention of detergent bile acids and subsequent hepatocellular damage, may be a feature of CAH[11]. In fact, in patients with necroinflammatory liver disease, high concentrations of hydrophobic hepatotoxic bile acids were found in liver tissue[11]. Moreover, relatively low concentrations of bile acids may potentiate heptotoxicity induced by other agents. Therefore, though UDCA administration has no effect on the most common aetiological agents of CAH, enrichment of the bile acid pool with this highly hydrophilic, non-toxic bile acid may counteract the detrimental effects of the retention of endogenous bile acids, thus improving the clinical expression of the disease. In addition, treatment with UDCA may be of particular interest in patients with autoimmune hepatitis, since UDCA was shown to have immunomodulatory effects also[12–14].

In this chapter, the results of the clinical studies carried out with UDCA in patients with CAH will be reviewed in order to give an indication of its potential use in clinical and experimental settings.

PILOT AND DOSE–RESPONSE STUDIES

After initial reports from Japan of improvement in serum transaminase levels during UDCA administration to patients with chronic liver disease[15–17], Leuschner *et al.* observed, for the first time in Europe, a consistent decrease of AST (by 42%) and ALT (by 39%) in 6 patients with CAH and concomitant radiolucent gallstones who were administered UDCA at a daily dose of 8–11 mg/kg for litholytic purposes[18]. Complete dissolution of gallstones was achieved in five of these patients after 5–20 months of treatment[18].

A significant improvement in transaminase and γ-GT serum levels was confirmed by a double-blind placebo-controlled randomized trial in which were enrolled 24 patients with chronic hepatitis[19].

A dose–response study, according to a randomized replicated Latin-square design, was performed by our group in 18 patients with a histological diagnosis of CAH, mainly related to HCV infection[20]. A significant decrease in serum transaminase levels was achieved with the lowest daily dose of 250 mg, corresponding to about 4 mg $kg^{-1} \cdot day^{-1}$, and no further significant improvements were observed with the two higher doses tested (500 and 750 mg/day). The finding of a quadratic relationship between UDCA dose and biliary levels of UDCA conjugates indicates that the maximum enrichment of the bile with UDCA is achieved with the daily dose of 8 mg/kg[20]. More recently, a dose–response study[21] was performed in patients with chronic hepatitis C and, based on the improvement induced on serum liver enzymes, it was suggested that the optimal dose that should be administered to those patients is 600 mg/day. In addition, a relationship between the decrease in serum transaminase levels and the decrease in the hydrophobicity index of the bile acid pool was reported[21].

Several controlled studies[19,21–24] have confirmed the biochemical improvement previously reported by uncontrolled studies[20,25–27]. In all published studies, the majority of patients enrolled had CAH of viral origin, mainly HCV infection. The extent of the decrease in serum ALT ranges from 25% to 58%. A concomitant decrease in γ-GT was consistently reported in patients with abnormal levels at enrollment. However, the low rate of complete normalization of serum liver enzyme levels renders these results unimpressive.

LONG-TERM CONTROLLED STUDIES WITH HISTOLOGICAL EVALUATION

Two randomized placebo-controlled long-term clinical trials aimed at assessing the effects on liver histology were performed with UDCA administered at the daily dose of 600 mg for 1 year[23,24]. Results from both studies indicate that the histological Knodell score was not improved by UDCA administration. However, in one study[24], a score reflecting the 'biliary component' of histology significantly improved compared with placebo, during UDCA administration. Such a 'biliary component' takes into account bile duct damage, ductular metaplasia of periportal hepatocytes, ductular proliferation, signs of cholangiolitis, and phenotypical changes from hepatocytic to biliary type of cytokeratins in liver cells[24]. Though the clinical relevance of such findings is unclear, it is suggested that there is a potential role for UDCA in the treatment of subsets of CAH patients with more evident biochemical and histological expression of cholestasis.

Results from a meta-analysis of all published trials[28] are consistent with improvement in AST, ALT and γ-GT, but no effect of UDCA on the histological expression of the disease was found.

UDCA FOR THE TREATMENT OF CAH OF AUTOIMMUNE AETIOLOGY

Recently, it was suggested that UDCA may have a potential role as primary or adjunctive therapy for the treatment of autoimmune hepatitis[29].

Although clinical experience on UDCA administration for the treatment of CAH of autoimmune aetiology is limited, preliminary data coming from two Japanese groups[30,31] are impressive. In one study, reported in abstract form, normalization of serum transaminase concentrations occurred in 7 of 8 treated patients and, in most of them, a decrease in serum levels of γ-globulins, IgG and antinuclear antibodies was observed[30]. At histology, improvement of intrahepatic inflammation was reported[30].

In the second study, 4 patients with autoimmune hepatitis who were non-responsive to treatment with prednisone (20 mg every other day) alone, were administered UDCA (600 mg/day) as combination therapy. After the addition of UDCA, ALT returned to normal levels; thus the dose of prednisone could be lowered to 5 mg every other day[31].

These data need to be confirmed by controlled studies in larger series of patients. The more realistic goal is obviously the reduction of corticosteroid dosage.

UDCA ASSOCIATED WITH INTERFERON-α FOR HCV-RELATED CAH

UDCA was suggested to have a role in the treatment of HCV-related CAH in association with interferon-α (IFN) with the aim of improving the response rate or of mantaining a sustained response to treatment. Results from two large studies have been published recently[32,33]. The designs of the two studies were identical: all patients were administered IFN for 6 months and one group was randomly assigned to additionally receive UDCA which was continued for three further months. No significant effect on the response rate was shown but UDCA appears to significantly prolong the period during which serum ALT remains within the normal range after the discontinuation of IFN (Figure 1). As expected, UDCA was shown to exert no effect on viraemia. A negligible additional improvement in histology, compared with IFN alone, was reported by one study[33].

In the proceedings of Falk Symposium No. 80, O'Brien *et al.*[34] reported data from 85 patients with chronic hepatitis C who were assigned to receive a 9-month course of IFN, at a dose of 3–5 MU, three times a week, either as monotherapy or in combination with UDCA at a daily dose of 600 mg/day. In the group receiving the combination therapy, they found a more rapid normalization of serum transaminase concentrations during treatment and a reduced relapse rate after discontinuation of treatment. Six months after discontinuation of treatment, 33% of patients who had received combination therapy and 8% of patients receiving IFN alone had normal liver function tests ($p<0.01$). In this study, however, treatment was not randomly assigned but 'patients were stratified into treatment groups based on patient selection of physician'. In addition, patients who were administered IFN alone were significantly older

($p<0.05$) and had more severe disease, i.e. significantly higher presence of liver cirrhosis ($p<0.05$), compared with patients administered the combination therapy.

CONCLUSIONS

Indications for treatment of CAH with UDCA are summarized in Table 1. The only indication which may be accepted at present is administration for the litholytic therapy of radiolucent gallstones concomitant to CAH. On the basis of data coming from long-term clinical trials, UDCA is unlikely to influence the

Table 1 Indications for treatment of CAH with UDCA

Indication	*Aim*
Accepted	
• CAH and associated radiolucent gallstones	Litholysis
To be confirmed	
• Autoimmune hepatitis	To reduce steroid dose
• CAH with cholestatic features	To contrast liver cell injury due to bile salt retention
Perspectives	
• HCV-related CAH in association with IFN	To increase response rate
• Recurrent HCV hepatitis in OLT patients	To prevent bile duct damage

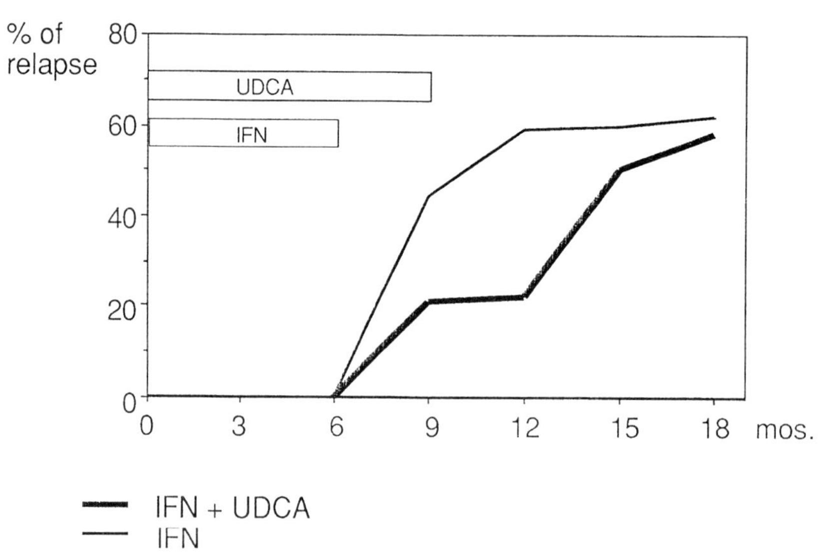

Fig. 1 Interferon-α and ursodeoxycholic acid for chronic active hepatitis related to hepatitis C infection: relapse rate after discontinuation of interferon-α. Modified from Boucher *et al.* 1995[32]

natural history of CAH. However, based on the documented improvement in histological parameters of cholestasis, it is possible that, in patients with cholestatic features, UDCA may play a therapeutic role. Therefore, long-term clinical trials, with clinically relevant end-points, in patients with such characteristics are warranted.

Only scanty but encouraging data are available for UDCA treatment in autoimmune hepatitis. In this case, the rationale for UDCA administration appears to be more solid since there is no identified virologic agent. The perspective of reducing steroid dose by the co-administration of UDCA is clinically relevant and should be tested, especially in view of the severe side-effects of long-term steroid therapy.

Based on the available published data, the association of UDCA with IFN for the treatment of CAH is not justified in terms of rationale, efficacy and cost effectiveness.

References

1. Podda M, Ghezzi C, Battezzati PM *et al.* Ursodeoxycholic acid for chronic liver diseases. J Clin Gastroenterol. 1988;10:s25–s31.
2. Podda M, Ghezzi C, Battezzati PM *et al.* Effect of different doses of ursodeoxycholic acid in chronic liver disease. Dig Dis Sci. 1989;34:59S–65S.
3. Poupon RE, Balkau B, Eschwege E, Poupon R and the UDCA–PBC Study Group. A multicenter, controlled trial of ursodiol for the treatment of primary biliary cirrhosis. N Engl J Med. 1991;324:1548–54.
4. Heathcote EJ, Cauch-Dudek K, Walker V *et al.* The Canadian multicentre double-blind randomized controlled trial of ursodeoxycholic acid in primary biliary cirrhosis. Hepatology. 1994;19:1149–56.
5. Lindor KD, Dickson ER, Baldus WP *et al.* Ursodeoxycholic acid in the treatment of primary biliary cirrhosis. Gastroenterology. 1994;106:1284–90.
6. Poupon RR, Poupon R, Balkau B and the UDCA–PBC Study Group. Ursodiol for long-term treatment of primary biliary cirrhosis. N Engl J Med. 1994;330:1342–7.
7. Heathcote EJ, Lindor KD, Poupon R *et al.* Combined analysis of French, American and Canadian randomized controlled trials of ursodeoxycholic acid therapy in primary biliary cirrhosis. Gastroenterology. 1995;108:1082A.
8. Armstrong MJ, Carey MC. The hydrophobic–hydrophilic balance of bile salts. Inverse correlation between reverse-phase high performance liquid chromatographic mobilities and micellar cholesterol-solubilizing capacities. J Lipid Res. 1982;23:70–80.
9. Hofmann AF, Popper H. Ursodeoxycholic acid for primary biliary cirrhosis. Lancet. 1987;11:398–9.
10. Attili AF, Angelico M, Cantafora A, Alvaro D, Capocaccia L. Bile acid induced liver toxicity: relation to the hydrophobic–hydrophilic balance of bile acids. Med Hypotheses. 1986;19:57–69.
11. Akashi Y, Miyazaki H, Yanagisawa J, Nakayama F. Bile acid metabolism in cirrhotic liver tissue: altered synthesis and impaired hepatic secretion. Clin Chim Acta. 1987;2:199–206.
12. Gianni L, Di Padova F, Zuin M, Podda M. Bile acid-induced inhibition of the lymphoproliferative response to phytohemagglutinin and pokeweed mitogen: an *in vitro* study. Gastroenterology. 1980;78:231–5.
13. Keane RM, Galacz TR, Mumster AM, Birmingham WB, Winchurch RA. Impairment of human lymphocyte function by bile salts. Surgery. 1983;95:439–42.
14. Calmus Y, Gane P, Poupon R. Hepatic expression of class I and class II major histocompatibility complex molecules in primary biliary cirrhosis: effect of ursodeoxycholic acid. Hepatology. 1990;11:12–15.
15. Ichida F. Clinical experience with ursodeoxycholic acid (S-Urso) for chronic hepatitis. Diagn Treat. 1961;36:388.
16. Yamanaka M. Study of curative effect of ursodeoxycholic acid for chronic hepatitis by double-blind trial. Diagn Treat. 1976;64:2150.

17. Ohya T. Long-term administration of ursodeoxycholic acid in patients with chronic hepatitis. A comparison of the effect of two doses on liver function. Jpn Pharmacol Ther. 1985;13:271–6.
18. Leuschner U, Leuschner M, Sieratzki J, Kurtz W, Hubner K. Gallstone dissolution with ursodeoxycholic acid in patients with chronic active hepatitis and two years follow-up. A pilot study. Dig Dis Sci. 1985;30:642–9.
19. Podda M, Ghezzi C, Battezzati PM, Crosignani A, Zuin M, Roda A. Effects of ursodeoxycholic acid and taurine on serum liver enzymes and bile acids in chronic hepatitis. Gastroenterology. 1990;98:1044–50.
20. Crosignani A, Battezzati PM, Setchell KDR *et al.* Effects of ursodeoxycholic acid on serum liver enzymes and bile acid metabolism in chronic active hepatitis; a dose–response study. Hepatology. 1991;13:339–44.
21. Takano S, Ito Y, Yokosuka O *et al.* A multicenter randomized controlled dose study of ursodeoxycholic acid for chronic hepatitis C. Hepatology. 1994;20:558–64.
22. Rolandi E, Franceschini R, Cataldi A, Cicchetti V, Carati L, Barreca T. Effects of ursodeoxycholic acid (UDCA) on serum liver damage indices in patients with chronic active hepatitis. Eur J Clin Pharmacol. 1991;40:473–6.
23. Bellentani S, Podda M, Tiribelli C *et al.* Ursodiol in the long-term treatment of chronic hepatitis: a double-blind multicenter clinical trial. J Hepatol. 1993:19:459–64.
24. Attili AF, Rusticali A, Varriale M, Carli L, Repice AM. The effect of ursodeoxycholic acid on serum enzymes and liver histology in patients with chronic active hepatitis. A 12-month double-blind, placebo-controlled trial. J Hepatol. 1994;20:315–20.
25. Osuga T, Tanaka N, Matsuzaki Y *et al.* Effect of ursodeoxycholic acid in chronic hepatitis and primary biliary cirrhosis. Dig Dis Sci. 1989;34:49S–51S.
26. Ideo G, Bellati G, Predraglio E *et al.* Efficacy of ursodeoxycholic acid in lowering alanine aminotransferase and gamma-glutamyl transpeptidase serum levels in patients with chronic active hepatitis and primary biliary cirrhosis. Curr Ther Res. 1990;47:62–6.
27. Buzzelli G, Moscarella S, Focardi G *et al.* Long-term treatment with ursodeoxycholic acid in patients with chronic active hepatitis. Curr Ther Res. 1991;50:635–42.
28. Simko V, Michael S, Prego V. Ursodeoxycholic therapy in chronic liver disease : a meta-analysis in primary billary cirrhosis and in chronic hepatitis. Am J Gastroenterol. 1994;89:392–8.
29. Czaja AJ. Autoimmune hepatitis. Current therapeutic concepts. Clin Immunother. 1994;1:413–29.
30. Nakamura K, Yoneda M, Tamori K *et al.* Effect of ursodeoxycholic acid (UDCA) on patients with type I autoimmune hepatitis. Gastroenterology. 1995;108:1129A.
31. Mima S, Sekiya C, Kanagawa H, Uchida T. Ursodeoxycholic acid (UDCA) therapy for autoimmune hepatitis. Int Hepatology Commun. 1994;2:207–12.
32. Boucher E, Jouanolle H, Andre P *et al.* Interferon and ursodeoxycholic acid combined therapy in the treatment of chronic viral C hepatitis: results from a controlled randomized trial in 80 patients. Hepatology. 1995;21:322–7.
33. Angelico M, Gandin C, Pescarmona E *et al.* Recombinant interferon-α and ursodeoxycholic acid *versus* interferon-α alone in the treatment and chronic hepatitis C: a randomized clinical trial with long-term follow-up. Am J Gastroenterol. 1995;90:263–9.
34. O'Brien CB, Helzel BS, Long WB, Wolfe L, Yoder A, Rubin RA. Ursodiol and interferon-α for the treatment of chronic hepatitis C. In: Hofmann AF, Paumgartner G, Stiehl A, eds. Bile acids in gastroenterology. Basic and clinical advances. Dordrecht, The Netherlands: Kluwer Academic Publishers; 1995:376–83.

35
Liver function tests for follow-up and assessment of prognosis of biliary diseases

J. REICHEN and H. ZIMMERMANN

INTRODUCTION

Chronic cholestatic diseases such as primary biliary cirrhosis or primary sclerosing cholangitis are characterized by a prolonged course and relatively long survival. The recent development of active, presumably disease-modifying drugs in the treatment of such diseases has made the search for surrogate markers, in particular those evaluating hepatic function, more pressing in order to assess the activity of drugs early, i.e. before hard end-points such as survival or need for transplantation become available[1]. Such surrogate markers could also be useful in assessing the timing of liver transplantation, which can be quite difficult in diseases with individual evolution such as primary sclerosing cholangitis. This review will attempt to answer the question of whether cholestasis *per se* affects liver function; if so whether this has an impact on prognosis; and finally, whether and which liver function tests can be used to assess novel forms of treatment of chronic cholestasis.

IMPACT OF CHOLESTASIS ON LIVER FUNCTION

Clinically, cholestasis ranges from mild biochemical abnormalities over symptomatic diseases to progressive, life-threatening disorders. It comes as no surprise that in the stage of biliary cirrhosis hepatic function should be impaired. The question remains of whether cholestasis *per se* impairs hepatic function; early results suggested that extra- but not intrahepatic cholestasis affected hepatic function as assessed by the clearance of antipyrine[2]. Using animal models we have developed three lines of evidence showing that cholestasis, in particular retention of cholephiles, adversely impacts on hepatic function. First, when comparing micronodular cirrhosis induced by chronic exposure to phenobarbital/CCl_4[3] with biliary cirrhosis induced by ligation/dissection of the common bile duct[4] it becomes apparent that the hepatocyte in the latter model is a 'sick cell' (Fig. 1). This becomes apparent when comparing hepatic function by the aminopyrine breath test with the stereologically determined hepatocyte volume: the former is more impaired in biliary than in micronodular cirrhosis, while hepatocyte volume is maintained in biliary but not in micronodular cirrhosis (Figs 1A and 1B). When hepatic cytochrome P450 content is expressed per millilitre of hepatocyte volume it becomes apparent that in biliary cirrhosis there is much less cytochrome P450 per hepatocyte than in micronodular cirrhosis (Fig. 1C) where this is maintained in agreement with the 'intact cell hypothesis'[5].

The second piece of evidence that cholestasis is responsible for hepatic functional impairment comes from the observation of the reversibility of functional and haemodynamic alterations after decompression of the biliary tree by Roux-en-Y anastomosis[6]. Finally, cholaemia without cholestasis, as induced by a choledocho-caval fistula in rats, induces portal hypertension (Fig. 2) and functional impairment in the absence of any relevant histological changes[7]. These observations lend further support to the hypothesis that retention of some cholephiles could be responsible for the functional impairment in chronic cholestasis.

Prime candidates for such a cholephile impacting on hepatic function are bile acids. Indeed, different mechanisms of action and different cellular targets have been proposed to be responsible for bile acid toxicity. Thus, bile acids lyse different plasma membranes *in vitro*[8,9]; in hepatocytes they induce blebbing of plasma membranes and release of cytosolic enzymes as a function of their hydrophobicity[10,11]. Another target of bile acid toxicity is the endoplasmic reticulum, in particular cytochrome P450[12]. Recently the mitochondrion has been identified as a major target of bile acid toxicity[13]. Earlier reports using bile acids at detergent concentrations found them to be uncouplers of oxidative phosphorylation[14]; however, at lower concentrations more likely found in chronic cholesta-

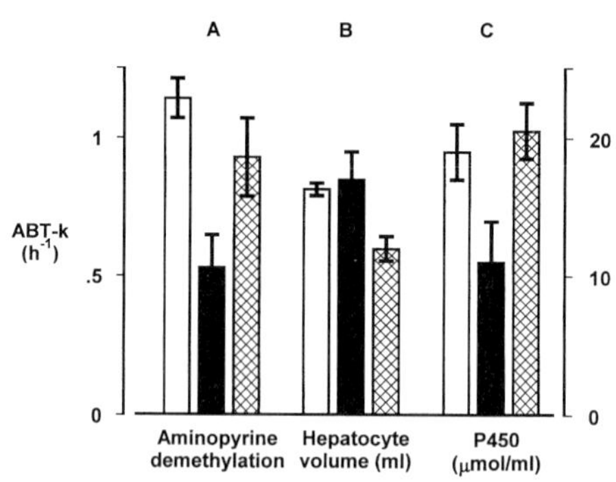

Fig. 1 Aminopyrine *N*-demethylation (**A**), hepatocyte volume (**B**) and cytochrome P450 content expressed per millilitre of hepatocyte (**C**) in control animals (open bars), rats with biliary (solid bars) and with micronodular cirrhosis (hatched bars). Aminopyrine *N*-demethylation was depressed in both groups ($p<0.001$ by ANOVA), while hepatocellular volume was depressed in micronodular but not biliary cirrhosis ($p<0.001$ by ANOVA). When cytochrome P450 was expressed per stereologically determined hepatocellular volume, it was markedly decreased in biliary but not micronodular cirrhosis ($p<0.001$ by ANOVA). Recalculated from refs. 3 and 4

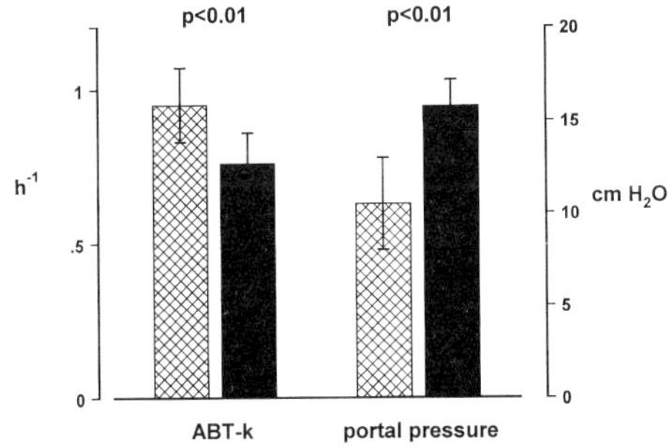

Fig. 2 Hepatic function assessed by the aminopyrine breath test (ABT-k) and portal pressure in control rats (hatched bars) and rats with cholaemia induced by a choledocho-caval fistula. Recalculated from ref. 7. The data show net impairment of hepatic function and portal hypertension in cholaemic rats in the absence of any relevant histological alteration

tic conditions, they impair sites I and III of the electron transfer chain[13]. This is of particular interest, since similar findings associated with mitochondrial proliferation have been described in chronic cholestasis induced by bile duct ligation in the rat[15,16]. Ursodeoxycholate, a more hydrophilic bile acid with protective properties against bile acid toxicity in different systems, is able to counteract these mitochondrial effects[17]. Recently it has been found that ursodeoxycholate reverses the membrane permeability transition in mitochondria induced by glycochenodeoxycholate[18]. Another potential target of bile acid toxicity is the Golgi apparatus: at least at high concentrations, bile acids are associated with the Golgi[19] and chronic bile acid feeding induces distention of Golgi vesicles[20]. Little is known about effects of bile acids in the nucleus, although they clearly are associated with this organelle[21]. The recent demonstration that bile acids induce nuclear proteases suggests that the nucleus could be an important target of bile acid toxicity[22].

The mechanism(s) of bile acid toxicity remain unclear. At high concentrations detergent effects clearly play a role[8,9], but it is unlikely that detergency is a major contributor to toxicity in cholestasis since such concentrations are never attained *in vivo*. It is conceivable, however, that even at submicellar concentrations bile acids remove strategically important lipids, thereby interfering with membrane function; such a mechanism has been clearly demonstrated in mitochondria, where hydrophobic bile acids selectively remove cardiolipin, an essential phospholipid of the inner mitochondrial membrane[13]. Bile acids are incorporated into different biomembranes; whether this alters membrane function remains to be unambiguously demonstrated[13,21]. An increase in cellular calcium has been proposed as a mechanism whereby bile acids induce cell death[23–27]. One potential mode of action is the finding that bile acids act as calcium ionophores[28]; however, in bile salt-induced cell damage it appears that most of the calcium comes from intracellular stores[29]. Bile acids clearly interfere with calcium signalling[30,31], but the role of calcium in bile acid-induced cell death needs to be redefined, since there is a dissociation between calcium fluxes and toxicity in the intact organ[32]. Bile acids increase hepatic oxygen consumption as a function of their hydrophobicity[33]; this raises the possibility that bile acids could act as redox cyclers, thereby inducing membrane damage. Indeed, there is evidence for oxygen radical damage induced by bile acids[34]. The most recent mechanism proposed for bile acid toxicity is induction of apoptosis by bile acids, in particular by glycochenodeoxycholate[22,35]; part of this is achieved by activation of nuclear proteases[22], but the exact molecular mechanism of this fascinating finding remains to be worked out.

These considerations by no means imply that bile acids are the sole candidates for cell damage and death in cholestasis. A list of such candidates with their potential mechanism(s) of actions is provided in Table 1. For a discussion of these compounds the reader is referred to a recent textbook for details[36].

IMPACT OF FUNCTIONAL IMPAIRMENT ON PROGNOSIS

The observation that in biliary cirrhosis induced by bile duct ligation in the rat there is a linear decay in hepatic function[4] suggested that functional impairment could impact on prognosis in chronic cholestasis (Fig. 3). Indeed, we have generated evidence that a similar concept could be applicable to patients with primary biliary cirrhosis using the galactose elimination capacity as a test of cytosolic hepatic function[37]. After a period – often lasting years – with constant hepatic function we observed a decline in galactose elimination capacity preceding any clinical deterioration; this decline allowed for the prediction of death with an accuracy in the range of a few months. Furthermore, this information was independent of the well-accepted Mayo Clinic criteria[38].

That cholestasis may have an impact of prognosis could well be applicable to other liver diseases also. Thus, the cholestatic form of alcoholic hepatitis carries a much worse prognosis than when cholestasis is absent[39]. In chronic hepatitis C, cholestasis as assessed by γ-glutamyl transpeptidase is a negative predictor of response to interferon-α[40,41]. The functional impairment in jaundiced patients as assessed by, for example, the antipyrine clearance, predicts surgical mortality[42].

In view of these findings it appears likely that the adverse impact of cholestasis on hepatic function bears on prognosis.

Table 1 Cholephiles with a potential for impacting on hepatic function and their potential mechanism(s) of action

Cholephile	*Mechanism of action*	*References*
Bilirubin	Mitochondrial uncoupling	61
Bile acids	Detergency	8,9
	Calcium release	24
	Induction of apoptosis	22
	Mitochondrial toxicity	13
	Redox cycling/lipid peroxidation	33,62
Leukotrienes	Haemodynamic and metabolic effects	63
Copper	Lipid peroxidation	64
Cholesterol	Membrane fluidity	65

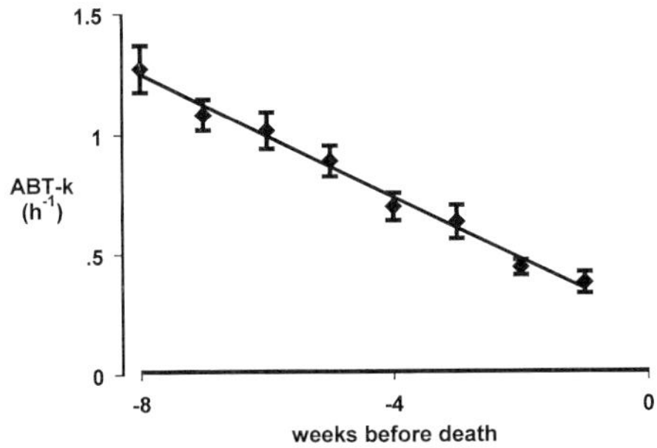

Fig. 3 Decline in hepatic function in rats with biliary cirrhosis induced by bile duct ligation/dissection. Aminopyrine *N*-demethylation decreased in a linear fashion when extrapolated back from the time of death ($y = 0.228–0.128\ x$; $r = 0.891$, $p<0.001$). Reprinted from ref. 4 with permission from the publisher

LIVER FUNCTION TESTS TO ASSESS NOVEL FORMS OF TREATMENT OF CHOLESTASIS

Among the conventional liver tests – enzymes, bilirubin, albumin and prothrombin time – only bilirubin has been shown to contain independent prognostic information in primary biliary cirrhosis[43]. The other tests have prognostic information only as part of general scores such as the Child–Pugh score[44] or of the different disease-specific scores[38,45,46].

When using these simple tests – as well as the more cumbersome test to be discussed below – one should be careful in avoiding tests which could be influenced by the pharmacological agent under study. This is particularly germane for ursodeoxycholate, which emerges as a premier drug in the treatment of chronic cholestatic diseases. The prognostic potential of different liver tests and their potential interference with ursodeoxycholate are listed in Table 2. Thus, ursodeoxycholate, like other bile acids, has direct effects on the excretion of organic anionic dyes[47,48]. At high concentrations it can interfere with hepatic bilirubin glucuronidation *in vitro*[49], while *in vivo* it appears to enhance extrahep-

Table 2 Different liver tests used in cholestatic conditions with an assessment of their prognostic potential and possible interference with ursodeoxycholate

Test	*Prognostic potential*	*Interference with UDCA*
Transaminases	None	No
Alkaline phosphatase	No*	No
Serum bilirubin	Yes	Yes
Serum bile acids	Uncertain	Yes
BSP clearance	Uncertain	Yes
Galactose elimination capacity	Yes	No
Aminopyrine breath test	Uncertain	No
Biliary scintigraphy	Uncertain	Probable

*Alkaline phosphatase has been shown to contain prognostic information in the King's College score for assessing prognosis in primary sclerosing cholangitis[45]

atic enzyme activity[50]. Thus, the prognostic value of the conventional liver tests, as well as that of the disease-specific scores, has to be re-evaluated under ursodeoxycholate treatment and under any other form of treatment.

Different clearance tests of one form or another have been used to assess treatment of cholestasis. The same caution as discussed above for the conventional tests apply to these tests, i.e. they have to be validated for the lack of direct interference with the therapeutic agent under investigation.

It appears logical to assess excretory function as a measure of the efficacy of therapeutic interventions. This can be achieved by clearance tests of compounds exclusively excreted into bile, such as sulphobromophthalein, diiminoacetates used in biliary scintigraphy or bile acids themselves. In their first description of ursodeoxycholate as a therapeutic agent in primary biliary cirrhosis, Poupon *et al.* demonstrated a marked improvement in sulphobromophthalein clearance in their patients[51]. We have generated similar data on the effects of ursodeoxycholate on sulphobromophthalein retention in cholestasis associated with cystic fibrosis[52]; an update on these data has been presented in this series of books[53], and is shown in Fig. 4. The same can be achieved by biliary scintigraphy. The diiminodiacetic compounds used in biliary scintigraphy are excreted by the same or similar canalicular carriers as sulphobromophthalein. Thus, biliary scintigraphy not only permits evaluation of hepatic clearance, but also visualization of partial obstruction, hepatic transit and entry into the small intestine. Colombo *et al.*[54] have used this approach to document marked improvement of hepatic excretory function in cholestatic patients with cystic fibrosis (Fig. 5). A similar approach consists of using γ-labelled bile acids such as [^{75}Se]homocholic acid taurine (SeHCAT), which behaves in quite a similar way to taurocholic acid[54]. Jazrawi and colleagues have used this synthetic bile acid to demonstrate improved clearance function of the liver in patients with primary biliary cirrhosis treated with ursodeoxycholic acid[55]. However, neither BSP clearance nor biliary scintigraphic parameters have ever been shown to carry prognostic information. Furthermore, as discussed above, there is direct interference with ursodeoxycholic acid at the level of the canalicular carrier. Thus, further studies on whether these biliary clearance tests carry prognostic information, and on

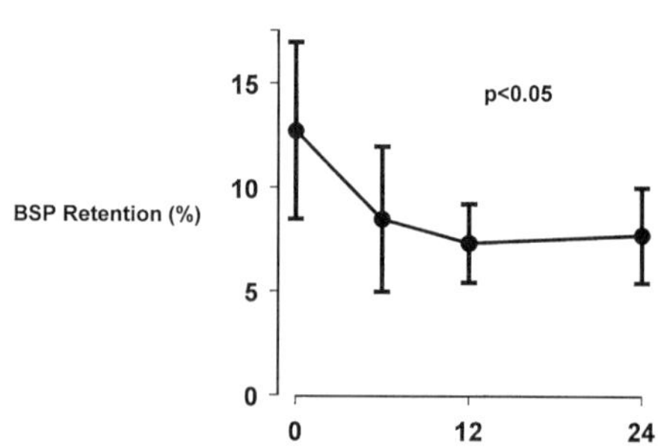

Fig. 4 Evolution of sulphobromophthalein (BSP) retention in cholestatic patients treated with ursodeoxycholate (15–20 mg/kg per day) for up to 2 years. The improvement in BSP retention was maintained up to 2 years and was significant as assessed by analysis of variance. Reprinted from ref. 53 with permission from the publisher

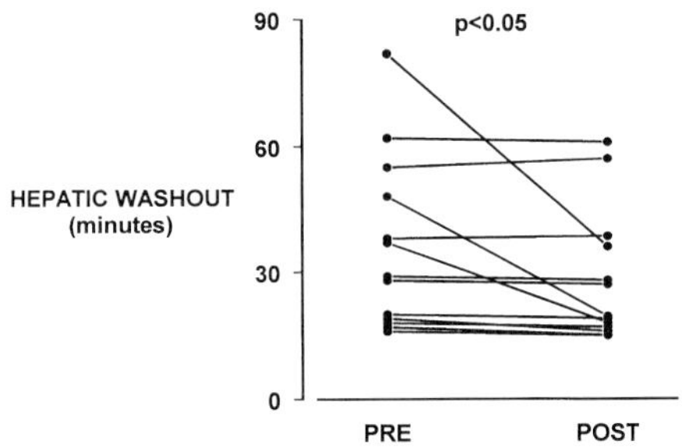

Fig. 5 Half-life of hepatic washout of cholestatic patients with cystic fibrosis assessed by biliary scintigraphy with ^{99m}Tc-tri-methyl-bromo-iminodiacetic acid before (pre) and during (post) treatment with ursodeoxycholic acid 10–15 mg/kg per day. Redrawn from ref. 54 with permission from the authors and publisher

whether this is maintained in treated patients, are required. In the meantime such tests are certainly useful to assess hepatic excretory function and its changes during anticholestatic treatment.

A variety of other clearance tests have been shown to carry prognostic information in chronic liver disease; for a thorough discussion of this topic the reader is referred to a recent review[56]. Among the most widely used clearance tests are the galactose elimination capacity, initially described by Tygstrup[57], the aminopyrine breath test[58], antipyrine clearance[59] and the appearance of MEGX, the major metabolite of lidocaine[60].

Recovery of hepatic function has been clearly demonstrated in obstructive jaundice in the rat[6]; however, none of these clearance tests has been formally evaluated to assess treatment of cholestatic conditions in humans. The galactose elimination capacity could be particularly interesting because of its prognostic information when performed serially in a given patient[37], its innocuousness and the lack of interference of cholestasis with the rate-limiting enzyme, galactose kinase. In an ongoing trial of treatment in primary biliary cirrhosis there was a consistent and statistically significant improvement in galactose elimination capacity under ursodeoxycholate treatment (Fig. 6). This trial investigates the addition of colchicine or placebo to a baseline treatment with ursodeoxycholate, 10–15 mg/kg per day. The finding that hepatic function improves in the majority of patients – a finding never seen in untreated patients – is strongly suggestive that a beneficial effect has been achieved; nevertheless, hard end-points will be required to ultimately prove this point.

In conclusion, further studies are needed to validate surrogate markers – be they conventional liver tests, scores or quantitative tests – under anticholestatic treatment. In the meantime it appears reasonable to include true measures of hepatic function into randomized trials, since they could be useful as surrogate markers. In the case of measures of hepatic excretory function they have already proven their utility; in the case of other clearance tests with proven prognostic information content, validation under treatment is needed, but it appears likely that they are useful surrogate markers at least in primary biliary cirrhosis.

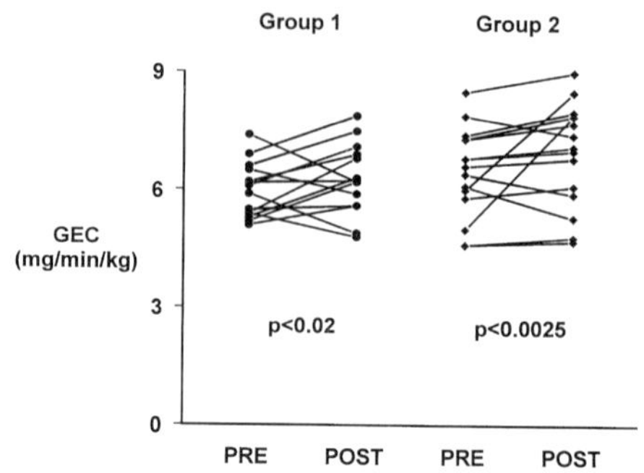

Fig. 6 Evolution of galactose elimination capacity (GEC) in primary biliary cirrhosis in an ongoing randomized clinical trial. All patients are treated with ursodeoxycholate (9–12 mg/kg per day); in addition they receive either placebo or colchicine (1 mg/kg per day). In both groups there is marked amelioration of cytosolic hepatic function after 1 year of treatment, suggesting that this is due to ursodeoxycholate

Acknowledgements

This work was supported by a grant from the Swiss National Foundation for Scientific Research (No. 32-30168.90).

References

1. Reichen J. Pharmacologic treatment of cholestasis. Semin Liver Dis. 1993;13:302–15.
2. Miguet JP, Vuitton D, Deschamps JP *et al.* Cholestasis and hepatic drug metabolism. Comparison of metabolic clearance rate of antipyrine in patients with intrahepatic or extrahepatic cholestasis. Dig Dis Sci. 1981;26:718–22.
3. Reichen J, Arts B, Schafroth U, Zimmermann A, Zeltner TB, Zysset T. Aminopyrine N-demethylation by rats with liver cirrhosis: evidence for the intact cell hypothesis. A morphometric–functional study. Gastroenterology. 1987;93:719–26.
4. Gross JB, Reichen J, Zeltner T, Zimmermann A. The evolution of changes in quantitative liver function tests in a rat model of cirrhosis: correlation with morphometric measurement of hepatocyte mass. Hepatology. 1987;7:457–63.
5. Wood AJJ, Villeneuve JP, Branch RA, Rogers LW, Shand DG. Intact hepatocyte theory of impaired drug metabolism in experimental cirrhosis in the rat. Gastroenterology. 1979;76:1358–62.
6. Zimmermann H, Reichen J, Zimmermann A, Saegesser H, Thenisch B, Hoeflin F. Reversibility of secondary biliary fibrosis by biliodigestive anastomosis in the rat. Gastroenterology. 1992;103:579–89.
7. Zimmermann H, Reichen J, Sägesser H, Tenisch B, Zimmermann A. Biliary retention in a chronic choledocho-venous fistula in the rat: induction of portal hypertension but not of biliary cirrhosis. J Hepatol. 1993;19:110–16.
8. Vyvoda OS, Coleman R, Holdsworth G. Effects of different bile salts upon the composition and morpholoy of a liver plasma membrane preparation. Biochim Biophys Acta. 1977;465:68–76.
9. Schölmerich J, Becher MS, Schmidt KH *et al.* Influence of hydroxylation and conjugation of bile salts on their membrane-damaging properties – studies on isolated hepatocytes and lipid membrane vesicles. Hepatology. 1984;4:661–6.
10. Miyazaki K, Nakayama F, Koga A. Effect of chenodeoxycholic and ursodeoxycholic acids on isolated adult human hepatocytes. Dig Dis Sci. 1984;29:1123–30.
11. Heuman DM, Pandank WM, Hylemon PB, Vlahcevic ZR. Conjugates of ursodeoxycholate protect against cytotoxicity of more hydrophobic bile salts: *in vitro* studies in rat hepatocytes and human erythrocytes. Hepatology. 1991;14:920–6.

12. Hutterer F, Denk H, Bacchin PG, Schenkman JB, Schaffner F, Popper H. Mechanism of cholestasis. 1. Effect of bile acids on microsomal cytochrome P-450 dependent biotransformation systems in vitro. Life Sci. 1970;9:977–87.
13. Krähenbühl S, Talos C, Fischer S, Reichen J. Toxicity of bile acids on the electron transport chain of isolated rat liver mitochondria. Hepatology. 1994;19:471–9.
14. Lee MJ, Whitehouse MW. Inhibition of electron transport chain and coupled phosphorylation in liver mitochondria by cholanic (bile) acids and their conjugates. Biochim Biophys Acta. 1965;100:317–28.
15. Krähenbühl S, Stucki J, Reichen J. Reduced activity of the electron transport chain in liver mitochondria isolated from rats with secondary biliary cirrhosis. Hepatology. 1992;15:1160–6.
16. Krähenbühl S, Krähenbühl-Glauser S, Stucki J, Gehr P, Reichen J. Stereological and functional analysis of liver mitochondria from rats with secondary biliary cirrhosis: impaired mitochondrial metabolism and increased mitochondrial content per hepatocyte. Hepatology. 1992;15:1167–72.
17. Krähenbühl S, Fischer S, Talos C, Reichen J. Ursodeoxycholate protects oxidative mitochondrial metabolism from bile acid toxicity: dose–response study in isolated rat liver mitochondria. Hepatology. 1994;20:1595–601.
18. Botla R, Spivey JR, Aguilar H, Bronk SF, Gores GJ. Ursodeoxycholate (UDCA) inhibits the mitochondrial membrane permeability transition induced by glycochenodeoxycholate: a mechanism of UDCA cytoprotection. J Pharmacol Exp Ther. 1995;272:930–8.
19. Lamri Y, Roda A, Dumont M, Feldmann G, Erlinger S. Immunoperoxidase localization of bile salts in rat liver cells. Evidence for a role of the Golgi apparatus in bile salt transport. J Clin Invest. 1988;82:1173–82.
20. Shefer S, Zaki FG, Salen G. Early morphologic and enzymatic changes in livers of rats treated with chenodeoxycholic and ursodeoxycholic acids. Hepatology. 1983;3:201–8.
21. Strange RC, Chapman BT, Johnston JD, Nimmoo IA, Percy Robb IW. Partitioning of bile acids into subcellular organelles and the in vivo distribution of bile acids in rat liver. Biochim Biophys Acta. 1979;573:535–45.
22. Kwo P, Patel T, Bronk SF, Gores GJ. Nuclear serine protease activity contributes to bile acid-induced apoptosis in hepatocytes. Am J Physiol. 1995;268:G613–21.
23. Oelberg DG, Dubinsky WP, Sackman JW, Wang LB, Adcock EW, Lester R. Bile salts induce calcium uptake in vitro by human erythrocytes. Hepatology. 1987;7:245–52.
24. Combettes L, Dumont M, Berthon B, Erlinger S, Claret M. Release of calcium from the endoplasmic reticulum by bile acids in rat liver cells. J Biol Chem. 1988;263:2299–303.
25. Anwer MS, Little JM, Oelberg DG, Zimniak P, Lester R. Effect of bile acids on calcium efflux from isolated rat hepatocytes and perfused rat livers. Proc Soc Exp Biol Med. 1989;191:147–52.
26. Hamada Y, Karjalainen A, Setchell BA, Millard JE, Bygrave FL. Acute effects of cholestatic and choleretic bile salts on vasopressin- and glucagon-induced hepato-biliary calcium fluxes in the perfused rat liver. Biochem J. 1992;283:575–81.
27. Marrero I, Sanchez-Bueno A, Cobbold PH, Dixon CJ. Taurolithocholate and taurolithocholate 3-sulphate exert different effects on cytosolic free Ca^{2+} concentration in rat hepatocytes. Biochem J. 1994;300:383–6.
28. Zimniak P, Little JM, Radominska A, Oelberg DG, Anwer MS, Lester R. Taurine-conjugated bile acids act as Ca^{2+} ionophores. Biochemistry. 1991;30:8598–604.
29. Combettes L, Berthon B, Doucet E, Erlinger S, Claret M. Bile acids mobilise internal Ca^{++} independently of external Ca^{++} in rat hepatocytes. Eur J Biochem. 1990;190:619–23.
30. Beuers U, Nathanson MH, Boyer JL. Effects of tauroursodeoxycholic acid on cytosolic calcium signals in isolated hepatocytes. Gastroenterology. 1993;104:604–12.
31. Bouscarel B, Fromm H, Nussbaum R. Ursodeoxycholate mobilizes intracellular calcium and activates phosphorylase a in isolated hepatocytes. Am J Physiol. 1993;264:G243–51.
32. Farrell GC, Duddy SK, Kass GEN, Llopis J, Gahm A, Orrenius S. Release of calcium from the endoplasmic reticulum is not the mechanism for bile acid-induced cholestasis and hepatotoxicity in the intact rat liver. J Clin Invest. 1990;85:1255–9.
33. Schölmerich J, Baumgartner U, Miyai K, Gerok W. Hepatic passage of bile acids increases oxygen uptake by perfused rat liver. Res Exp Med. 1990;190:69–75.
34. Sokol RJ, Devereaux M, Khandwala R, O'Brien K. Evidence for involvement of oxygen free radicals in bile acid toxicity to isolated rat hepatocytes. Hepatology. 1993;17:869–81.
35. Patel T, Bronk SF, Gores GJ. Increases of intracellular magnesium promote glycodeoxycholate-induced apoptosis in rat hepatocytes. J Clin Invest. 1994;94:2183–92.

36. Reichen J, Simon FR. Cholestasis. In: Arias IM, Boyer JL, Fausto N, Jakoby WB, Schachter D, Shafritz DA, editors. The liver: biology and pathobiology, 3rd edn. New York: Raven Press; 1994:1291–326.
37. Reichen J, Widmer T, Cotting J. Accurate prediction of death by serial determination of the galactose elimination capacity in primary biliary cirrhosis – a comparison with the Mayo model. Hepatology. 1991;14:504–10.
38. Dickson ER, Grambsch PM, Fleming TR, Fisher LD, Langworthy A. Prognosis in primary biliary cirrhosis: model for decision making. Hepatology. 1989;10:1–7.
39. Nissenbaum M, Chedid A, Mendenhall C, Gartside P. Prognostic significance of cholestatic alcoholic hepatitis. Dig Dis Sci. 1990;35:891–6.
40. Serfaty L, Giral P, Loria A, Andreani T, Legendre C, Poupon R. Factors predictive of the response to interferon in patients with chronic hepatitis C. J Hepatol. 1994;21:12–17.
41. Bellentani S, Podda M, Tiribelli C *et al.* Ursodiol in the long-term treatment of chronic hepatitis – a double-blind multicenter clinical trial. J Hepatol. 1993;19:459–64.
42. McPherson GAD, Benjamin IS, Boobis AR, Brodie MJ, Hampden C, Blumgart LH. Antipyrine elimination as a dynamic test of hepatic functional integrity in obstructive jaundice. Gut. 1982;23:734–8.
43. Shapiro JM, Smith H, Schaffner F. Serum bilirubin: a prognostic factor in primary biliary cirrhosis. Gut. 1979;20:137–40.
44. Conn HO. A peek at the Child–Turcotte classification. Hepatology. 1981;1:673–6.
45. Farrant JM, Hayllar KM, Wilkinson ML *et al.* Natural history and prognostic variables in primary sclerosing cholangitis. Gastroenterology. 1991;100:1710–17.
46. Dickson ER, Murtaugh PA, Wiesner RH *et al.* Primary sclerosing cholangitis: refinement and validation of survival models. Gastroenterology. 1992;103:1893–901.
47. Ishii K, Wolkoff AW. Inhibition of rat hepatocyte organic anion transport by bile acids. Am J Physiol. 1994;267:G458–64.
48. Torres AM, Galan AI, Tiribelli C. Competition of bile acids on the sulfobromophthalein uptake in basolateral rat liver plasma membrane vesicles. Biochem Pharmacol. 1994;48:1301–4.
49. Pozzi EJS, Luquita MG, Catania VA, Garay EAR, Mottino AD. Inhibition of rat liver microsomal bilirubin UDP-glucuronosyltransferase by ursodeoxycholic acid. Life Sci. 1994;55:111–20.
50. Pozzi EJS, Catania VA, Luquita MG, Roma MG, Garay EAR, Mottino AD. Effect of oral administration of ursodeoxycholic acid on rat hepatic and intestinal UDP-glucuronosyltransferase. Can J Physiol Pharmacol. 1994;72:1265–71.
51. Poupon R, Chretien Y, Poupon RE, Ballet F, Calmus Y, Darnis F. Is ursodeoxycholic acid an effective treatment for primary biliary cirrhosis? Lancet. 1987;1:834–6.
52. Cotting J, Lentze MJ, Reichen J. Effects of ursodeoxycholic acid therapy on nutrition and liver function in patients with cystic fibrosis and long-standing cholestasis. Gut. 1990;31:918–21.
53. Cotting J, Dufour JF, Lentze MJ, Paumgartner G, Reichen J. Ursodeoxycholate in the treatment of cholestasis in cystic fibrosis – a 2 year experience and review of the literature. In: Lentze MJ, Reichen J, editors. Paediatric cholestasis: novel approaches to treatment. Dordrecht: Kluwer; 1992:345–53.
54. Colombo C, Castellani MR, Balistreri WF, Seregni E, Assaisso ML, Giunta A. Scintigraphic documentation of an improvement in hepatobiliary excretory function after treatment with ursodeoxycholic acid in patients with cystic fibrosis and associated liver disease. Hepatology. 1992;15:677–84.
55. Jazrawi RP, Decaestecker JS, Goggin PM *et al.* Kinetics of hepatic bile acid handling in cholestatic liver disease – effect of ursodeoxycholic acid. Gastroenterology. 1994;106:134–42.
56. Reichen J. Assessment of hepatic function with xenobiotics. Semin Liver Dis. 1995 (In press).
57. Tygstrup N. Determination of the hepatic galactose elimination capacity after a single intravenous injection in man. Acta Physiol Scand. 1963;58:162–72.
58. Lauterburg BH, Bircher J. Expiratory measurement of maximal aminopyrine demethylation in vivo: effect of phenobarbital–partial hepatectomy–portacaval shunt and bile duct ligation in the rat. J Pharmacol Exp Ther. 1976;196:501–9.
59. Brodie BB, Axelrod J. The fate of antipyrine in man. J Pharmacol Exp Ther. 1950;98:97–104.
60. Oellerich M, Raude E, Burdelski M *et al.* Monoethylglycinexylidide formation kinetics: a novel approach to assessment of liver function. J Clin Chem Biochem. 1987;25:845–53.
61. Zetterstrom R, Ernster L. Bilirubin – an uncoupler of oxidative phosphorylation in isolated mitochondria. Nature. 1956;178:1335–7.

62. DeLange RJ, Glazer AN. Bile acids: antioxidants or enhancers of peroxidation depending on lipid concentration[2]. Arch Biochem Biophys. 1990;276:19–25.
63. Krell H, Dietze E. Hemodynamic and metabolic responses to leukotriene C4 in isolated perfused rat liver. Hepatology. 1989;10:300–5.
64. Sokol RJ, Devereaux M, Mierau GW, Hambidge KM, Shikes RH. Oxidant injury to hepatic mitochondrial lipids in rats with dietary copper overload. Gastroenterology. 1990;99:1061–71.
65. Reichen J, Buters JTM, Sojic Z, Roos FJ. Abnormal lipid composition of microsomes from cirrhotic rat liver – does it contribute to decreased microsomal function? Experientia. 1992;48:482–6.

Index

43. Reutter W, Popper H, Arias IM, Heinrich PC, Keppler D, Landmann L, eds.: *Modulation of Liver Cell Expression.* Falk Symposium No. 43. 1987 ISBN: 0-85200-677-2*
44. Boyer JL, Bianchi L, eds.: *Liver Cirrhosis.* Falk Symposium No. 44. 1987 ISBN: 0-85200-993-3*
45. Paumgartner G, Stiehl A, Gerok W, eds.: *Bile Acids and the Liver.* Falk Symposium No. 45. 1987 ISBN: 0-85200-675-6*
46. Goebell H, Peskar BM, Malchow H, eds.: *Inflammatory Bowel Diseases – Basic Research & Clinical Implications.* Falk Symposium No. 46. 1988 ISBN: 0-7462-0067-6*
47. Bianchi L, Holt P, James OFW, Butler RN, eds.: *Aging in Liver and Gastrointestinal Tract.* Falk Symposium No. 47. 1988 ISBN: 0-7462-0066-8*
48. Heilmann C, ed.: *Calcium-Dependent Processes in the Liver.* Falk Symposium No. 48. 1988 ISBN: 0-7462-0075-7*
50. Singer MV, Goebell H, eds.: *Nerves and the Gastrointestinal Tract.* Falk Symposium No. 50. 1989 ISBN: 0-7462-0114-1
51. Bannasch P, Keppler D, Weber G, eds.: *Liver Cell Carcinoma.* Falk Symposium No. 51. 1989 ISBN: 0-7462-0111-7
52. Paumgartner G, Stiehl A, Gerok W, eds.: *Trends in Bile Acid Research.* Falk Symposium No. 52. 1989 ISBN: 0-7462-0112-5
53. Paumgartner G, Stiehl A, Barbara L, Roda E, eds.: *Strategies for the Treatment of Hepatobiliary Diseases.* Falk Symposium No. 53. 1990 ISBN: 0-7923-8903-4
54. Bianchi L, Gerok W, Maier K-P, Deinhardt F, eds.: *Infectious Diseases of the Liver.* Falk Symposium No. 54. 1990 ISBN: 0-7923-8902-6
55. Falk Symposium No. 55 not published

55B. Hadziselimovic F, Herzog B, Bürgin-Wolff A, eds.: *Inflammatory Bowel Disease and Coeliac Disease in Children.* International Falk Symposium. 1990 ISBN 0-7462-0125-7

56. Williams CN, eds.: *Trends in Inflammatory Bowel Disease Therapy.* Falk Symposium No. 56. 1990 ISBN: 0-7923-8952-2
57. Bock KW, Gerok W, Matern S, Schmid R, eds.: *Hepatic Metabolism and Disposition of Endo- and Xenobiotics.* Falk Symposium No. 57. 1991 ISBN: 0-7923-8953-0
58. Paumgartner G, Stiehl A, Gerok W, eds.: *Bile Acids as Therapeutic Agents: From Basic Science to Clinical Practice.* Falk Symposium No. 58. 1991 ISBN: 0-7923-8954-9
59. Halter F, Garner A, Tytgat GNJ, eds.: *Mechanisms of Peptic Ulcer Healing.* Falk Symposium No. 59. 1991 ISBN: 0-7923-8955-7
60. Goebell H, Ewe K, Malchow H, Koelbel Ch, eds.: *Inflammatory Bowel Diseases – Progress in Basic Research and Clinical Implications.* Falk Symposium No. 60. 1991 ISBN: 0-7923-8956-5
61. Falk Symposium No. 61 not published
62. Dowling RH, Folsch UR, Löser Ch, eds.: *Polyamines in the Gastrointestinal Tract.* Falk Symposium No. 62. 1992 ISBN: 0-7923-8976-X
63. Lentze MJ, Reichen J, eds.: *Paediatric Cholestasis: Novel Approaches to Treatment.* Falk Symposium No. 63. 1992 ISBN: 0-7923-8977-8
64. Demling L, Frühmorgen P, eds.: *Non-Neoplastic Diseases of the Anorectum.* Falk Symposium No. 64. 1992 ISBN: 0-7923-8979-4

64B. Gressner AM, Ramadori G, eds.: *Molecular and Cell Biology of Liver Fibrogenesis.* International Falk Symposium. 1992 ISBN: 0-7923-8980-8

*These titles were published under the MTP Press imprint.

Falk Symposium Series

65. Hadziselimovic F, Herzog B, eds.: *Inflammatory Bowel Diseases and Morbus Hirschprung*. Falk Symposium No. 65. 1992 ISBN: 0-7923-8995-6
66. Martin F, McLeod RS, Sutherland LR, Williams CN, eds.: *Trends in Inflammatory Bowel Disease Therapy*. Falk Symposium No. 66. 1993 ISBN: 0-7923-8827-5
67. Schölmerich J, Kruis W, Goebell H, Hohenberger W, Gross V, eds.: *Inflammatory Bowel Diseases – Pathophysiology as Basis of Treatment*. Falk Symposium No. 67. 1993 ISBN: 0-7923-8996-4
68. Paumgartner G, Stiehl A, Gerok W, eds.: *Bile Acids and The Hepatobiliary System: From Basic Science to Clinical Practice*. Falk Symposium No. 68. 1993 ISBN: 0-7923-8829-1
69. Schmid R, Bianchi L, Gerok W, Maier K-P, eds.: *Extrahepatic Manifestations in Liver Diseases*. Falk Symposium No. 69. 1993 ISBN: 0-7923-8821-6
70. Meyer zum Büschenfelde K-H, Hoofnagle J, Manns M, eds.: *Immunology and Liver*. Falk Symposium No. 70. 1993 ISBN: 0-7923-8830-5
71. Surrenti C, Casini A, Milani S, Pinzani M , eds.: *Fat-Storing Cells and Liver Fibrosis*. Falk Symposium No. 71. 1994 ISBN: 0-7923-8842-9
72. Rachmilewitz D, ed.: *Inflammatory Bowel Diseases – 1994*. Falk Symposium No. 72. 1994 ISBN: 0-7923-8845-3
73. Binder HJ, Cummings J, Soergel KH, eds.: *Short Chain Fatty Acids*. Falk Symposium No. 73. 1994 ISBN: 0-7923-8849-6
74. Keppler D, Jungermann K, eds.: *Transport in the Liver*. Falk Symposium No. 74. 1994 ISBN: 0-7923-8858-5

74B. Stange EF, ed.: *Chronic Inflammatory Bowel Disease*. Falk Symposium. 1995 ISBN: 0-7923-8876-3

75. van Berge Henegouwen GP, van Hoek B, De Groote J, Matern S, Stockbrügger RW, eds.: *Cholestatic Liver Diseases: New Strategies for Prevention and Treatment of Hepatobiliary and Cholestatic Liver Diseases*. Falk Symposium 75. 1994. ISBN: 0-7923-8867-4
76. Monteiro E, Tavarela Veloso F, eds.: *Inflammatory Bowel Diseases: New Insights into Mechanisms of Inflammation and Challenges in Diagnosis and Treatment*. Falk Symposium 76. 1995. ISBN 0-7923-8884-4
77. Singer MV, Ziegler R, Rohr G, eds.: *Gastrointestinal Tract and Endocrine System*. Falk Symposium 77. 1995. ISBN 0-7923-8877-1
78. Decker K, Gerok W, Andus T, Gross V, eds.: *Cytokines and the Liver*. Falk Symposium 78. 1995. ISBN 0-7923-8878-X
79. Holstege A, Schölmerich J, Hahn EG, eds.: *Portal Hypertension*. Falk Symposium 79. 1995. ISBN 0-7923-8879-8
80. Hofmann AF, Paumgartner G, Stiehl A, eds.: *Bile Acids in Gastroenterology: Basic and Clinical Aspects*. Falk Symposium 80. 1995 ISBN 0-7923-8880-1
81. Riecken EO, Stallmach A, Zeitz M, Heise W, eds.: *Malignancy and Chronic Inflammation in the Gastrointestinal Tract – New Concepts*. Falk Symposium 81. 1995 ISBN 0-7923-8889-5
82. Fleig WE, ed.: *Inflammatory Bowel Diseases: New Developments and Standards*. Falk Symposium 82. 1995 ISBN 0-7923-8890-6

82B. Paumgartner G, Beuers U, eds.: *Bile Acids in Liver Diseases*. International Falk Workshop. 1995 ISBN 0-7923-8891-7

83. Dobrilla G, Felder M, de Pretis G, eds.: *Advances in Hepatobiliary and Pancreatic Diseases: Special Clinical Topics*. Falk Symposium 83. 1995. ISBN 0-7923-8892-5

Falk Symposium Series

84. Fromm H, Leuschner U, eds.: *Bile Acids – Cholestasis – Gallstones: Advances in Basic and Clinical Bile Acid Research.* Falk Symposium 84. 1995 ISBN 0-7923-8893-3
85. Tytgat GNJ, Bartelsman JFWM, van Deventer SJH, eds.: *Inflammatory Bowel Diseases.* Falk Symposium 85. 1995 ISBN 0-7923-8894-1